The Christian's Guide to Holistic Health

A Theological Approach to Holistic Health for Body, Mind, and Spirit

DR. MAXWELL SHIMBA

Published in Manhattan, New York by Shimba Publishing, LLC.

Shimba Publishing LLC

Table of Contents

Preface

To the esteemed reader, the diligent student of theology, the weary pastor, the questioning saint, and any who find themselves at the intersection of faith and flesh, of pulpit and practice, I address you not as one who has mastered this subject, but as a fellow pilgrim on the arduous, often perplexing, journey of embodied existence. What you hold in your hands is the fruit of decades of theological inquiry, pastoral anguish, and personal struggle—a systematic attempt to articulate a vision of human life that takes with utmost seriousness the profound, often neglected, biblical declaration: *Your body is a temple of the Holy Spirit.*

We live, I contend, in an age of profound anthropological confusion. From one direction, we are assailed by a gnosticism more pervasive and subtle than that which confronted the early church. This modern gnosticism does not always manifest as a formal heresy denying the goodness of creation; rather, it operates as a practical, lived dualism that functionally relegates the physical body to the status of a mere container, a temporary shell for the "real" self—the soul. Within this framework, what one eats, how one rests, the state of one's nervous system, the management of one's physical energy—these are considered matters of secular concern, peripheral at best to the life of faith, and at worst, a dangerous distraction from "spiritual" matters. The sanctuary of the soul, in this view, has no necessary connection to the condition of its earthly dwelling. The result is a faith that is intellectually robust yet physically depleted, emotionally volatile, and often incapable of sustained, tangible service in a world that groans for redemption.

From the opposite direction, we face the siren song of a therapeutic, aesthetic, and technological materialism that worships the body not as a temple, but as an idol. Here, the physical form is curated, optimized, and displayed for its own sake, for the sake of pleasure, performance, or social capital. Health becomes an end in itself—a pseudo-salvation project pursued through the rituals of the gym, the altar of the organic grocery store, and the sacraments of supplements. This is not stewardship; it is narcissism dressed in the language of wellness. It is the very inversion of Paul's warning in 1 Corinthians 6:12-13, where freedom becomes license and the body, rather than being *for the Lord*, becomes a slave to its own appetites and appearances.

It is between this Scylla of gnostic neglect and Charybdis of materialistic idolatry that this volume seeks to navigate a third way: the ancient and yet ever-new path of *Embodied Stewardship*. This is not a "Christian health book." You will find within these pages no seven-step programs to your best life now, no guaranteed formulas for longevity, no simplistic proof-texting that reduces the complex wisdom of Scripture to a list of dietary rules. Such approaches, I fear, often represent a baptized version of the very self-help culture they purport to transcend.

No, the aim of this treatise is far more ambitious, and I pray, far more foundational. My purpose is to construct a comprehensive *theological framework*—a dogmatic structure—within which the daily, mundane realities of our physical existence can be understood, evaluated, and enacted as acts of worship. We must, as a people of the Book, develop a *theology of eating* that is more profound than saying grace before a meal. We must cultivate a *theology of rest* that understands Sabbath and sleep as acts of radical faith and defiance against the idolatry of productivity. We must forge a *theology of the mind* that sees the renewal of our cognitive patterns not as a secular therapeutic technique but as a spiritual warfare mandated in 2 Corinthians 10:5. We must recover a *theology of physical discipline* that views the strengthening of our bodies not as a pursuit of vanity but as a preparation for service, a tangible outworking of the command to "love our neighbor as ourselves."

This task requires us to return, with exegetical patience and systematic rigor, to the very foundations of our faith. We must begin, as we do in Part I, with the doctrine of Creation. We must ask: What does it mean that God formed Adam from the dust of the ground and breathed into his nostrils the *breath of life*? The Hebrew concept of *nephesh*—the living being—shatters our Hellenistic predispositions toward body-soul dualism. The human person, from the very beginning, was an *animated body*, a psychosomatic unity. To be human is to be *embodied*. This creational goodness, however, is now viewed through the tragic lens of the Fall. Our exploration in Chapter 4 is therefore not a diversion into pessimism, but a necessary diagnosis of the disorder we all experience. The curse in Genesis 3 is not merely spiritual; it is profoundly physical, introducing toil, pain, disease, and death into the fabric of our bodily existence. A theology of health that ignores the reality of the Fall is a theology of denial. It is only upon this foundation of Creation and Fall that the glorious light of Redemption can shine with its full brilliance. The doctrine of the Incarnation stands as the ultimate refutation of all gnosticism. The eternal Word did not merely *appear* to become flesh; He *became* flesh (John 1:14). He took upon Himself our physical nature, with its vulnerabilities, its need for food and sleep, its capacity for pain. In His ministry, Jesus healed sick bodies, fed hungry crowds, and wept at a tomb. His resurrection was not a disembodied escape from matter, but the transformation and vindication of the physical, the firstfruits of what is to come for all who are in Him (1 Corinthians 15:20-23). And it is this resurrected Christ who, through the agency of the Holy Spirit, now takes up residence within the believer. The staggering implication of 1 Corinthians 6:19 is that the same divine power that raised Christ from the dead now indwells our mortal bodies. The temple, though marred by the Fall, has become a construction site for the New Creation.

This redemptive reality propels us into the practical domains of Parts II, III, and IV. Our exploration of nutrition, therefore, is not a search for a "biblical diet" but a recovery of a *theology of food*—from the creational menu of Genesis 1 to the manna in the wilderness, from the Levitical laws to Jesus' declaration that all foods are clean, culminating in the Eucharistic feast where simple bread and wine become vehicles of grace. We must ask not only "What should I eat?" but "What does my eating *say* about my trust in God as Provider? What does it say about my relationship to His creation and to my global neighbor?"

Our foray into mental and emotional well-being is not an uncritical adoption of secular psychology, but a robust articulation of what it means to have the "mind of Christ" (1 Corinthians 2:16). We will delve into the dark night of the soul with Elijah, the profound lament of the Psalms, and the agonizing prayer of Christ in Gethsemane. We will wrestle with the reality of clinical depression and anxiety, not as a sign of weak faith, but as a complex affliction that may have somatic, spiritual, and psychological dimensions, requiring a multi-faceted ministry of the church that embraces both prayer and medicine, both Scripture and therapy.

And finally, our consideration of physical discipline is a call to reclaim the body for its creational and missional purpose. When Paul uses the language of athletic training in 1 Timothy 4:7-8, he is not being dismissive of the physical. He is appropriating a powerful cultural metaphor and sanctifying it. Bodily training has "some value"—limited, temporal value—but when that training is re-oriented toward the goal of godliness and service, its value is taken up into the economy of the Kingdom. A strong, healthy, well-rested body is not a trophy; it is a tool—a tool for longer, more effective service, for greater endurance in suffering, for the tangible love of our neighbor that often requires physical presence and exertion.

The journey upon which we are about to embark is therefore a deeply theological one. It is an exercise in thinking God's thoughts after Him about the entirety of our human existence. It is a call to repent of our gnostic tendencies that neglect the physical, and of our materialistic idolatries that worship it. It is an invitation to see every meal, every night's sleep, every walk, every moment of managed stress, and every conscious thought as an opportunity to participate in the ongoing redemption of our whole persons, to the glory of God.

I invite you, therefore, to read with a Bible open, with a critical mind, and with a prayerful heart. Engage with the patristic sources, wrestle with the exegetical arguments, and consider the practical implications for your own life and for the ministry of the church. The task is urgent. The world is watching a church that often preaches a gospel of salvation for the soul while its members are too tired, too sick, too anxious, and too undisciplined to be the hands and feet of Christ in a broken world. May this work be a small contribution toward a reformation of our understanding—a recovery of the sacred truth that we are fearfully and wonderfully made, and that the call to "glorify God in your body" is the most practical, the most holistic, and the most profoundly spiritual mandate for the people of God.

Introduction
The Doctrine of Embodied Stewardship

Beloved in Christ, fellow heirs of the grace of life, I invite you to embark with me upon a theological expedition of the most intimate and consequential kind—an exploration of the very flesh and blood, the synapses and sinews, the cravings and consumptions that constitute our earthly sojourn. We stand today at a critical juncture in the history of Western Christianity, where the conversation surrounding human health has been largely abdicated to the secular marketplace, a marketplace that speaks with the forked tongue of hedonism and asceticism, of instant gratification and delayed reward, yet remains utterly mute concerning the *telos*—the ultimate purpose and end—of the human body. It offers us a gospel of longevity without eternity, performance without purpose, and wellness without wholeness. It is a gospel that, for all its promises, leaves the soul parched and the spirit adrift, for it fails to answer the most fundamental of questions: *For whom and for what does this body exist?*

It is into this cacophony of competing salvific narratives that we must speak with clarity and courage, recovering a vision that is at once ancient and explosively relevant. This treatise represents a sustained argument, a dogmatic plea, for what I have termed the doctrine of **Embodied Stewardship**. This is not a new doctrine, mind you, but a forgotten chord in the great symphony of biblical truth, a chord that when struck, resonates through every facet of our created existence. We posit that the care of one's body—from the macronutrients we ingest to the neurochemicals we balance, from the muscles we strengthen to the passions we discipline—is not a secondary or tertiary spiritual concern, but rather, is inextricably woven into the very fabric of Christian discipleship. It is a sacred trust, a priestly responsibility bestowed upon us by the Creator, who, after forming Adam from the dust of the ground, did not discard the clay as worthless, but breathed into it His own breath, sanctifying the material forever.

The central thesis that will undergird every page of our exploration is this: **The physical body is ontologically and functionally inseparable from the life of the spirit.** This assertion stands as a bulwark against the persistent and pernicious heresy of Gnosticism, which, like a theological phantom, has haunted the Church for two millennia. This ancient error, in its modern, sophisticated forms, does not always explicitly deny the goodness of creation, but it operates as a practical, functional dualism. It creates a spiritual caste system where prayer, Bible study, and evangelism are considered "spiritual work," while meal planning, exercise, and the pursuit of emotional health are relegated to the realm of "secular maintenance." This is a diabolical lie that has crippled the witness of the Church and impoverished the lives of countless believers. It is a lie that ignores the fundamental truth that we do not *have* bodies; we *are* bodies. We are, in the rich Hebrew conception, *nephesh chayyah*—living beings, psychosomatic unities, whose spiritual worship is rendered through material means.

Our foundational text, the bedrock upon which this entire edifice is constructed, comes from the Apostle Paul's first letter to the Corinthian church, a community drowning in a culture of sexual license and philosophical dualism not unlike our own. In 1

Corinthians 6:19-20, he poses a question that should shake us from our anthropological slumber: "Or do you not know that your body is a temple of the Holy Spirit within you, whom you have from God? You are not your own, for you were bought with a price. So glorify God in your body."

I want you to feel the weight of these words. This is not a vague spiritual metaphor. This is a radical, ontological claim about the nature of your present, physical reality. The Greek word used here for temple is *naos*, which does not refer to the entire temple complex (*hieron*), but to the inner sanctuary, the Holy of Holies, the most sacred space on earth, where the very Shekinah glory of God dwelt in the midst of His people. This is what you are. Your body—with its aches and its appetites, its strengths and its weaknesses—is the *naos*, the dwelling place of the Third Person of the Trinity. This is not a future promise for the resurrection; this is a present-tense reality for every person indwelt by the Spirit of Christ.

Consider the implications of this with me. In the Old Testament, the temple was a place set apart exclusively for the worship of Yahweh. Its materials were chosen with intentionality—the finest gold, purest linen, most fragrant incense. Its maintenance was a sacred duty; its defilement was a capital offense. The priests were consecrated, their bodies washed and anointed, their garments holy, for they served in the presence of Holiness itself. Now, transpose that reality onto your own physical existence. To treat this body as a mere vehicle for personal pleasure, a machine for performance to be optimized for selfish gain, or a canvas for self-expression untethered from its Divine Architect, is a profound category error. It is to take the Holy of Holies and turn it into a common marketplace, a den of thieves, or a vanity fair.

Conversely, to neglect this temple—through the slow suicide of gluttony, the passive resignation of sloth, the willful ignorance of medical science, or the anxious refusal to entrust our cares to God—is not merely a lack of self-discipline. It is an act of desecration. It is to allow the walls of the sanctuary to crumble, the gold to tarnish, and the altar to grow cold. We would be rightfully appalled if our local church building were left to rot, its roof leaking and its walls covered in graffiti. How much more should we be appalled when we, the living temples of God, engage in practices that systematically dismantle the very dwelling place of the Almighty?

Therefore, the structure of this work is designed to systematically unpack the multifaceted dimensions of this sacred stewardship. We begin, as all sound theology must, **in Part I: Foundational Principles of Holistic Stewardship**, by laying the groundwork in the fertile soil of biblical doctrine. We will delve into the creation narratives to understand the original design for the human body as part of God's "very good" creation. We will explore the profound mystery of the *Imago Dei*—the Image of God—and its inescapable embodiment. We will then gaze unflinchingly into the abyss of the Fall, developing a theology of affliction that can account for the reality of disease, disorder, and death without attributing all suffering to personal sin, yet without absolving us of our responsibility as stewards. And we will anchor our hope in the doctrines of Incarnation and Redemption, for in the person of Jesus Christ, God took on flesh, thereby sanctifying material existence forever, and through His bodily resurrection, He has secured the future redemption of these very bodies that now house His Spirit.

From this doctrinal foundation, we will move to the practical outworkings of stewardship. **Part II: Nutritional Stewardship: Nourishing the Temple** will reframe our understanding of food from mere fuel to a theological category. We will explore the biblical narrative of food, from the creational menu in Eden to the manna in the wilderness, from the Levitical dietary laws to Jesus' declaration that all foods are clean, culminating in the Eucharistic feast where simple bread and wine become vehicles of grace. We will develop a theology of eating that encompasses gratitude, discipline, justice, and community, arguing that every meal is an act of communion with God's provision and a rehearsal for the Marriage Supper of the Lamb.

Part III: Mental and Emotional Well-being: The Renewed Mind will confront the modern epidemic of mental affliction with both theological precision and pastoral compassion. We will examine the mental and emotional lives of biblical figures, from the despair of Elijah to the laments of David, recognizing that the path of faith often traverses the valley of shadows. We will explore the Apostle Paul's prescription in Philippians 4:8 for cognitive stewardship, learning to take every thought captive to the obedience of Christ. And we will delve into the spiritual disciplines of prayer, meditation, and contemplation, not as esoteric exercises, but as God-ordained means of grace for grounding the soul and building emotional resilience in a world of chaos.

Finally, **Part IV: Physical Discipline: The Faithful Body in Action** will redeem the concept of physical training from the realms of vanity and performance. We will explore a theology of work and physical labor, rooted in Adam's original vocation to "work and keep" the Garden. We will examine Paul's use of the athletic metaphor in 1 Timothy 4:7-8, arguing that "bodily training" is of value when its end is godliness and enhanced capacity for service. And we will develop a theology of rest, exploring the profound spiritual significance of Sabbath and sleep as acts of faith and trust in a sovereign God.

Our methodology throughout will be unapologetically academic and scholarly. We will engage in rigorous exegesis, drawing from the original languages of Scripture. We will sit at the feet of the Church Fathers and the Reformers, learning from their insights and their errors. And we will engage with contemporary scientific research—from neurobiology to nutritional science to kinesiology—operating from the presupposition that all truth is God's truth. General Revelation, the book of nature, will be read in the light of Special Revelation, the book of Scripture, and where they speak to the same reality, they will never ultimately conflict.

The goal of this treatise is to equip you—pastors, theologians, educators, and earnest disciples—to think critically and biblically about the entirety of your embodied life. It is a call to move beyond the fragmented, therapeutic self-help that dominates the landscape and to embrace a grand, unifying vision of human flourishing—a vision of *Shalom*. This Hebrew concept of peace is not merely the absence of conflict, but the presence of holistic well-being, right relationships, and harmonious order that reflects the very character of God's kingdom. It is a state where the body is nourished, the mind is clear, the emotions are ordered, the spirit is vibrant, and all are directed toward the glory of God and the service of neighbor.

This, then, is the path of Embodied Stewardship. It is the recognition that the great commandment to love the Lord our God with all our heart, soul, mind, and strength is an utterly comprehensive command, encompassing every facet of our being. It is the understanding that the second commandment, to love our neighbor as ourselves, requires us to have a self that is well-stewarded, capable of sustained, tangible love. We are called to tend the garden of our own embodied existence, not as an act of self-worship, but as an act of priestly devotion, a daily offering of our whole selves as a living sacrifice, holy and acceptable to God, which is our spiritual worship.

PART I

FOUNDATIONAL PRINCIPLES OF HOLISTIC STEWARDSHIP

CHAPTER 01

The Biblical Mandate for Physical Health: An Exegesis of 1 Corinthians 6:19-20

1.1 Introduction: The Modern Disconnect Between Spirituality and Physicality

My dear brothers and sisters, we gather today not merely as students of theology, but as inhabitants of a world fractured by a profound and pervasive anthropological heresy—a heresy so deeply embedded in our cultural consciousness, so subtly woven into the fabric of our religious practice, that we often fail to recognize its presence, even as we breathe its toxic air. I speak of the great and terrible divorce between the spiritual and the physical, a schism in the human person that has left our theology disembodied and our bodies de-theologized. We have, perhaps unknowingly, erected an altar to a God who is concerned with souls but seems curiously indifferent to the sinew and bone, the gut and gland, the very fleshly existence in which those souls are inextricably enmeshed.

This is not the biblical witness! This is the ghost of ancient heresies—the specter of Gnosticism, the shadow of Neo-Platonism—haunting the hallways of the modern church. We have created a false hierarchy of value, a spiritual caste system where activities deemed "spiritual"—prayer, fasting, Bible study, evangelism—are afforded the highest premium, while the so-called "secular" or "mundane" acts of physical maintenance—the careful selection of food, the disciplined pursuit of rest, the intentional stewardship of our physical energy, the management of our emotional and mental states—are relegated to a lower tier of spiritual concern, if they are considered at all. We have, in effect, created a sacred-secular divide that runs straight through the center of the human person, and we are reaping the whirlwind of this theological error.

Look around you. Behold the faithful Christian, zealous for the Lord, who spends hours in intercessory prayer yet systematically destroys the very temple in which the Holy Spirit resides through a diet of processed foods, chronic sleep deprivation, and unmanaged stress. Witness the pastor, a shepherd of souls, whose body is breaking down under the weight of ministerial demands, who preaches of the peace that passes understanding while his own nervous system is a frayed wire, crackling with anxiety. Consider the small group that gathers weekly for deep theological discussion, fueled by sugary snacks and caffeine, their fellowship simultaneously enriching their spirits and malnourishing their bodies. Do we not see the profound dissonance here? Do we not recognize that we are, in practice if not in creed, functional Gnostics?

This Gnostic impulse manifests in two primary, and equally destructive, forms. On one hand, we see the **Ascetic Impulse**, a descendant of the ancient heresy that viewed the material world as inherently evil or, at best, a temporary prison for the pure soul. This impulse leads to a neglect, even a disdain, for the physical body. The body's needs are seen as a distraction from spiritual pursuits, its appetites as temptations to be suppressed rather than gifts to be stewarded. This is a faith that is suspicious of pleasure, uncomfortable with physicality, and ultimately, docetic in its Christology—unable to fully embrace a Savior who ate, drank, slept, sweated, and bled. This impulse says, "It doesn't matter what I do with my body; only the soul is eternal." It is a theology of abandonment, where the body is left to decay while the soul soars to heaven.

On the other hand, we face the **Therapeutic-Utilitarian Impulse**, the dominant religion of our secular age. This is not a denial of the body, but a worship of it for all the wrong reasons. Here, the body is not a temple, but an idol. It is an object to be curated, optimized, and displayed. Its value is measured in aesthetics, performance, and pleasure. Health becomes a salvific project, a pursuit of longevity and vitality for their own sake, severed from any transcendent purpose. The gym becomes a cathedral of self-worship, the organic grocery store its communion rail, and the wellness influencer its high priest. This impulse says, "My body is mine to do with as I please, to shape according to my will, to use for my own gratification and glory." It is a theology of autonomy, a declaration of independence from the Creator's design.

And caught between these two falsehoods—the neglect of the Ascetic and the idolatry of the Therapeutic—the average Christian lives in a state of quiet confusion. We feel a vague sense of guilt when we neglect our health, yet we also feel a sense of vanity when we attend to it. We lack a coherent, robust, *biblical* framework that can sanctify the physical, that can transform the daily acts of eating, sleeping, moving, and resting from secular chores into sacred rituals, from acts of self-interest into acts of worship.

This is why we must begin our journey here, at the very foundation. We must return to the apostolic word, to a text that cuts through this fog of confusion with the surgical precision of divine revelation. We must plant our feet on the solid rock of 1 Corinthians 6:19-20 and allow its tectonic truth to shake the foundations of our compromised anthropology. For the Apostle Paul, writing to a church drowning in a culture of sexual license and philosophical dualism strikingly similar to our own, does not offer a gentle corrective. He delivers a theological bombshell, a statement so radical, so comprehensive in its implications, that if we truly grasped its meaning, it would revolutionize everything from our grocery lists to our gym memberships, from our sleep schedules to our stress management.

He asks a question that should echo in our minds and convict our hearts: "Or do you not know...?" This is not a question seeking new information, but a rhetorical dagger aimed at our willful ignorance. It implies that this is a truth they *should* have known, a foundational reality that should have been shaping their behavior all along. They were living in a state of forgetfulness, a spiritual amnesia regarding the true nature of their own bodies. And I fear, my friends, that we in the modern church are suffering from the same amnesia. We have forgotten who we are. We have forgotten *what* we are.

The core of our modern disconnect, therefore, is an identity crisis. We have lost the stunning, terrifying, glorious reality of our ontological status as revealed in Scripture. We do not see ourselves as sacred vessels, as animated sanctuaries. We see ourselves as ghosts in a machine, and we either ignore the machine or worship it, but we do not understand its divine purpose. We have divorced the Great Commandment—to love the Lord with all our heart, soul, mind, and *strength*—from the physical reality of that strength. We have severed the second commandment—to love our neighbor as ourselves—from the physical capacity required to enact that love in sustained, tangible service.

This introductory exploration, then, is a call to remembrance. It is a summons to return to first principles. It is an invitation to have our minds renewed and our paradigms shattered by the simple, profound, and life-altering question: "Do you not know that your body is a temple of the Holy Spirit?" Everything that follows in this treatise—our theology of nutrition, our psychology of mental health, our philosophy of physical discipline—rests upon our answer to this question. For if we answer in the affirmative, if we truly *know* this to be true, then the care of this body can no longer be a matter of personal preference or cultural trend. It becomes a non-negotiable, sacred obligation, the most basic and practical outworking of our faith. It becomes, in the truest sense, our spiritual worship.

1.2 Exegetical Analysis of 1 Corinthians 6:12-20

Beloved, we now turn our attention to the sacred text itself, to the very words breathed out by God that form the foundation of our doctrine of Embodied Stewardship. To understand the explosive force of verses 19 and 20, we must first immerse ourselves in their immediate context, for the Apostle Paul's radical declaration about the body as a temple does not emerge from a vacuum. It is a divine thunderclap aimed at dispersing the thick fog of two competing philosophical errors that had engulfed the Corinthian church: the error of libertinism and the error of asceticism. These were not merely abstract ideas; they were lived realities, competing spiritualities that were shaping the community's behavior in profound and destructive ways. And I tell you today, these same ancient errors, dressed in modern garb, continue to wage war for the soul of the Church and for our understanding of our own bodies.

Let us first set the stage. The city of Corinth was a bustling, wealthy, and notoriously immoral port city, a crossroads of cultures and philosophies. It was a center for the worship of Aphrodite, whose temple employed a thousand sacred prostitutes, making sexual immorality not just a personal vice but a religious act. Into this context, the gospel of Jesus Christ had come as a radical invasion of light into darkness. But the darkness, as it so often does, sought to compromise the light, to blend it with the prevailing worldview. Some Corinthian believers, intoxicated by their new-found freedom in Christ and influenced by a proto-Gnostic worldview that despised the material realm, had taken up a dangerous slogan: **"All things are lawful for me."** This was the cry of the libertine, the spiritual antinomian. Their logic was perverse yet compelling: If Christ has set us free from the law, and if the physical body is temporary and ultimately unimportant, then what I *do* with this body is a matter of moral indifference. I can indulge its every appetite—including visiting prostitutes—because these physical acts cannot touch my redeemed spirit. This was a theology of grace divorced from holiness, of freedom divorced from love, of spirit divorced from body. It was, in essence, the ancient version of the Therapeutic-Utilitarian impulse, using Christian language to justify hedonism.

But Paul will have none of it. He takes their own slogan and, with the skill of a master theologian, turns it back on them. **"All things are lawful for me,"** he concedes, **"but not all things are helpful."** The Greek word here is *symphero*—it means to bear together, to be profitable, to be advantageous. Paul introduces a new criterion for Christian behavior that transcends mere permissibility. The question is not, "Is this allowed?" but "Is this *beneficial*? Does this action, this habit, this consumption, contribute to the overall health, wholeness, and functional purpose of my entire being—body and spirit—as a vessel for God's glory?" He immediately follows with a second, devastating rebuttal: **"All things are lawful for me, but I will not be dominated by anything."** Here is the crux of the matter. The libertine, in their pursuit of absolute freedom, becomes the absolute slave. What begins as an act of autonomy—"I can do this"—ends in a state of addiction, compulsion, and bondage. The body and its appetites are no longer servants to be stewarded; they become masters to be obeyed. The one who boasts of their freedom to eat anything becomes a slave to gluttony. The one who claims sexual license becomes a slave to lust. This is not freedom; it is a different, more insidious form of slavery. Paul is arguing that true spiritual freedom is the capacity to choose the good, to refuse to be enslaved by any created thing, because we are bound only to Christ.

He then moves to a positive theological assertion that shatters the libertine framework at its foundation. In verse 13, he declares, **"The body is not meant for sexual immorality, but for the Lord, and the Lord for the body."** This is a direct refutation of the Gnostic and Hellenistic dualism that underpinned their behavior. The Greek philosophers saw the body as a prison, a tomb, a temporary shell to be escaped. But Paul proclaims a stunning, holistic truth: The Lord is *for* the body. The Creator has a purpose, a destiny, for this physicality. The body is *for* the Lord. Its very design, its functions, its capacities, are intended for His service and His glory. This is not a temporary arrangement; it is an eternal reality, sealed by the fact that **"God raised the Lord and will also raise us up by his power."** The resurrection of Jesus Christ is the ultimate vindication of the body. It is God's definitive "Yes!" to the material world He created. The libertine's disregard for the body is, therefore, a denial of the gospel itself—a denial of the incarnation, the crucifixion, and the resurrection.

But Paul is not finished. He drives the theological stake even deeper in verse 15, with a statement so staggering that we must pause to let its full weight crush our individualistic tendencies: **"Do you not know that your bodies are members of Christ?"** The word "members" here is *mele*, meaning limbs or organs. This is not a loose metaphor of association. This is an ontological claim about our union with Christ. When you became a Christian, you were not just added to a mailing list or signed up for a club. You were grafted, by the Spirit, into the very life of the resurrected Christ. Your physical body became a limb of His cosmic, glorified body. Your hand is His hand in the world. Your foot is His foot. Your eyes are His eyes. This is the doctrine of the *unio mystica*, the mystical union, and it has devastating ethical implications. Shall I then take a member of Christ—a limb of the Son of God—and make it one with a prostitute? The question is meant to be absurd, horrifying. It is a spiritual and physical profanity of the highest order.

He reinforces this in verse 16 by quoting Genesis 2:24: **"The two shall become one flesh."** The libertine, viewing sex as a casual physical act with no spiritual significance, is operating with a profoundly unbiblical anthropology. The biblical view is that sexual union constitutes a profound, one-flesh unity—a mysterious fusion of two lives at the deepest level of their being. It is not merely a biological transaction; it is a theological reality, a covenant act that shapes the soul. To engage in sexual immorality is to violently tear a member from Christ and fuse it to another in a way that defiles, dis-integrates, and destroys the sacred unity for which we were designed.

And now, having laid this meticulous theological groundwork—having established the principles of beneficial stewardship, the danger of enslaving dominion, the Lord's purpose for the body, the reality of the resurrection, and the profound mystery of our union with Christ—Paul arrives at his climactic, crowning argument in verses 19 and 20. He returns to his refrain, **"Or do you not know...?"** and this time, he unveils the ultimate reason, the final and unanswerable motive for the stewardship of the body.

"Do you not know that your body is a temple of the Holy Spirit within you, whom you have from God?" Let us parse this with the reverence it deserves. The word for "temple" here is not the general term *hieron*, which refers to the entire temple complex. It is *naos*—the inner sanctuary, the Holy of Holies. This was the most sacred space in all of creation for a first-century Jew. It was the dwelling place of the Shekinah glory, the terrifying and glorious presence of Yahweh Himself. Only the High Priest could enter, once a year, with blood and trembling. This, Paul says, is what you have become. Not a common building, not an outer court, but the Holy of Holies itself. The Spirit of the living God, the same Spirit who hovered over the waters of creation and who raised Jesus from the dead, has taken up permanent, personal residence within your physical body. Every cell, every neuron, every hormone, every heartbeat exists within the precincts of this most holy sanctuary. This means that your digestive system is part of the *naos*. Your circulatory system is part of the *naos*. Your endocrine system and your nervous system are part of the *naos*. There is no part of your physical existence that is not now sacred space, set apart for the manifest presence of God.

This reality leads to the final, crushing, and glorious point: **"You are not your own, for you were bought with a price."** This is the language of the slave market. We were not merely wandering lost; we were prisoners of war, slaves to sin, with a price on our heads that we could never pay. But God, in Christ, paid that price. The blood of His own Son was the redemption price. We have been purchased, acquired. We are now *douloi*, bond-servants of Christ. The libertine's cry, "All things are lawful for me," is exposed as the ultimate fiction. I am not my own. My body is not my own to abuse, to neglect, or to idolize. It is Christ's purchased possession. I am a steward, a caretaker, a priest assigned to maintain a sanctuary that belongs to Another.

Therefore, the ultimate motivation for caring for our bodies is not self-preservation, not vanity, not even the pursuit of wellness for its own sake. It is **gratitude**. It is the loving, worshipful response of a redeemed slave who, having been purchased at an incalculable cost, now desires with every fiber of their being to honor and glorify the Master who bought them. **"So glorify God in your body."** This is the final, imperative conclusion. How do we glorify God? We glorify Him by maintaining His temple in a state of holiness and wholeness. We glorify Him by ensuring that this sanctuary is a fit dwelling for His Spirit, not a dilapidated, defiled, or dysfunctional ruin. We glorify Him by using the strength, health, and vitality of these redeemed bodies to do His work, to love our neighbors, and to proclaim the gospel of the Kingdom in both word and deed. This, my friends, is the biblical mandate. This is the foundation upon which all else is built.

1.3 Theological Implications of the "Temple" Metaphor: Sacred Space, Indwelling Presence, and Place of Worship

Beloved, having stood upon the solid rock of Paul's exegetical argument, we must now allow the tectonic shifts of its truth to reshape the very landscape of our lives. The declaration that our bodies are the *naos* of the Holy Spirit is not a mere theological datum to be filed away; it is a living, breathing, transformative reality that demands a radical reorientation of our entire existence. This metaphor of the temple is not a casual illustration; it is a dense, multi-faceted theological lens through which we are commanded to view our physical selves. Let us then, with fear and trembling, polish this lens and peer deeply into its implications, for we are engaging with nothing less than the architectural blueprint of our identity in Christ.

First, and most fundamentally, the temple metaphor establishes our bodies as **Sacred Space**. In the ancient world, and supremely in the consciousness of Israel, a temple was not merely a building; it was a place set apart, a zone of intense and concentrated holiness, a beachhead of heaven on earth. It was defined by its *purity*, its *purpose*, and the *reverence* it demanded. Consider the meticulous regulations of the Levitical code. The materials—the finest gold, the purest linen, the most carefully selected stones—were all chosen for their quality and durability, their ability to reflect the majesty of the Divine Resident. The priests underwent rigorous rituals of cleansing and consecration before they could enter to perform their duties. Specific objects and activities were strictly prohibited from the premises because they would defile the sacred space. There was a profound understanding that the nature of the space was determined by the nature of the God who inhabited it.

Now, transpose this reality onto your physical being. Your body is that consecrated ground. This has immediate and uncomfortable implications for the principle of *purity*. The question of what we consume—whether food, drink, media, or entertainment—is fundamentally a question of temple maintenance. Are we bringing that which is pure, wholesome, and excellent into the sanctuary of God, or are we, like the corrupt priests of Malachi's day, offering polluted food upon His altar (Malachi 1:7)? When we ingest substances that cloud our minds, inflame our fleshly passions, or slowly poison our systems, we are not merely making a poor health choice; we are desecrating the inner court. When we feed our eyes and minds with images and narratives that promote lust, violence, greed, or cynicism, we are hanging profane tapestries on the walls of the Holy of Holies. The Gnostic impulse that says, "What I watch or eat doesn't affect my spirit," is here exposed as a lie. The physical and the spiritual are one integrated sanctuary; to defile one is to defile the whole.

This sacred space also has a defined *purpose*. The Jerusalem temple was not a multi-purpose community center. It was designed for one primary function: to facilitate the worship of Yahweh and to mediate His presence to His people. Its architecture, its rituals, its very existence were teleological—they were oriented toward a specific end. So too, our bodies have a divine *telos*. They are not for self-gratification, as the libertine would have it. They are not for self-mutilation or neglect, as the ascetic implies. They are *for the Lord* (1 Corinthians 6:13). The purpose of your digestive system is to fuel a life of worship and service. The purpose of your musculoskeletal system is to provide the strength for kneeling in prayer and for lifting the burdens of your neighbor. The purpose of your nervous system is to process information from God's world in a way that leads to wonder and wisdom. Every biological system, every physiological function, finds its ultimate meaning and fulfillment when it is oriented toward the glory of God. To use this body for a purpose contrary to its design—for habitual sin, for vengeful violence, for selfish indulgence—is a profound perversion of its sacred architecture.

And this leads, inevitably, to the required posture of *reverence*. We do not tromp through a sanctuary with muddy boots and a loud voice. We enter with hushed tones, with a bowed head, with a sense of awe. Do we approach our own physical existence with such reverence? The modern world encourages a posture of either entitlement or disdain toward the body—it is a toy for our pleasure or a problem to be solved. But the biblical view calls for a sacred reverence. This means listening to its God-given signals of hunger, fatigue, and pain, not as annoyances to be suppressed with caffeine and pills, but as the temple's alarm system, signaling a need for care and attention. It means treating it with respect through hygiene, through rest, through compassionate medical care, and through protection from harm. It is to see this physical frame not as "meat," but as a miraculously wrought dwelling place, worthy of honor and diligent upkeep precisely because of the glory of its Inhabitant.

This brings us to the second staggering implication: the reality of the **Indwelling Presence**. The *naos* is not a museum, an empty monument to a departed deity. It is a residence. The Holy

Spirit is not a occasional visitor; He has taken up permanent, personal residency within you. The same *Ruach Elohim* that brooded over the primordial waters, the same *Ruach HaKodesh* that empowered the prophets and anointed the kings, the same Spirit that raised Jesus Christ from the dead, now tabernacles in your mortal flesh. Let the weight of that truth settle upon you. The infinite, holy, creative power of God is dwelling within the finite, fragile confines of your body.

This residency is the source of our sanctification and our power. The Old Testament temple was sanctified by God's presence; it was His glory that made the space holy. In the same way, it is the indwelling Spirit who sanctifies us, who sets us apart as holy unto the Lord. Our stewardship, then, is not a project of self-sanctification through sheer willpower. It is a cooperative venture with the Divine Resident. We work out our salvation with fear and trembling, *because it is God who works in us*, both to will and to work for his good pleasure (Philippians 2:12-13). The power to say "no" to the defiling influences and "yes" to the purifying ones comes from His enabling presence within the temple.

But this residency also implies an intimate and constant communion. The Spirit is not a silent tenant. He intercedes for us with groanings too deep for words (Romans 8:26). He guides us into all truth (John 16:13). He bears His fruit in our lives—love, joy, peace, and more (Galatians 5:22-23). Our response to this intimate Indwelling Presence must be one of *sensitive attentiveness*. We are called to live in a state of conscious, moment-by-moment awareness of His presence within us. This is the practice of the presence of God in its most intimate form. It is to cultivate a listening heart, to be quick to confess anything that grieves Him (Ephesians 4:30), and to create an internal environment of worship and surrender that is pleasing to our Divine Guest. Every act of bodily care, then, becomes an act of hospitality to the Holy Spirit. We are cleaning the house, preparing the meal, and maintaining the grounds for our most honored and beloved Resident.

Finally, the temple metaphor defines our bodies as the primary **Place of Worship**. The ultimate purpose of the Jerusalem temple was to be the center of Israel's worship, the place where sacrifices were offered and God's praises were sung. In a stunning eschatological shift, Jesus declared to the Samaritan woman that a time was coming when true worship would not be confined to Mount Gerizim or Jerusalem, but would be a matter of "spirit and truth" (John 4:21-24). Paul, building on this, reveals that the new locale for this true worship is the human body itself. "So glorify God in your body" (1 Corinthians 6:20). The imperative is clear: your body is the new altar, the new sanctuary, the new holy ground where the sacrifice of praise is to be continually offered.

This transforms worship from a scheduled event to a continuous lifestyle. It sacralizes the entirety of our physical existence. When you choose a nourishing meal over a degrading one, that is an act of worship. When you go for a walk, stewarding the cardiovascular system God gave you, that is an act of worship. When you discipline yourself to get adequate sleep, honoring the body's need for restoration, that is an act of worship. When you manage your stress through prayer instead of panic, demonstrating trust in God's sovereignty, that is an act of worship. And yes, when you gather with other living temples to sing praises, that is the corporate expression of what is to be the daily, private reality of each member.

This worship is expressed through the presentation of our bodies as a *living sacrifice* (Romans 12:1). In the old temple, dead animals were placed on the altar. In the new temple, we place our living, breathing, working, resting bodies upon the altar of God's service. This is our "spiritual worship," our *logikos latreia*—the rational, logical, and fitting service of a creature redeemed entirely by grace. The worship God desires is not merely the songs we sing with our lips, but the totality of our physical lives offered back to Him in grateful obedience. Every act of stewardship, every choice for purity, every moment of rest, every exertion of strength—when done for the Lord and through the power of His indwelling Spirit—becomes a fragrant offering, a spiritual sacrifice acceptable to God through Jesus Christ. The temple is not a place we go to; it is what we are. And the worship is not something we do; it is what we were created to be.

1.4 Corroborating Scriptural Witness: The Triune Testimony to Embodied Stewardship

Beloved, the foundational truth of 1 Corinthians 6:19-20 does not stand as a solitary pillar in the landscape of Scripture. To view it as such would be to risk construing it as a novel Pauline innovation or an isolated spiritual maxim. No, this radical anthropology is woven into the very fabric of the biblical narrative, from the first verses of Genesis to the final greetings of the apostolic letters. It is a chord that resonates throughout the canon, and to hear its full, rich harmony, we must listen for its echoes in the Law, the Prophets, and the Writings. The doctrine of the body as the temple of the Holy Spirit is not an outlier; it is the logical and theological consummation of a story that begins with dust and divine breath. Let us, therefore, trace this golden thread through three pivotal passages that corroborate, illuminate, and expand upon this central mandate.

First, we turn to the great Pauline treatise on the application of redemption, the Epistle to the Romans. In chapter 12, verses 1 and 2, we find what is perhaps the most comprehensive and programmatic statement on the Christian life ever penned: **"I appeal to you therefore, brothers, by the mercies of God, to present your bodies as a living sacrifice, holy and acceptable to God, which is your spiritual worship. Do not be conformed to this world, but be transformed by the renewal of your mind, that by testing you may discern what is the will of God, what is good and acceptable and perfect."**

Here, the temple metaphor of 1 Corinthians finds its explicit ethical and liturgical counterpart. Paul's "therefore" reaches back across eleven chapters of profound theological exposition—of human depravity, of justification by faith, of union with Christ in his death and resurrection, of the struggle with indwelling sin, and of the sovereign purposes of God in election. It is upon the solid bedrock of these "mercies of God" that he builds his appeal. The response to such grace is not merely an internal feeling or a verbal assent; it is the physical, tangible presentation of our *bodies* as a *living sacrifice*.

Consider the radical nature of this command. In the Old Testament sacrificial system, the animal was killed *before* it was placed on the altar. Its death was the prerequisite for its acceptance. But Paul calls us to offer ourselves as living sacrifices. This means that our entire physical existence—our breathing, our working, our eating, our resting—is to be continuously placed upon the altar of God's service. The altar is no longer a stone structure in Jerusalem; it is the ongoing, daily reality of a life offered to God. This sacrifice is to be *holy*—set apart from common use, consecrated exclusively for God's purposes—and *acceptable* to Him, meaning it aligns with His character and will as revealed in His Word.

And then Paul delivers the stunning punchline: this bodily offering is your *logiken latreian*. This Greek phrase is dense with meaning. *Latreia* is the word for religious service or worship, often used of the priestly temple service. *Logiken* can mean "spiritual" in the sense of being wrought by the Spirit, but its primary meaning is "rational," "logical," or "true to reason." This is not an ecstatic, disembodied spiritualism. It is the most rational, logical, and fitting response a redeemed creature can offer to its Creator-Redeemer. To withhold your body from this sacrificial offering is, from a Pauline perspective, profoundly illogical. It is a contradiction of the gospel itself. The body, therefore, is not an impediment to worship; it is the necessary instrument of true, spiritual worship. The mind's renewal (the transformation of our thinking) is intrinsically linked to the body's presentation. We cannot have one without the other. A renewed mind will necessarily lead to a consecrated body, and a consecrated body becomes the vehicle through which a renewed mind discerns and performs the will of God in the world.

But to fully appreciate this New Testament fulfillment, we must journey back to the very beginning, to the pristine origins of humanity. In **Genesis 1:26-28 and 2:7, 15**, we find the creational blueprint that establishes the inherent goodness and sacred purpose of the physical body. The text declares that God created humanity in His own image, *tselem Elohim*. This *Imago Dei* is not merely a spiritual quality; it is embodied. The divine image is stamped upon physical, gendered beings—"male and female he created them." Our physicality is not an afterthought or a lower nature; it is part of the divine likeness itself.

This is powerfully underscored in Genesis 2:7: **"then the LORD God formed the man of dust from the ground and breathed into his nostrils the breath of life, and the man became a living creature."** The Hebrew word for "formed" is *yatsar*, a potter's term, conveying intimate, hands-on craftsmanship. The body (*basar*) is skillfully fashioned from the dust of the earth (*aphar*). It is material, earthly. But it is not merely material. God breathes His own *nishmat chayyim*—the breath of life—into this clay form, and the result is a *nephesh chayyah*—a living being. The human is an *ensouled body*, an *embodied soul*. There is no dualism here. The physical and the spiritual are fused together in a holistic unity from the moment of creation. The body is, therefore, inherently good, a masterpiece of the divine Artisan.

Furthermore, this embodied image-bearer is immediately given a physical, cultural mandate. In Genesis 1:28, they are commanded to "be fruitful and multiply and fill the earth and subdue it, and have dominion." This requires physical bodies. In Genesis 2:15, Adam is placed in the garden "to work it and keep it." The Hebrew words *avad* (to work, serve) and *shamar* (to keep, guard) imply purposeful, physical labor. The body was designed for creative, productive, stewarding work within the created order. Its original purpose was not passivity or escape, but active, engaged, physical dominion under God's authority. The Fall corrupted this labor, turning it into painful toil (Genesis 3:17-19), but it did not annul the mandate. The New Testament vision of presenting our bodies as a living sacrifice is, in a profound sense, the redemption and restoration of this original creational purpose. We are reclaiming our bodies for the work of "subduing" and "keeping" the little plot of creation that is our own life, offering it back to God as our priestly service.

Finally, we see this holistic vision reflected in the pastoral heart of the apostolic community. The aged apostle John writes in his third letter, verse 2: **"Beloved, I pray that all may go well with you and that you may be in good health, as it goes well with your soul."** This is a breathtakingly comprehensive pastoral blessing. The Greek word for "go well" is *euodousthai*, which means to prosper on a journey, to succeed in one's endeavors. The word for "health" is *hugiainein*, from which we get "hygiene," meaning to be sound, healthy, and well-functioning in one's physical being.

John makes no artificial separation. He does not pray only for the prosperity of Gaius's soul. He explicitly yokes the prosperity and health of his physical life to the prosperity of his spiritual life. The "as" (*kathos*) indicates a correspondence, a harmony that is desired between the outer and the inner man. This apostolic wish demolishes any lingering sacred-secular divide. It is a prayer for holistic *shalom*—for the total well-being of the person. John recognizes that a soul flourishing in truth and love (3 John 3-4) should be accompanied by a body that is functioning in health and vitality, and vice-versa. He is praying that the external circumstances of Gaius's life, including his physical health, would be in harmonious alignment with the internal reality of his spiritual vitality. This is not a prayer for the "prosperity gospel" in the modern, materialistic sense; it is a prayer for integrated, holistic flourishing that enables maximum effectiveness and testimony for the gospel. It is an implicit affirmation that caring for one's physical health is a spiritual concern, worthy of apostolic intercession.

Thus, from the creation narrative's declaration of embodied goodness, to the Romans 12 mandate for bodily worship, to the apostolic prayer for holistic health, the scriptural witness forms a consistent and powerful chorus. The body is good, the body is for God's glory, the body is the instrument of our worship, and the body's well-being is a matter of profound spiritual significance. The temple theology of 1 Corinthians 6 is not a strange new teaching; it is the glorious unveiling of what has been true from the beginning and what remains the hopeful prayer of God's people until the final redemption of our physical frames.

1.5 Historical Theology: Views of the Body in Early Church Fathers (e.g., Augustine, Clement of Alexandria)

Beloved, as we continue to erect the theological framework for our doctrine of Embodied Stewardship, we must now turn our gaze backward, to the foundational centuries of the Church's pilgrimage. For we do not interpret Scripture in a vacuum, but as members of a great cloud of witnesses, standing upon the shoulders of those who first wrestled with the implications of the Gospel in a world saturated with competing philosophies. The Patristic era, the age of the Church Fathers, was a crucible in which Christian orthodoxy was forged in the fires of controversy and reflection. And central to these controversies was the question of the body. How were these early theologians, these shepherds of souls and defenders of the faith, to understand the flesh that the Word had become? Their answers, their struggles, their profound insights, and their tragic missteps, have left an indelible mark upon the Christian tradition, creating a complex legacy that we must navigate with both gratitude and critical discernment.

To understand the Patristic landscape, we must first appreciate the powerful intellectual currents against which the early Church had to swim. The dominant philosophical atmosphere of the Greco-Roman world was profoundly dualistic, shaped by the enduring influence of Platonism and its various offshoots. In this worldview, reality was divided into two realms: the higher, immaterial, unchanging realm of the Forms—the realm of true being, goodness, and light—and the lower, material, changing realm of becoming—the world of shadows, illusion, and decay. The human person was seen as a divine spark, an immortal soul, tragically imprisoned in a mortal, material body. Salvation, in this schema, was the soul's liberation from the body, its ascent from the cave of material existence back to the pure, intellectual contemplation of the Divine. This was the air that the Apologists and Fathers breathed, and it posed a constant, seductive threat to a fully biblical anthropology.

It is within this context that we encounter the formidable figure of **Clement of Alexandria (c. 150 – c. 215)**, a theologian of the Alexandrian school who sought to baptize Greek philosophy into the service of Christ. Clement, in works like his *Paedagogus* (The Tutor), provides one of the most detailed early Christian treatments of daily life, including extensive discussions on food, drink, dress, and sleep. His approach is that of a spiritual director guiding the believer toward *apatheia*—a state of tranquility and freedom from disordered passions.

Clement's view of the body is, in many ways, a nuanced and pastoral attempt at a *via media*. He vehemently rejects the crass libertinism that would indulge the body's every whim. For Clement, the Christian is called to a life of moderation and self-control. He offers practical, even proto-hygienic advice: he recommends simple, nourishing food over rich delicacies, warns against drunkenness, and advocates for moderation in all things. He sees the body as an instrument that must be kept in good working order for the sake of the soul's pursuits. In this, he aligns with the biblical principle of stewardship. The body is the horse, and the soul is the rider; a well-trained and cared-for horse is essential for the rider to reach his destination.

However, the pervasive influence of Platonic dualism casts a long shadow over Clement's thought. While he does not see the body as inherently evil, he consistently views it with suspicion, as the primary source of the passions that war against the soul. His goal is not the positive sanctification of the body as a good creation, but its *subjugation* and *management* for the sake of spiritual advancement. The body's needs are concessions to its weakness. For instance, he permits marriage but clearly views celibacy as a higher, more spiritual state. He allows food, but primarily as a necessary fuel, warning against taking any real pleasure in it, lest it inflame desire. The body, in Clement's framework, is less a temple and more a potential adversary that must be held in check by the rational soul. This creates a tension, a tendency toward an asceticism that, while not as extreme as that of the desert monks, still leans toward a spirituality of negation and control rather than one of affirmation and consecration. The "temple" is maintained, but more as a fortress under siege than a dwelling place filled with glory.

This trajectory finds its most profound and psychologically complex expression in the towering figure of **Saint Augustine of Hippo (354-430)**. No single figure, perhaps, has done more to shape Western Christianity's understanding of the human person, and his wrestling with the body is central to his entire theological project. Augustine's anthropology cannot be understood apart from his own dramatic conversion, as recounted in his *Confessions*, a text that sears itself into the reader's memory with its raw honesty about the power of bodily desire, particularly lust.

For Augustine, the body is unequivocally part of God's good creation. He is a staunch anti-Manichean, rejecting the heresy that taught the material world was the creation of an evil deity. The body, in its original, pre-lapsarian state, was perfectly subject to the will. In Paradise, Augustine imagines, Adam and Eve could command their bodily members with the same effortless authority with which we command our hands to move. Sexual desire, like all other physical functions, would have been a calm act of the will, devoid of the tumultuous, involuntary *libido* that characterizes it after the Fall.

And herein lies the heart of the Augustinian view: the catastrophic nature of the Fall. Sin, for Augustine, is not merely a legal transgression; it is a fundamental dislocation of the human person, a wounding of our very nature. Its most evident symptom is the rebellion of the body against the soul. We now experience what he famously called the *libido dominandi*, the lust for domination, and this is manifested physically in the phenomenon of *concupiscentia carnis*—concupiscence of the flesh. This is not merely sexual desire, but a fundamental disorder of all our appetites, a state of inner division where the flesh lusts against the spirit (Galatians 5:17) in a way that was never God's original intention.

Thus, in Augustine's mature thought, the body itself is not evil, but it has become a field of battle, a constant reminder of our fallen state. The involuntary stirrings of desire, the weakness of the flesh, the insubordination of our members—these are the evidence of original sin inscribed upon our very biology. This perspective leads to a profound theological realism, but it also carries a powerful, and some would argue, damaging, psychological weight. The body becomes associated with shame, with a loss of control, with the "law of sin" that dwells in our members (Romans 7:23). While Augustine would affirm the resurrection of the body, his focus in the *saeculum*—this present age—is often on the body's role as an instrument of sin and a source of spiritual struggle. The call to stewardship, then, becomes a call to a militant asceticism, a constant warfare to bring the rebellious body into subjection through grace, lest its disordered desires lead the soul to perdition. The temple is a battlefield, and the indwelling Spirit is the divine General in a war against the traitorous flesh.

When we place Clement and Augustine in dialogue, we see the early Church's profound struggle to hold creation and redemption together in tension with the reality of the Fall. Both, in their own ways, affirm the body's origin in a good creation. Both vehemently reject the libertine indulgence of the body. Yet, both are profoundly shaped by a philosophical milieu that viewed materiality as inferior to spirit, leading them to emphasize the subjugation of the body for spiritual ends. The positive, creational vision of the body as the essential instrument for fulfilling the cultural mandate, the holistic *shalom* of 3 John 1:2, often recedes into the background, overshadowed by a defensive, post-lapsarian focus on the body as a problem to be managed.

This Patristic legacy is our inheritance. It has given us a rich vocabulary for understanding the dynamics of sin and the necessity of grace in the spiritual life. It has rightly warned us against the idolatry of the flesh. But it has also, at times, bequeathed to us a spirituality tinged with a suspicion of the physical that can hinder a full-orbed celebration of the body as the *naos* of the Holy Spirit. Our task, as modern stewards of this tradition, is to receive its wisdom while critically refining it in the brighter light of a more comprehensive biblical theology—one that, without denying the reality of concupiscence, can also proclaim with joy that these very bodies, in all their materiality, are fearfully and wonderfully made, indwelt by Deity, and destined for glorious, physical resurrection. The journey of historical theology reveals that we are still learning, still recovering, the breathtaking implications of the Incarnation for these jars of clay.

1.6 The Body as a Non-Negotiable Locus of Christian Obedience and Witness

Beloved, as we draw this foundational chapter to its close, we must now gather up the threads of our exegetical, theological, and historical exploration and weave them into a single, unshakable conviction that must henceforth govern our every breath, our every meal, our every movement, our every moment of rest. The cumulative weight of the biblical witness, from Genesis to the Apostolic writings, and even through the complex legacy of the Church Fathers, presses upon us one inescapable conclusion: **the physical body is a non-negotiable, indispensable, and primary locus of Christian obedience and witness.** It is not an optional addendum to the spiritual life; it is the very theater in which the drama of redemption is enacted, the essential instrument through which our faith finds its tangible expression in the world.

Let us be unequivocally clear: to relegate the care and discipline of the body to the realm of secondary issues, matters of Christian liberty, or personal preference is to commit a grave theological error. It is to fundamentally misunderstand the gospel. The great heresy of our age is not a formal denial of the Trinity or the deity of Christ, though those abound, but a *practical, lived* heresy of anthropological dualism that severs the spiritual from the physical, creating a schism in the human person that the Incarnation came to heal. We have been seduced into believing that we can pursue God with our hearts and minds while simultaneously neglecting, abusing, or idolizing the physical vessel that contains them. This is a demonic deception, for it neutralizes the potency of our witness and dilutes the integrity of our discipleship.

Consider the profound implications of this for the nature of **Christian obedience**. Obedience to God is never abstract or disembodied. The Ten Commandments are not ten suggestions for spiritual contemplation; they are directives for embodied living: "You shall not murder" regulates the physical act of taking life. "You shall not commit adultery" governs the physical and relational union of sexuality. "You shall not steal" concerns the physical property of our neighbor. When Jesus summarizes the Law as loving God with all our heart, soul, mind, and *strength*, and loving our neighbor *as ourselves*, He is issuing a command that is irreducibly physical. Love is not a sentiment; it is an action. It requires the expenditure of caloric energy, the use of vocal cords, the employment of muscular strength, the engagement of the senses. We love our neighbor by feeding the hungry, which requires hands to prepare food and legs to carry it. We love our neighbor by visiting the sick and imprisoned, which requires a body to travel and to sit in presence. We love our neighbor by sheltering the homeless, which requires physical labor and the sharing of material resources.

Therefore, the disciplined stewardship of our physical strength, our health, and our energy is not a self-centered pursuit. It is an act of preparation for love. It is the sharpening of the tool for its intended work. A body weakened by chronic neglect, a mind fogged by poor nutrition and sleep deprivation, a nervous system frayed by unmanaged stress—these are not merely personal problems; they are impediments to the Great Commandment. They diminish our capacity for sustained, costly, tangible love. When we choose the salad over the gluttonous feast, we are not just making a healthy choice; we are choosing to have more energy for our family, our ministry, our neighbor. When we discipline ourselves to go to bed on time, we are not just avoiding fatigue; we are ensuring that we will be mentally and emotionally present for the people who need us tomorrow. When we engage in physical exercise, we are not merely building muscle; we are building the physical resilience required to endure in long-term service, to bear one another's burdens, to run the race set before us without collapsing before the finish line. This is why bodily stewardship is a non-negotiable of obedience: because you cannot love your neighbor with a body you are actively destroying or passively allowing to decay.

Furthermore, the body is the indispensable instrument of our **sacramental life**. The God who created matter uses matter as a means of grace. In the waters of Baptism, a physical body is washed, signifying a spiritual reality. In the Eucharist, we physically eat bread and drink wine, and through these material elements, by faith, we partake of the body and blood of Christ. These are not spiritual metaphors alone; they are physical actions with spiritual consequences. They teach us that God meets us in and through our physicality. To disdain the body is to disdain the very channels through which God has chosen to communicate His grace. Our participation in these sacraments is a profound affirmation of the goodness of the physical and a rehearsal for the day when we will sit at the physical, material Marriage Supper of the Lamb.

This leads us directly to the body's role in **Christian witness**. In a world that is simultaneously obsessed with and confused by the body—treating it as everything from a canvas for self-expression to a machine for optimization—the Church is called to display a radically different anthropology. Our testimony is not merely verbal; it is incarnational. The world needs to see a people who treat their bodies with reverence, not with the anxious control of the narcissist or the pious neglect of the false ascetic. They need to see a people who eat with gratitude and discipline, who rest without guilt and work without compulsion, who age with grace and face illness with hope, who steward their health not as a god but as a gift for God's service.

This kind of embodied witness is profoundly counter-cultural. It preaches a silent sermon about a God who is Lord of all creation, including our physical frames. It testifies to a hope that is not an escape *from* the body, but the redemption *of* the body. When we treat our bodies as temples, we are making a visible, tangible statement about the value of the One who dwells within. A neglected, chronically stressed, malnourished, or undisciplined Christian is a walking contradiction. Their life preaches a gospel that is powerful enough to save the soul but not to sanctify the body. But a believer whose life is marked by the peaceful, disciplined, joyful stewardship of their physical existence is a powerful apologia for the faith. They demonstrate that the Gospel is holistic, that it addresses the whole person, and that the Lordship of Christ extends to every calorie consumed, every hour of sleep, every moment of exercise, and every thought taken captive.

Therefore, my brothers and sisters, the call to embodied stewardship is a call to radical, integrated discipleship. It demands that we repent of our functional Gnosticism. It requires that we bring our grocery lists, our workout routines, our sleep schedules, and our medical appointments under the searching light of Scripture and the lordship of Christ. It is here, in the mundane, physical details of our daily existence, that we prove the reality of our faith. It is here that we offer our bodies as living sacrifices. It is here that we glorify God in our bodies.

This is not a call to a new legalism, a fresh set of rules to be anxious about. It is an invitation into a new freedom—the glorious freedom of the children of God, who are no longer slaves to the tyranny of appetite, the idolatry of appearance, or the neglect of the physical. It is the freedom to use this body, this temple, for its ultimate and highest purpose: to know God, to enjoy Him forever, and to love our neighbor as ourselves. Let us then go forth from this place, not as disembodied spirits, but as whole, integrated persons, determined to live out the truth that our bodies are not our own, they were bought with a price, and therefore, we will glorify God in these, our physical frames.

CHAPTER 02

Theological Anthropology: The Unity of Body, Soul, and Spirit

2.1 Introduction: The Architecture of Human Being

Beloved, we now embark upon what may be the most critical theological expedition of our entire study—a journey into the very mystery of human personhood. For if our doctrine of Embodied Stewardship, so powerfully established upon the temple metaphor of 1 Corinthians 6, is to stand firm against the relentless tides of cultural confusion and spiritual error, it must be built upon the unshakable foundation of a right understanding of what—or rather, *who*—a human being actually is. We must move now from the powerful *metaphor* of the temple to the intricate *architecture* of the human being as revealed in the grand narrative of Scripture. We are engaging here in the sacred science of **Theological Anthropology**—that branch of divinity which studies humanity from the perspective of its origin, its nature, its destiny, and its relationship to God.

I tell you today that the prevailing models of the human person offered to us by the modern world are not merely incomplete; they are pathogenic. They are soul-sickening visions that lead either to despair or to a dangerous, inflated pride. On one hand, we are presented with the stark, sterile vision of **Reductive Materialism**. This is the dominant dogma of our scientific age, which insists that the human person is nothing more than a complex assemblage of biochemical processes, a fortuitous collocation of atoms, an advanced neural computer. In this view, consciousness is an epiphenomenon, love is a synaptic illusion, and the soul is a myth. You are your body, and when your body ceases to function, *you* cease to exist. This is a anthropology of dust, and to dust it shall return. It offers no foundation for inherent dignity, no basis for ultimate meaning, and no hope beyond the grave. It reduces the glorious symphony of human experience to the random clattering of particles in the void.

In reaction to this barren materialism, many, even within the church, have instinctively retreated into a form of **Dualistic Spiritualism**. This is the ancient, persistent error that fundamentally divides the human person into two separate, often warring, substances: a higher, immortal, spiritual soul and a lower, temporary, material body. In this schema, popularized by Greek philosophy and often unwittingly baptized into Christian piety, the *real* you is the soul. The body is at best a temporary vehicle, a spacesuit for the soul's journey through the material world, and at worst, a prison, a tomb, a source of temptation and corruption from which the soul longs to be liberated. This view creates a spiritual hierarchy where activities of the mind and spirit are valued above the needs and disciplines of the body. It leads to a neglect of physical health, a suspicion of physical pleasure, and a failure to see the body's role in salvation and sanctification.

Both of these models—the reductionist and the dualist—are profound heresies against the biblical witness. They represent a catastrophic failure to understand the divine architecture of the human being. The Scriptures present us with a third way, a vision of breathtaking wholeness and integration. The biblical view is neither a monism that collapses spirit into matter, nor a dualism that tears them asunder. It is, rather, a holistic **psychosomatic unity**—a dynamic, complex, and glorious integration in which the physical and the spiritual are inextricably co-inherent, mutually conditioning, and essential to the totality of what it means to be a human person created in the *Imago Dei*.

This holistic anthropology is not a secondary or abstract doctrine. It is the essential framework, the architectural blueprint, without which our pursuit of holistic health becomes just another form of secular wellness, devoid of its ultimate meaning and power. If we get our anthropology wrong, our entire approach to stewardship will be skewed. If we are merely souls, then bodily discipline is at best a helpful tool and at worst a distraction. If we are merely bodies, then health is the highest good, and death is the ultimate defeat. But if we are, as Scripture reveals, *ensouled bodies* and *embodied souls*, then the care of this physical frame is a sacred duty integral to our spiritual worship, and the hope of the resurrection is the glorious completion of our creation and redemption.

Therefore, in this chapter, we will delve into the deep structures of biblical personhood. We will wrestle with the exegetical complexities of the tripartite and bipartite views, seeking to understand what the Scripture means when it speaks of spirit (*pneuma*), soul (*psyche*), and body (*soma*). We will recover the profound Hebraic concept of *nephesh*—the living being—which stands as a bulwark against all forms of Hellenistic dualism. We will explore the functional distinctions between pneuma and psyche in the New Testament, understanding how the spirit relates us to God and how the soul constitutes our natural life. We will reaffirm the essential goodness and integral nature of the body (*soma*) as part of our personal identity, a truth sealed by the doctrine of the bodily resurrection. And we will see how all of this is grounded in and flows from our status as bearers of the Divine Image.

This is not an academic exercise for the sake of curiosity. This is a pastoral and practical necessity. For when a believer struggling with anxiety understands that their panic is not just a "spiritual" failure but a disruption of the psychosomatic unity that may have physiological, psychological, and spiritual dimensions, they can seek holistic help without shame. When a Christian seeking to glorify God realizes that their choice of food affects not only their physical health but also their mental clarity and spiritual receptivity, they are empowered to eat as an act of worship. When the church grasps that we are not meant to escape our bodies but to offer them as living sacrifices, our entire approach to worship, mission, and community is transformed.

So, I invite you, dear friends, to open your minds and hearts to the profound mystery of your own being. We are about to explore the architecture of the human person as designed by the Master Architect. We will see that we are fearfully and wonderfully made, not as a collection of separate parts, but as a complex, dynamic, and integrated whole, created for relationship with God and destined for a glory that will encompass both body and spirit for all eternity. Let us begin this exploration with humility and awe, for to study the human person is to gaze upon a masterpiece of the Divine Artisan.

2.2 Tripartite and Bipartite Views: An Exegetical Survey

Beloved, as we delve deeper into the architecture of the human person, we must now confront a question that has occupied the finest theological minds of the Church for two millennia: what is the fundamental constitution of a human being? Are we composed of two essential parts, or three? This is not a mere academic parlor game, a speculative debate for theologians with too much time on their hands. No, this question strikes at the very heart of how we understand our relationship with God, the nature of sin and salvation, and indeed, the practical outworking of our embodied stewardship. The way we answer this question will shape our spirituality, our approach to discipleship, and our understanding of what it means to be made whole in Christ.

The history of Christian thought reveals a persistent, nuanced, and often contentious debate concerning the number of constituent parts in a human. This debate generally crystallizes around two primary models: the **Tripartite** view (body, soul, and spirit) and the **Bipartite** view (material and immaterial, or body and soul/spirit). We must approach this topic not with a spirit of divisiveness, but with a humble desire to be faithful to the whole counsel of God, recognizing that pious and learned saints have found compelling evidence for both perspectives within the sacred text. Our task is to listen carefully to the biblical witness, to weigh the exegetical evidence, and to arrive at a formulation that best captures the integrated complexity of the human person as presented in Scripture.

Let us begin with the **Tripartite View**, which posits that a human being is composed of three distinct, though intimately related, components: the body (*soma*), the soul (*psyche*), and the spirit (*pneuma*). Proponents of this view, which includes a significant stream of early Church Fathers and finds resonance in much of the early Greek patristic tradition, point to several key texts that appear to delineate these three aspects with intentional precision.

The cornerstone of the tripartite position is **1 Thessalonians 5:23**: "*Now may the God of peace himself sanctify you completely, and may your whole spirit and soul and body be kept blameless at the coming of our Lord Jesus Christ.*" Here, the Apostle Paul offers a benediction that seems to encompass the entire human person. He uses a threefold structure: pneuma (spirit), psyche (soul), and soma (body). The tripartite advocate argues that this is not a casual or poetic listing, but a deliberate, theological description of the holistic nature of human sanctification. The word "whole" (*holokleron*) implies an integrity and completeness that includes every facet of our being. If "soul" and "spirit" were merely synonymous terms, Paul would be guilty of a redundant tautology, an unnecessary repetition that weakens the force of his comprehensive prayer. Instead, he appears to be praying for the sanctification of the believer in every dimension: the spiritual dimension that relates directly to God, the psychological dimension that constitutes the natural life and personality, and the physical dimension of bodily existence. This, for the tripartite view, is a clear biblical warrant for a trichotomous anthropology.

Further compelling support is drawn from **Hebrews 4:12**, which speaks of the living and active Word of God, sharper than any two-edged sword, "*piercing to the division of soul and of spirit, of joints and of marrow.*" The author of Hebrews presents a powerful image of the penetrating, discerning power of Scripture. It does not merely separate the grossly physical from the immaterial; it performs a more subtle and profound surgery, making a distinction even between that which is most intimately connected—the *psyche* and the *pneuma*. The analogy is drawn from the human body: just as a sword can separate joints (*harmon*, the meeting points of bones) and marrow (*myelos*, the innermost, life-producing substance within the bones), so the Word of God can divide between the soul and the spirit. The tripartite interpretation sees here a recognition that the *psyche* (the natural, self-conscious life, the seat of the emotions and will) and the *pneuma* (the God-conscious faculty, the capacity for communion with the Divine), while closely united, are not identical. The Word of God can discern the motivations, revealing whether an action springs from the natural soul (which can be noble but ultimately self-directed) or from the redeemed spirit (which is oriented toward God). This ability to divide presupposes a real, functional distinction between the two.

However, standing in contrast to this view is the **Bipartite View**, which has been the dominant position in Western theology, particularly within the Reformed and Thomistic traditions. This view sees the human person as composed of two fundamental parts: the material body (*soma*) and the immaterial soul or spirit, with "soul" (*psyche*) and "spirit" (*pneuma*) being largely synonymous terms used to describe the single, immaterial aspect of human nature from different perspectives.

The bipartite view finds strong exegetical support in numerous passages where "soul" and "spirit" appear to be used interchangeably. A key text is **Matthew 10:28**, where Jesus instructs His disciples: "*And do not fear those who kill the body but cannot kill the soul. Rather fear him who can destroy both soul and body in hell.*" Here, the fundamental dichotomy is clear:

the body (*soma*) and the soul (*psyche*). The soul is presented as that which survives physical death and faces eternal judgment. There is no mention of a third, distinct "spirit" in this ultimate contrast between the physical and the eternal fate of the person.

Similarly, in the poignant scene of Gethsemane, Jesus confesses to His disciples in **Matthew 26:38**, "*My soul (*psyche*) is very sorrowful, even to death.*" He is describing the deepest anguish of His inner being, the core of His personhood, and He uses the term *psyche.* In Luke's account of the crucifixion, Jesus cries out, "*Father, into your hands I commit my spirit (*pneuma*)!*" (Luke 23:46). The bipartite advocate argues that these are not descriptions of different parts of Christ's immaterial being, but synonymous terms for His inner self, His life principle, offered up to the Father. The *psyche* is sorrowful, the *pneuma* is committed—both refer to the one, immaterial center of His person.

Another powerful line of evidence for the bipartite view comes from the Pauline corpus itself, specifically **2 Corinthians 5:1-8**. Here, Paul contrasts our present earthly existence with our future heavenly one. He describes our current state as being in an "earthly tent" (*skenous*, the physical body) that is being destroyed. Our longing is not to be "unclothed" (a disembodied state), but to be "further clothed" with our heavenly dwelling. The entire passage operates with a two-part framework: the physical body ("tent") and the self that inhabits it, which he refers to variously as "we" ourselves, and which, when absent from the body, is "at home with the Lord" (v.8). The fundamental contrast is between embodied existence and disembodied existence with the Lord, with no intermediate, third component delineated.

Furthermore, the bipartite view argues that the tripartite proof-texts can be understood differently. In 1 Thessalonians 5:23, the listing of "spirit, soul, and body" can be seen as a rhetorical device known as a triad, a common Hebraic way of expressing totality (e.g., "heart, soul, and might" in Deuteronomy 6:5). Paul is not outlining a metaphysical blueprint but praying for the sanctification of the *whole person* in every conceivable aspect. Similarly, in Hebrews 4:12, the division of "soul and spirit" is not a metaphysical separation of two distinct entities, but a powerful metaphor for the penetrating discernment of God's Word, which can separate the deepest, most hidden intentions and thoughts of the *heart* (a single, inner source)—much like dividing joints and marrow, which are not separate substances but different aspects of a single physical structure.

This survey reveals that the biblical witness is rich and complex, presenting a picture of the human person that resists simplistic reduction. We are faced with texts that, on the surface, seem to support both a two-part and a three-part model. The resolution, as we shall see, is not to force a rigid either/or but to seek a more holistic synthesis that does justice to the Hebraic worldview underlying the Scriptures—a worldview that thinks in terms of functional, dynamic unity rather than static, structural parts.

2.3 A Holistic Synthesis: The Hebraic Concept of *Nephesh*

Beloved, having carefully surveyed the exegetical landscape of the tripartite and bipartite views, we now find ourselves at a critical juncture. To remain entrenched in a debate framed by the very categories of Greek philosophical substance metaphysics is to risk missing the profound, life-giving unity of the biblical witness. The resolution to this ancient debate is not found in choosing one set of proof-texts over another, but in a fundamental paradigm shift—a return to the rich, holistic, and dynamic Hebraic worldview that forms the foundational soil of divine revelation. We must learn to think like Hebrew poets and prophets, not like Greek philosophers. And at the very heart of this Hebrew anthropology lies the pivotal, often misunderstood, concept of ***nephesh*** (נֶפֶשׁ).

Let us be clear: the common English translation of *nephesh* as "soul" is one of the most consequential and misleading translational choices in the entire Bible. For the average Christian, conditioned by two millennia of Hellenistic influence, the word "soul" immediately conjures the image of an immortal, immaterial, spiritual substance temporarily inhabiting a physical body—a ghost in the machine. This is the Platonic soul, the psyche of Greek philosophy, a divine spark yearning for release from its material prison. But this is not what nephesh means. To impose this foreign concept upon the Hebrew text is to do violence to the biblical understanding of the human person and to create the very dualistic schism we are seeking to heal.

So, what, then, is *nephesh*? The term is used over 750 times in the Old Testament, and its meaning is robust, concrete, and embodied. Fundamentally, a *nephesh* is a **whole, living being**. It is the "self," the "life," the "person," the vital, animating force that constitutes a creature as alive. Crucially, *nephesh* is not something a person *has*; it is what a person *is* when they are alive. We see this from the very beginning of creation. In Genesis 1:20, 24, God creates the great sea creatures and every *nephesh chayyah*—every "living creature"—that moves. Animals are *nephesh*. They are living beings, whole and complete in their animated, physical existence.

But the defining moment for human anthropology comes in Genesis 2:7, a verse that should be the cornerstone of all our thinking about the body: "*Then the LORD God formed the man of dust from the ground and breathed into his nostrils the breath of life (*nishmat chayyim*), and the man became a living creature (*l'nephesh chayyah*)."* Let us parse this with the utmost care. The process is deliberate and profound. First, God *forms* (*yatsar*). This is the language of a potter, an artisan, working with a material substance—the *aphar*, the dust of the ground. This is the body (*basar*), the physical, material component, skillfully crafted from the earth. It is, at this point, inert, lifeless clay.

Then, God *breathes*. He imparts the *nishmat chayyim*—the breath of life. This "breath" (*neshamah*) is closely related to the word *ruach*, meaning wind, spirit, or breath. It is the animating principle, the power of life that comes directly from God Himself. It is divine energy.

And now, the critical climax: the text does *not* say, "and God put a soul into the body." It declares the result of this divine in-breathing: "*the man became a living nephesh.*" The dust *became* a living being. The inanimate material, when filled with God's life-giving breath, was transformed into a new, holistic reality: a *nephesh chayyah*. The human is not a composite of a body *plus* a soul. The human is an *animated body*, a *physical being filled with the breath of God*. The physical and the spiritual are not two separate things that are joined together; they are two necessary aspects that, when united by divine fiat, constitute a single, irreducible reality: a living human person.

This is why the Hebrew conception of personhood is fundamentally holistic and anti-dualistic. You cannot have a *nephesh* without a body, and a body without the breath of life is not a *nephesh*; it is a corpse. This is the death described in Ecclesiastes 12:7: "the dust returns to the earth as it was, and the spirit (*ruach*) returns to God who gave it." The *nephesh* ceases to exist as a living, integrated whole when the body and the life-breath are separated. The hope of the Old Testament saint, therefore, was not for the immortality of a disembodied soul, but for the resurrection of the body—the restoration of the *nephesh*—as the full and final victory over death. This is the hope of Job: "And after my skin has been thus destroyed, yet in my flesh I shall see God" (Job 19:26).

This holistic anthropology is powerfully demonstrated in what we might call Hebrew psychology. In our modern, Western view, we locate our inner life—our thoughts, emotions, and will—in the brain, in the mind, an abstract, non-physical space. But the Hebrew worldview, consistent with its view of the *nephesh*, located these faculties in specific physical organs. This was not primitive ignorance; it was a profound theological statement about the psychosomatic unity of the person.

- The **heart** (*lev*) was not merely the pump for blood; it was the center of the intellect, the will, and the moral life. To "set your heart" on something was to direct your entire cognitive and volitional capacity toward it (Exodus 7:23).
- The **bowels** (*rachamim*, related to the word for womb) were the seat of deep, visceral compassion and mercy. When Jeremiah speaks of his "bowels being troubled" (Jeremiah 31:20), he is describing a physical-emotional experience of profound pity.
- The **kidneys** (*kelayot*) were considered the seat of the deepest inner thoughts, the conscience, and the

emotions. The Psalmist speaks of God examining his "heart and mind" (literally, "kidneys and heart") in Psalm 7:9 and of God testing his *kelayot* in Psalm 26:2.

- The **bones** (*atsamot*) could express joy ("our bones vibrate like grass," Job 4:14) or anguish ("my bones are troubled," Psalm 6:2).

This was not a belief that thoughts were manufactured in the kidneys, but a powerful, embodied way of expressing that the entire person—the whole *nephesh*—thinks, feels, and wills. There is no purely "mental" event that is disconnected from the physical, and no purely "physical" event that is disconnected from the inner self. A guilty conscience causes physical discomfort. Deep love is felt in the gut. Joy makes the bones vibrate. This is the language of a people who understood that they were, from top to bottom, integrated, psychosomatic unities.

Therefore, when we return to the New Testament debate with this Hebraic foundation of *nephesh*, we can propose a holistic synthesis. The New Testament terms *soma* (body), *psyche* (soul), and *pneuma* (spirit) are not describing separate, metaphysical *parts* that can be neatly dissected. Rather, they are describing different *modes of being*, different *faculties or relationships* of the one, whole person.

- ***Soma*** is the person in their physical, embodied existence, their mode of being as a creature in the world, relating to other creatures and to the material creation.
- ***Psyche*** is the person as a living, self-conscious individual, the seat of natural life, will, emotion, and personality—the New Testament counterpart to the *nephesh*.

- ***Pneuma*** is the person in their capacity for relationship with God, the faculty that is receptive to the Holy Spirit, the dimension of the person that is oriented toward the transcendent.

A human being is not a spirit *and* a soul *and* a body. A human being is a single, unified *nephesh* who *has* a physical mode of existence (*soma*), a natural, self-aware mode of existence (*psyche*), and a God-oriented mode of existence (*pneuma*). In the unregenerate person, the *pneuma* is deadened, inoperative, cut off from God (Ephesians 2:1). In regeneration, the Holy Spirit quickens the human *pneuma*, restoring its capacity for communion with God, and begins the process of sanctifying the entire *nephesh*—renewing the *psyche* (Romans 12:2) and redeeming the *soma* (Romans 8:23).

This holistic synthesis, grounded in the Hebraic *nephesh*, allows us to affirm the valid insights of both the bipartite and tripartite views without succumbing to a destructive dualism. It tells us that we are not souls trapped in bodies, but glorious, God-breathed unities of heaven and earth. And it is this whole person—this living *nephesh*—that is called to be a temple of the Holy Spirit and offered as a living sacrifice to God.

2.4 The Functional Distinction of Pneuma and Psyche

Beloved, having established the foundational Hebraic concept of the human person as a unified *nephesh*—a psychosomatic whole—we must now navigate the nuanced terrain of the New Testament's development of this anthropology. The apostolic writings, while firmly rooted in this holistic soil, introduce a refinement, a functional distinction that is critical for understanding the dynamics of salvation, sanctification, and the spiritual life. While the human is an indivisible unity, the New Testament, under the inspiration of the Holy Spirit and engaging with a Hellenistic world, develops a clearer functional distinction between *pneuma* (spirit) and *psyche* (soul). This is not a retreat into Greek dualism, but a pastoral and theological clarification of the different capacities and orientations of the one, whole person. To misunderstand this distinction is to confuse the natural with the spiritual, to mistake psychological well-being for spiritual vitality, and to misunderstand the very nature of the Holy Spirit's work in redemption.

Let us begin with a deep exegetical and theological exploration of the ***Pneuma*** (πνεῦμα). In the New Testament, the human *pneuma* is that unique dimension or faculty of the human person that is specifically fashioned for relationship with the transcendent, the holy, the divine. It is the capacity for God-consciousness. It is the receptor, the antenna, the innermost sanctuary of the human being designed for communion with the Holy Spirit. This is not a "part" that can be isolated, but it is the fundamental orientation of the whole person toward God as their ultimate source, reference point, and destination.

The Apostle Paul provides the definitive description of this function in **Romans 8:16**: "*The Spirit himself bears witness with our spirit (*pneumati hēmōn*) that we are children of God.*" Here we see the divine-human interaction that defines the regenerated *pneuma*. The Holy Spirit (*Pneuma Hagion*) does not bear witness to our *psyche*—our emotional center or our intellect—but directly to our *pneuma*. This is a profound, non-conceptual, ontological communication that establishes our core identity as sons and daughters. It is the *pneuma* that is the seat of this filial knowledge, a knowing that transcends emotional feeling or rational deduction. It is the faculty of direct spiritual perception and communion. It is through the *pneuma* that we "know" God, not merely know about Him. It is through the *pneuma* that we cry "Abba! Father!" (Romans 8:15), an utterance that springs from a depth far below the conscious operations of the *psyche*.

This God-ward orientation of the *pneuma* is what distinguishes humanity from the animals. While animals are *nephesh chayyah* (living beings), possessing a *psyche* that constitutes their individual, animating life, they do not possess a *pneuma* in this distinct, relational sense. The human *pneuma* is what makes us *capax Dei*—capable of God. It is the imprint of the Divine, the locus of the *Imago Dei* that makes relational fellowship with our Creator possible. It is the "heart" in its deepest, most theological sense—the core of the person where the ultimate "yes" or "no" to God is spoken.

In stark contrast, the ***Psyche*** (ψυχή) represents the totality of the natural, self-conscious life of the individual. If the *pneuma* is the person in their vertical orientation toward God, the *psyche* is the person in their horizontal orientation toward the world and themselves. It is the seat of the will, the emotions, the mind, the desires, and the personality. It is the animating principle of the individual life, the "self" as it expresses itself in time and space. This is the direct New Testament counterpart to the Old Testament *nephesh*.

We see the *psyche* in its full range in the Gospels. In **Matthew 26:38**, Jesus declares, "*My soul (*psyche*) is very sorrowful, even to death.*" Here, *psyche* encompasses the deepest emotional and psychological anguish. It is the seat of His sorrow, the core of His human experience in the face of suffering. Conversely, in the parable of the rich fool, the man says to his *psyche*, "*Soul, you* *have ample goods laid up for many years; relax, eat, drink, be merry*" (**Luke 12:19**). Here, the *psyche* is the object of his self-talk, the center of his identity that he believes can be satisfied with security and pleasure. The *psyche* is the life that can be saved or lost (Matthew 16:25-26), the natural life that feels, thinks, chooses, and experiences the world.

This brings us to the critical spiritual dynamics that unfold based on the condition of the *pneuma*. In the unregenerate person, the one dead in trespasses and sins (**Ephesians 2:1-2**), a catastrophic spiritual condition exists. The *pneuma*, the God-conscious faculty, is deadened, inoperative, "dead" as Paul explicitly states. It is severed from its life-source, like a electrical socket with no connection to the power grid. It may have the form, but it has no function. It is incapable of true spiritual perception or communion.

In this state, the *psyche* is left to operate autonomously from God. It becomes the commanding center of the human person. The mind, will, and emotions, untethered from the orienting influence of a functioning *pneuma*, become self-referential and curved in on themselves. The intellect may be brilliant, but it cannot submit to God's truth (Romans 8:7). The emotions may be powerful, but they are not governed by the peace of Christ. The will may be strong, but it is bent toward self-gratification. This is the state of "the natural person" (*psychikos anthrōpos*) who "does not accept the things of the Spirit of God, for they are folly to him, and he is not able to understand them because they are spiritually discerned" (1 Corinthians 2:14). The *psyche*, operating alone, cannot comprehend the *pneuma*-realm.

But hallelujah, in the miracle of regeneration, this spiritual corpse is brought to life! When a person is born again by the

Spirit of God (John 3:5-8), the human *pneuma* is resurrected, quickened, made alive together with Christ (Ephesians 2:5). The Holy Spirit takes up residence and instantly establishes a living connection with this now-vitalized human *pneuma. This is the moment of spiritual birth, the creation of a new capacity for knowing and loving God that was not there before.

And this is where the glorious, lifelong process of sanctification begins. The Holy Spirit, now in residence and in communion with the regenerated *pneuma*, begins the great work of sanctifying the *psyche*. The renewed *pneuma* becomes a beachhead of divine life from which the Holy Spirit launches His campaign to reclaim the entire territory of the human person. This is what Paul describes in **Romans 12:2**: "*Do not be conformed to this world, but be transformed by the renewal of your mind (*nous*).*" The *nous*, the mind, is a key faculty of the *psyche*. Its renewal is not a self-help project; it is the direct result of the Holy Spirit working from the regenerated *pneuma* outward, retraining the *psyche* to think, feel, and choose in accordance with the truth of God. The desires of the *psyche* are gradually re-oriented from self-gratification to the glory of God and the love of neighbor. The emotions are increasingly brought under the dominion of the fruit of the Spirit.

This process has direct and profound implications for our embodied stewardship. A thought life (*psyche*) that is being renewed by the Spirit will inevitably lead to different choices regarding the *soma* (body). It will discern that gluttony is not just bad for the heart but a sin against the temple. It will understand that physical discipline is not vanity but a preparation for service. It will see that adequate sleep is an act of trust, not laziness. The sanctification of the *psyche* directly governs the stewardship of the *soma*.

And this entire process looks forward to its glorious consummation: the final redemption of the *soma* itself (**Romans 8:23**). We, who have the firstfruits of the Spirit—the renewed *pneuma*—groan inwardly as we wait for the adoption as sons, the redemption of our bodies. The healing that begins in the *pneuma* and extends to the *psyche* will one day be completed in the resurrection of the *soma*, when the whole, integrated *nephesh* is fully and finally reconstituted in glory, a perfect vessel for the indwelling Spirit for all eternity. Thus, the functional distinction between *pneuma* and *psyche* is not a static map of parts, but a dynamic description of the pathway of holiness, from the quickening of our God-consciousness to the transformation of our natural life, all for the ultimate glory of God in our entire, redeemed being.

2.5 The Body (Soma) as Essential to Personal Identity

Beloved, we now arrive at a truth so foundational, so counter-intuitive to the prevailing spirit of our age, and so glorious in its implications that it must be seared into our theological consciousness: **The body is not a disposable container, a temporary costume, or a mere instrument for the soul. It is integral to your very identity.** To speak of "me" is to speak of my embodied self. The "I" that thinks, feels, chooses, and loves is an "I" that does so from within and through this particular, physical form. This is not a temporary arrangement for our earthly pilgrimage; it is the eternal destiny of humanity as revealed in the gospel. The resurrection of the body—not a disembodied, ghostly eternal existence—is the cornerstone of the Christian hope. To misunderstand this is to risk a form of practical Gnosticism that devalues the very creation God called "very good" and for which the Son of God suffered, died, and rose again.

Let us begin by confronting the pervasive cultural and even religious assumption that the "real you" is your soul, and your body is simply the house you live in for a while. This is the language of Platonic philosophy, not of biblical revelation. This view leads to one of two errors: either a neglect of the body as spiritually irrelevant, or an idolatrous obsession with the body as a project for personal vanity. The biblical witness offers a radically different and more profound vision. When God formed Adam from the dust of the ground, He was not crafting a prison for a pre-existing soul; He was creating *Adam*. The dust, animated by the divine breath, *became* a living *nephesh*. The physicality was not an add-on; it was constitutive of his very being. Your body is not something you *have*; in a most fundamental sense, it is something you *are*. Your personal history is written in its scars, your habits are etched in its neural pathways, your joys and sorrows are encoded in its very chemistry. To despise the body is to despise the self that God created.

This truth is sealed for all eternity by the doctrine of the **Resurrection**. The entire fifteenth chapter of 1 Corinthians is Paul's magnificent, sustained argument against a spirituality that would deny the body's eternal significance. To the Corinthians, influenced by philosophies that saw salvation as an escape from materiality, Paul declares the resurrection of the body to be of first importance. He stakes the entire truth of the gospel on it: "*If Christ has not been raised, your faith is futile and you are still in your sins*" (1 Corinthians 15:17). But why is a physical resurrection so essential? Because the salvation God offers is not an escape from creation, but the *redemption of* *creation*. Sin brought corruption and death to the entire human person—spirit, soul, *and body*. The gospel, therefore, must address the whole person. If Christ only saved our souls, then death, the "last enemy" (1 Corinthians 15:26), would have the final victory over our bodies. But Christ is the "firstfruits of those who have fallen asleep" (1 Corinthians 15:20). His resurrection is the prototype, the guarantee, of our own.

And what was the nature of Christ's resurrection? It was unequivocally, undeniably, *bodily*. In Luke 24:39, the resurrected Jesus stands before His terrified disciples and says, "*See my hands and my feet, that it is I myself. Touch me, and see. For a spirit does not have flesh and bones as you see that I have.*" This is one of the most theologically significant statements in all of Scripture. The resurrected Lord is not a disembodied spirit, a ghost, or a vague spiritual presence. He is the same Jesus who was crucified, now transformed and glorified, but still possessing a physical, tangible body. He eats fish with them (Luke 24:42-43). He invites Thomas to place his finger in the wounds of His hands and side (John 20:27). The resurrection body is continuous with the earthly body, yet it is also transformed—no longer subject to suffering, decay, or the ordinary limitations of space and time. It is a *soma pneumatikon* (a spiritual body), as Paul describes it (1 Corinthians 15:44), not a body *made of* spirit, but a physical body perfectly animated by and submitted to the Holy Spirit.

This has a staggering implication for you and for me: our eternal destiny is not to be disembodied souls floating on clouds, strumming harps. Our destiny is to be resurrected, embodied persons, inhabiting a resurrected, physical creation—the New Heavens and the New Earth. The hope of the Christian is not to *leave* our bodies behind, but to *receive them back*, glorified and perfected, as the final act of our adoption as sons and daughters (Romans 8:23). This means that the body you have now is not a temporary shell to be discarded. It is the raw material, the seed (1 Corinthians 15:37-38), of your eternal self. God is not going to create a new body for you out of nothing; He is going to raise and transform *this* body. There is a continuity between the mortal body and the resurrection body, just as there is a continuity between a seed and the full-grown plant that springs from it.

Therefore, how you treat your body in the present is a matter of profound theological significance. It is not a question of mere prudence or preference. It is a statement about what you believe concerning God's creation, Christ's redemption, and your own eternal destiny. To neglect the body through gluttony, sloth, or willful ignorance is to treat with contempt the future vessel of glory. To abuse the body through addictive substances or immoral practices is to deface the masterpiece that God intends to display for all eternity. Conversely, to care for the body—to nourish it, to strengthen it, to rest it, to manage its stress—is an act of hope. It is a tangible expression of faith in the resurrection. It is to cooperate with the Holy Spirit in the here and now, preparing the "seed" for its future glorification. We are, in a sense, curating our own resurrection bodies. We are tending the soil from which the new creation will spring forth.

This understanding elevates every act of physical stewardship to an act of eschatological significance. When you choose to eat a meal that truly nourishes your cells, you are participating in God's creational and redemptive purposes for your physical being. When you engage in exercise that strengthens your heart and muscles, you are preparing a body that, in its resurrected form, will be capable of untold service and exploration in the

New Creation. When you discipline your sleep to allow for cellular repair and cognitive restoration, you are honoring the divine design for a body that will one day be fully and perfectly energized by the light of God's presence. The body is not a barrier to spiritual life; it is the essential instrument and the eternal object of that life.

This also provides a desperately needed Christian response to the modern crises of body image and identity. In a world that tells you your body is a canvas for self-invention to be manipulated according to your will, or a machine to be optimized for performance, the gospel tells you a more beautiful story. Your body is a sacred trust, a unique and irreplaceable aspect of your God-given identity, destined for glory. Its limitations, its particularities, its very metabolism are part of the "fearful and wonderful" craftsmanship of God (Psalm 139:14). To hate your body is to hate a fundamental aspect of how God has chosen to make *you*. Our calling is not to conform our bodies to the fleeting ideals of the world, but to present them as living sacrifices, holy and acceptable to God, which is our spiritual worship (Romans 12:1). We steward them not for our own glory, but for His, looking forward with eager anticipation to the day when He will "transform our lowly body to be like his glorious body, by the power that enables him even to subject all things to himself" (Philippians 3:21). The body, therefore, is not an accident of biology or a temporary residence. It is you. And it is forever.

2.6 The *Imago Dei* and its Embodied Implications

Beloved, we now ascend to the very pinnacle of human dignity and purpose—the profound and mysterious doctrine of the *Imago Dei*, the Image of God. Recorded in the majestic prologue of Genesis, we read: "*Then God said, 'Let us make man in our image, after our likeness.'... So God created man in his own image, in the image of God he created him; male and female he created them*" (Genesis 1:26-27). This declaration is the non-negotiable foundation for all Christian anthropology, ethics, and, I contend, for our understanding of embodied stewardship. To be human is to be *imago Dei*. But what does this mean? For centuries, theologians have rightly discerned that this image encompasses functional, relational, and substantive aspects. Yet, we have often spiritualized this concept to the point of abstraction, failing to grasp its radical, inescapable *embodiment*. The *Imago Dei* is not stamped upon a disembodied soul; it is stamped upon a physical, gendered, breathing, working, relating creature of dust and divine breath. We reflect God in and *through* our physicality.

Let us first explore the **Functional Aspect** of the image. God immediately follows the declaration of His intent with a command that defines humanity's vocation: "*And let them have dominion over the fish of the sea and over the birds of the heavens and over the livestock and over all the earth and over every creeping thing that creeps on the earth*" (Genesis 1:26). This is the "Cultural Mandate." Humanity is created as God's vice-regent, His royal representatives, tasked with stewarding, cultivating, and ruling over the earth. This is a function that is irreducibly physical. It requires bodies. It requires hands to till the soil, voices to name the animals, minds to invent and build, and feet to walk the length and breadth of the creation. Our creative capacity—our drive to make art, music, technology, and culture—is a physical expression of our imaging of the Creator God. When a carpenter builds a table, a composer writes a symphony, or a farmer tends a field, they are enacting the *Imago Dei* through their physical labor. They are extending God's wise and loving order into the world through the instrument of their bodies. Therefore, to neglect the strength, health, and capability of our bodies is to impair our capacity to fulfill this creational mandate. A body weakened by chronic neglect is a poorly maintained tool for exercising godly dominion. Our physical stewardship is directly linked to our functional imaging of God in the world.

Secondly, the *Imago Dei* has a profound **Relational Aspect**. The God who is, in His own triune being, a perfect, eternal community of Father, Son, and Holy Spirit, creates humanity for relationship. The divine assessment, "It is not good that the man should be alone" (Genesis 2:18), precedes the creation of the woman. The image of God is reflected not merely in the individual, but in the relational nexus of "male and female." Our physicality is fundamental to this relationality. We relate through physical presence: a handshake, an embrace, a shared meal, the intimate union of marriage. The human face, with its capacity for countless expressions, is a primary vehicle of relational communication, reflecting something of the divine prosopon (person). Our ability to form communities, to show compassion through physical acts of service, to weep with those who weep and rejoice with those who rejoice—all of this requires a body. The degradation of the body through abuse or neglect directly harms our capacity for relationship. Chronic illness, self-induced fatigue, or a body wracked by the consequences of poor stewardship can isolate us, diminish our emotional availability, and hinder our ability to love our neighbor as ourselves. Conversely, a body that is cared for—that has the energy for conversation, the vitality for service, and the health for presence—becomes a more effective instrument for reflecting the relational nature of the God who is Love.

Thirdly, we consider the **Substantive Aspect** of the image. This refers to the innate capacities with which God has endowed humanity, capacities that reflect His own nature. These include our moral conscience, our rational intellect, our capacity for language, and our eternal spirit. But we must never forget that these "immaterial" faculties are inextricably housed in and expressed through the material brain and nervous system. Our ability to reason, to discern good from evil, to contemplate eternity, and to commune with God—all of these activities have a physical substrate. The health of the body, particularly the brain, directly impacts the function of the mind. Malnutrition, sleep deprivation, and unmanaged stress can cloud our judgment, dull our moral sensitivity, and hinder our prayer life. This is not to reduce spiritual life to biochemistry, but to acknowledge the psychosomatic unity God has created. To care for the body through proper nutrition, rest, and stress management is to maintain the physical temple in which these God-reflecting capacities reside. It is an act of stewardship over the very instruments of our rationality, morality, and spirituality.

This embodied understanding of the *Imago Dei* reaches its breathtaking climax in the **Incarnation of Jesus Christ**. He is, as Paul declares, "*the image of the invisible God*" (Colossians 1:15). In Jesus of Nazareth, the perfect and complete *Imago Dei* is, for the first time since the Fall, fully manifest in a human life. And He is *embodied*. The infinite God is made visible in a particular human body with a specific face, a recognizable voice, and a tangible presence. In Christ, we see what it means to be truly human. He exercises dominion by calming storms and healing bodies. He embodies relational love by touching lepers, eating with sinners, and weeping at a tomb. He demonstrates perfect moral and rational clarity in His teaching and His resistance to temptation. The entire ministry of Jesus validates the essential goodness and theological significance of the physical body. He redeems the *Imago Dei* not by escaping the body, but by sanctifying it through His sinless life, His atoning death, and His bodily resurrection.

Therefore, the implications for our daily lives are profound and inescapable. The degradation of the body through gluttony, sloth, chemical abuse, or immorality is not merely a personal health issue or a private vice. It is an active *distortion* of the *Imago Dei*. It is like taking a masterpiece portrait of the King and smearing mud upon it. It misrepresents God to the world. It declares that the Creator's handiwork is unimportant, that the temple of the Spirit is worthless, and that the vessel destined for glory is contemptible.

Conversely, the faithful care for the body—the disciplined eating, the purposeful exercise, the pursuit of rest, the management of stress—is far more than self-improvement. It is an act of *imaging God*. It is a reflective act that mirrors God's own care for His creation. Just as God tenderly sustains and provides for the world He made, so we are called to tenderly sustain and provide for the bodies He has entrusted to us. It is a declarative act that proclaims to the world the inherent dignity and sacred purpose of every human life. It is an act of hope that anticipates the resurrection, treating the body as the seed of a future glory. And it is an act of worship, a tangible "Amen" to God's own pronouncement that His creation—including our physical frames—is "very good." Our bodies are not merely *our* bodies; they are living, breathing icons of the Divine, and our stewardship of them is one of the primary ways we glorify God in this present age.

2.7 Pastoral and Practical Applications of Holistic Anthropology

Beloved, we have journeyed through the high country of theological anthropology, exploring the architecture of the human person as a psychosomatic unity, a living *nephesh*, bearing the *Imago Dei*. But doctrine that does not descend from the mountain to transform the valley of our daily existence is mere abstraction. This integrated, holistic view of the human person is not an intellectual curiosity; it is a pastoral imperative with seismic implications for how we live, how we minister, and how we understand the entirety of the Christian life. It demands a fundamental reorientation of our practice, shattering the sacred-secular divide that has long crippled the Church's witness and the believer's wholeness. Let us now explore the profound practical outworkings of this theology in three critical areas: our spiritual disciplines, our approach to mental health, and our navigation of complex ethical issues.

First, consider the transformative implications for our understanding and practice of the **Spiritual Disciplines**. For too long, we have operated with a hidden Gnosticism that treats disciplines like prayer, fasting, and Communion as purely "spiritual" activities, their physical components being at best incidental and at worst a distraction. A holistic anthropology reveals this to be a grave error. These disciplines are God-ordained means of grace that precisely because we are psychosomatic unities, engaging the whole person—body, soul, and spirit—in the process of sanctification.

Take **prayer**, for instance. The Bible is replete with examples of prayer assuming physical postures. People kneel (1 Kings 8:54), bow down (Psalm 95:6), lift their hands (Psalm 141:2), and fall on their faces (Matthew 26:39). This is not theatrical performance. It is a theological statement enacted through the body. Kneeling physically enacts humility and submission before the sovereignty of God. Lifting hands embodies receptivity and surrender. The posture of the body can shape the posture of the soul. To confine prayer to the disembodied thoughts of a mind lying in bed is to ignore a God-given tool for focusing our entire being on communion with Him. The physical act disciplines the wandering mind and directs the affections of the heart.

Then there is **fasting**. What is fasting, if not the most direct and practical application of our holistic anthropology? Fasting is the voluntary, temporary abstinence from food for a spiritual purpose. It is a tangible, physical act of declaring that "*Man shall not live by bread alone, but by every word that comes from the mouth of God*" (Matthew 4:4). The bodily hunger pangs become a trigger for prayer, a physical reminder of our ultimate dependence not on physical sustenance, but on God Himself. The body's craving is transformed into the soul's crying out. Furthermore, modern science confirms what the saints have long known: fasting can clear mental fog, reset metabolic systems, and enhance cognitive function. This is not a coincidence; it is General Revelation confirming Special Revelation. The physical discipline of fasting creates a psychosomatic environment of heightened spiritual awareness, where the body's deprivation fuels the spirit's intensity. It is a powerful rebuke to both the ascetic who despises the body's needs and the glutton who is enslaved by them.

And what of the Lord's **Supper, Holy Communion**? This is the ultimate sanctification of the physical. In this sacrament, God takes the most mundane of physical acts—eating and drinking—and makes it the vehicle of the most profound spiritual reality. We do not merely *think* about Christ's sacrifice; we physically taste the bread and wine. Our teeth crush the grain, our throats swallow the fruit of the vine. This physical consumption is, by the mystery of faith, a spiritual partaking of Christ (1 Corinthians 10:16). The sacrament screams to us that God saves and sustains us not by bypassing our physicality, but by redeeming it. It tells us that our daily meals can also be acts of communion and gratitude, and that to treat our bodies with contempt is to disregard the very logic of the Gospel enacted at the Table.

Secondly, a holistic anthropology revolutionizes our pastoral approach to **Mental Health**. The modern church has often found itself trapped in a destructive dichotomy. On one side, there is a harmful spiritualization that labels conditions like clinical depression or anxiety disorders as solely the result of unconfessed sin, a lack of faith, or demonic oppression. This heaps shame upon suffering and drives people away from the help they desperately need. On the other side, there is an uncritical adoption of a purely secular, medical model that reduces these struggles to mere chemical imbalances, offering pharmaceutical and therapeutic solutions while ignoring the spiritual dimensions of despair, meaning, and hope.

Our theology of the integrated *nephesh* provides a third way, a more compassionate and comprehensive framework. Anxiety and depression are not *either* spiritual *or* physical/psychological problems; they are disruptions of the *psychosomatic unity*. They are maladies of the whole person. A panic attack, for example, is a terrifying cascade of spiritual fear, catastrophic thoughts (*psyche*), and a flood of adrenaline causing a racing heart, sweating, and shortness of breath (*soma*). To tell someone only to "pray more" while ignoring the physiological component is as foolish as prescribing only a beta-blocker while ignoring the spiritual roots of fear and the need for the peace of Christ that surpasses understanding (Philippians 4:6-7).

A holistic pastoral approach, therefore, requires a multi-faceted ministry of care. It involves:

1. **Spiritual Direction and Prayer:** Gently exploring the state of the person's relationship with God, leading them to Scriptures of comfort and promise, practicing the presence of Christ, and engaging in prayer that acknowledges the struggle without simplistic condemnation.
2. **Psychological Care:** Encouraging, without stigma, the pursuit of competent Christian counseling that can help identify and retrain maladaptive cognitive patterns, process trauma, and develop healthy emotional coping skills.
3. **Somatic Care:** Asking practical questions about sleep, nutrition, exercise, and caffeine intake. Is the person's body being properly stewarded, or are their physical habits exacerbating their mental state? The state of the body is not incidental to the state of the mind.

This integrated approach treats the person with the dignity of their God-given complexity, addressing the disruption in their spirit, soul, *and* body, and pointing them to the Christ who is the source of healing for the whole person.

Finally, this anthropology provides a robust foundation for Christian **Ethics**, particularly in areas intensely focused on the body. Our culture treats the body as a machine to be optimized or a canvas for self-expression—a piece of property over which the individual has absolute autonomy. The biblical view declares the body is a sacred trust, an integral part of the person, created for God's glory.

Consider **sexuality**. The modern world severs sexual activity from its creational purpose, treating it as recreational, a matter of personal preference devoid of inherent meaning. But our holistic anthropology, confirmed by Scripture, teaches that sexual union constitutes a "one-flesh" reality (Genesis 2:24; 1 Corinthians 6:16)—a profound psychosomatic union that is not merely physical but encompasses the whole person. This is why sexual immorality is so destructive; it tears at the very fabric of the integrated self, creating a dissonance between the physical act and the spiritual-psychological commitment for which it was designed. Christian sexual ethics, therefore, is not a repressive list of rules, but a protective framework for honoring the sacredness of the whole person and the God-ordained context—covenantal marriage—where this powerful union can flourish.

In issues of **substance abuse**, we see not just a "bad habit" but a profound enslavement that warps the *Imago Dei*. Addictive substances hijack the brain's reward system (*soma*), cloud judgment and will (*psyche*), and create a spiritual alienation as the pursuit of the substance replaces the pursuit of God. Treatment, therefore, must be holistic: addressing the physical dependency through detoxification, the psychological patterns through therapy, and the spiritual void through the gospel's power to break strongholds and offer a new master in Christ.

And in the complex field of **bioethics**—from transgenderism to genetic engineering to end-of-life issues—a holistic anthropology provides our guiding star. The body is not a neutral object to be manipulated according to our will. It is a divine given, a fundamental aspect of our created identity. The attempt to sever gender identity from biological sex is a direct assault on the psychosomatic unity God has created. The pursuit of technological enhancement that treats the body as a machine to be upgraded reflects a failure to see it as a sacred temple. Our ethical reasoning must begin with the question: "Does this action honor the body as an essential, God-given part of the human person, created in His image and destined for resurrection?" This question protects human dignity and guides us through the most challenging ethical dilemmas of our time.

The truth of our holistic anthropology, therefore, is not a doctrine to be filed away. It is a lens through which we view everything. It transforms our worship from a mental exercise into a full-bodied offering. It reframes our suffering as an opportunity for whole-person care. It grounds our ethics in the sacredness of the embodied self. Let us then live, and minister, as those who truly believe that we are fearfully and wonderfully made—body, soul, and spirit—for the glory of God.

2.8 Conclusion: The Unified Vessel of Stewardship

Beloved, as we draw this profound chapter on theological anthropology to its culmination, we find ourselves standing before a vision of the human person so majestic, so integrated, and so sacred that it must fundamentally and permanently reorder our entire approach to life and godliness. The journey we have undertaken—from the exegetical debates surrounding our constituent parts to the profound Hebraic synthesis of the nephesh, from the functional distinctions of pneuma and psyche to the eternal significance of the soma—has led us to one inescapable, glorious conclusion. Theological anthropology reveals, with the clarity of divine revelation, that the human person is not a collection of loosely affiliated components, but a complex, dynamic, and profound **unity of body, soul, and spirit**. We are a single, God-breathed masterpiece, a living tapestry in which the threads of the physical, the psychological, and the spiritual are so intricately woven together that to pull on one is to tension the entire fabric of our being.

This is not a mere philosophical proposition. It is the foundational reality that makes the very concept of Embodied Stewardship not only possible but necessary. To care for one's health, therefore, is to bow in humble acknowledgment of this God-ordained unity. It is to recognize that the Creator, in His infinite wisdom, did not create disposable containers for eternal souls, but fashioned living, integrated beings whose physicality is essential to their identity and their destiny. The steward who has grasped this truth understands a profound and transformative secret: he or she does not merely maintain a physical shell, a temporary housing unit for the "real" self. No, the faithful steward tends to the *integrated whole*. This is the sacred vocation that flows directly from our anthropology.

Consider what this means in the daily rhythm of a life lived coram Deo, before the face of God. The act of **nourishing the body**—the conscious choice to consume foods that are life-giving, to hydrate with water, to provide the building blocks for cellular repair and energy—is never a merely biological act. It is an act of sustaining the physical foundation upon which the soul depends. The brain, an organ of the body, is the seat of the mind, a faculty of the soul. When we nourish the body with quality fats, proteins, and complex carbohydrates, we are literally providing the physical substrate for clear thinking, emotional stability, and moral discernment. When we poison the body with excess sugar, processed chemicals, and inflammatory agents, we are not just harming a machine; we are clouding the very instrument through which the soul perceives truth, manages emotion, and exercises will. The quality of your prayer life, the clarity of your theological reflection, the resilience of your patience in trial—all are intimately connected to the glucose stability in your bloodstream, the inflammation levels in your neural tissue, and the restorative quality of your sleep. To nourish the body is to honor the soul that is inextricably housed within it.

But this integrated care moves in both directions. The steward also recognizes that this body-housed soul is itself **enlivened by the spirit**. This is the dynamic work of the Holy Spirit, the *Pneuma Hagion*, who, upon the regeneration of the human *pneuma*, begins His sanctifying work from the inside out. A soul that is being renewed by the Spirit—a mind being transformed (Romans 12:2), emotions being filled with the fruit of the Spirit (Galatians 5:22-23), a will being aligned with God's will—will inevitably issue in different choices for the body. A soul filled with the love of Christ will find the motivation to overcome the sloth that neglects the body. A soul indwelt by the peace of Christ will develop the discipline to manage stress in ways that do not ravage the nervous system. A soul experiencing the joy of the Lord will find the strength to resist the fleeting pleasures of gluttony or substance abuse. The enlivened spirit, through the soul, directs and empowers the care of the body. The state of your spirit, your connection to the Divine, is the ultimate wellspring of motivation and power for the physical discipline required to steward the temple well.

And all of this—the nourishing of the body, the renewal of the soul, the quickening of the spirit—converges on a single, magnificent, all-encompassing purpose: **the glorification of**

the Triune God. This is the *telos*, the ultimate end and goal, of our unified existence. We glorify God *in our bodies* (1 Corinthians 6:20) because they are His artwork. We glorify God with our souls—our minds, wills, and emotions—as we love Him with all our heart, soul, and mind (Matthew 22:37). We glorify God through our spirits as they commune with His Spirit in worship that is both rational and profound (John 4:24). The holistic stewardship of the unified human person is, therefore, the most comprehensive act of worship we can offer. It is our "spiritual worship," our *logiken latreian*, to present our *bodies* as a living sacrifice (Romans 12:1).

This transforms every mundane act into a potential doxology. The choice to go for a walk is no longer just about cardiovascular health; it is an act of preparing a stronger, more enduring vessel for the service of the Kingdom. The decision to turn off the screen and go to sleep is not merely about avoiding fatigue; it is an act of faith, trusting God with the world for a few hours while we participate in the nightly sacrament of rest, acknowledging our creatureliness. The discipline of saying "no" to a third helping is not just about weight management; it is a tangible declaration that our comfort is not our god, and that we are mastering our appetites so that we will not be mastered by anything (1 Corinthians 6:12).

The unified vessel of your personhood—body, soul, and spirit—is the primary instrument given to you for the great symphony of glorifying God. A musician does not maintain only the strings of a violin while letting the wood crack and the varnish peel. He cares for the entire instrument, because its wholeness is essential to the beauty of the music it was created to produce. So it is with us. We are the instruments, and our lives are the music. To care for the unified vessel is to ensure that the music of our lives is a beautiful, resonant, and faithful anthem to the glory of the Great Composer, the Triune God—Father, Son, and Holy Spirit—to whom be all praise, now and forevermore. Let us therefore go forth from this place as whole-person stewards, living testaments to the glorious integration for which we were created and redeemed.

CHAPTER 03

The Concept of *Shalom*: Wellness as Divine Harmony

3.1 Introduction: Beyond the Absence of Conflict

Beloved, as we continue to construct our theology of Embodied Stewardship, we must now ascend to a higher vantage point. We have laid the anthropological foundation, understanding the human person as an integrated unity of body, soul, and spirit. But to what end? For what ultimate purpose do we steward this sacred trust? The modern world offers us a plethora of answers, all of which are tragically myopic and reductionist. It speaks of "wellness," a term that has been co-opted by consumer culture and often signifies little more than the absence of diagnosable disease, coupled with a self-centered pursuit of feeling good, looking good, and performing optimally. This modern "wellness" is primarily individualistic, therapeutic, and functional—it is about *my* vitality, *my* longevity, *my* mental clarity. It is a vision of health that often ends with the self.

But the biblical witness unveils a vision so much more magnificent, so much more comprehensive, and so much more demanding that it utterly transcends and transforms our petty, self-referential notions of wellness. This vision is encapsulated in the profound Hebrew concept of ***Shalom*** (שלום). To translate *Shalom* simply as "peace" is to do a profound disservice to its cosmic scope and depth. In our modern, Western understanding, "peace" is often a negative concept—the absence of conflict, the cessation of war, a state of quiet and tranquility. While *Shalom* includes this, it is so much more. *Shalom* is a positive, dynamic, and robust state of being. It is the state of wholeness, completeness, integrity, harmony, and flourishing that permeates every level of existence—from the inner life of the individual to the vast expanse of the cosmos. It is the divine ecosystem for which all creation yearns, and it is the ultimate goal of all holistic stewardship.

To understand *Shalom*, we must first deconstruct our impoverished modern paradigms. The therapeutic individualism of our age tells us that health is a personal project. Your wellness is your responsibility, your achievement, your possession. It is a commodity to be purchased through gym memberships, superfoods, and meditation apps. This paradigm is inherently isolating and fragile. It fractures the essential connectedness of human life, making your health a private affair, disconnected from the health of your community, your environment, and your relationship with God. It is a vision of wellness that can be enjoyed by the wealthy in gated communities while the world outside groans under the weight of injustice, poverty, and ecological decay. This is not *Shalom*.

In stark contrast, the biblical concept of *Shalom* is inherently relational, communal, and cosmic. It cannot be achieved in isolation. Your personal health is inextricably linked to the health of the body of Christ, the well-being of your neighbor, and the flourishing of the created order. *Shalom* is the webbing of right relationships. It is the state of affairs where everything is rightly ordered under the sovereign lordship of God, functioning in perfect harmony according to its created design. It is the vision of the Psalmist who declares, "Steadfast love and faithfulness meet; righteousness and peace (*Shalom*) kiss each other" (Psalm 85:10). Here, *Shalom* is not a standalone virtue; it is the beautiful, flourishing reality that emerges when covenant loyalty (*hesed*), truth (*emet*), and justice (*tsedeq*) are in perfect, relational alignment.

This divine harmony operates on multiple, interconnected planes, and a breach in one area inevitably causes dissonance in all others. There is:

- **Vertical *Shalom***: A state of right relationship between the creature and the Creator. This is the foundational peace of being reconciled to God through the blood of the cross (Colossians 1:20), where we no longer live as enemies or estranged subjects, but as beloved children who cry "Abba, Father."
- **Internal *Shalom***: A state of integration and wholeness within the individual person. It is the harmony between body, soul, and spirit we explored in the previous chapter. It is the state where the mind, will, and emotions are aligned under the lordship of Christ, and the body is a willing instrument of righteousness, rather than a source of rebellion or decay.
- **Horizontal *Shalom***: A state of right relationships within the human community. It is justice in the courts, generosity to the poor, integrity in commerce, and love

within the family. It is the community life depicted in Acts, where there was "not a needy person among them" (Acts 4:34)—a tangible expression of social and economic *Shalom*.

- **Environmental *Shalom***: A state of harmonious relationship between humanity and the rest of creation. It is the fulfillment of the creation mandate to "work and keep" the garden (Genesis 2:15), exercising a priestly dominion that cultivates and protects, rather than a tyrannical dominion that exploits and destroys.

This comprehensive vision of *Shalom* is the true "divine ecosystem" in which human health finds its fullest meaning and purpose. Your pursuit of physical health is not an end in itself. It is a participation in God's restorative work. When you discipline your body through exercise, you are not just building muscle; you are cultivating the strength necessary to bear your brother's burden (Galatians 6:2), thus contributing to horizontal *Shalom*. When you choose a nutritious diet, you are not just optimizing your biochemistry; you are honoring the body as a temple of the Spirit and respecting the agricultural systems of God's world, touching on environmental *Shalom*. When you manage your stress through prayer and Scripture, you are not just seeking personal calm; you are fostering the internal *Shalom* that allows you to be a peacemaker and a source of stability for others (Matthew 5:9), and you are deepening your vertical *Shalom* through dependence on God.

Therefore, the goal of our Embodied Stewardship is not merely personal wellness. It is to become conduits and cultivators of *Shalom*. We steward our own health so that we have the spiritual, psychological, and physical capacity to actively participate in God's mission of restoring all things to Himself. A tired, sick, malnourished, and anxious Christian has little reserve with which to love their neighbor, pursue justice, care for creation, or engage in sacrificial ministry. A whole, healthy, and integrated person is a powerful instrument of *Shalom* in a fractured world. Our personal stewardship is the necessary foundation for our missional calling. In the chapters that follow, we will explore the rupture of this *Shalom* through the Fall and its glorious restoration in Christ, the true Prince of *Shalom*. But for now, let this vision captivate you: you are called to more than self-care. You are called to be an agent of divine harmony, a living, breathing, embodied signpost of the coming Kingdom where *Shalom* will be all in all.

3.2 Exegetical Foundations of *Shalom*

Beloved, if we are to build our lives upon the robust framework of *Shalom*, we must anchor our understanding not in our own sentimental longings for peace, but in the unshakable rock of God's self-revelation in Scripture. *Shalom* is not a vague, spiritualized feeling; it is a concrete theological reality that pulses through the entire biblical narrative, appearing over 250 times from Genesis to Revelation. To grasp its true meaning, we must become careful students of the text, allowing the Word itself to define the contours of this divine harmony. Let us, therefore, turn our attention to three foundational passages that illuminate the essence of *Shalom* from distinct yet complementary angles: its nature as covenantal wholeness, its inextricable link to relational righteousness, and its source in divine wisdom.

First, we must understand *Shalom* as **Covenantal Wholeness**. The most pristine and powerful definition is given to us by God Himself, encoded in the sacred words of the Aaronic blessing in

Numbers 6:24-26: "*The LORD bless you and keep you; the LORD make his face to shine upon you and be gracious to you; the LORD lift up his countenance upon you and give you* ***shalom***."

Please notice the majestic structure of this priestly benediction. It is a tripartite invocation that builds to a glorious climax. It begins with the foundational petition for provision and protection: "The LORD bless you and keep you." This encompasses all material needs and physical safety—the basic requirements for earthly existence. Then, it ascends to the relational and spiritual dimension: "The LORD make his face to shine upon you and be gracious to you." Here, we move beyond mere provision to the desire for God's favorable presence, His smile, His unmerited favor. It is the prayer for a restored relationship, for the light of divine affection to dispel the darkness of alienation.

And then, we reach the summit, the culmination of all divine favor: "*and give you shalom*." This is not an addendum. This is the ultimate gift. In this context, *Shalom* is the comprehensive state of well-being that flows from being a people who are *both* provided for *and* living in the gracious, shining presence of Yahweh. It is the total package of human flourishing. It includes health, but is more than health. It includes safety, but is more than safety. It includes prosperity, but is more than material wealth. It is the state of a community whose every dimension—physical, social, spiritual, economic—is functioning in harmonious alignment because God is in their midst. This *Shalom* is not something they achieve; it is something they *receive* as a gift from the Covenant-Keeper. It is the definitive mark of a people who are right with God, and therefore, are whole in themselves and in their common life. This covenantal *Shalom* is the ultimate goal of God's redemptive plan for His people.

But this wholeness has a specific moral character, which leads us to our second exegetical foundation: **Relational Righteousness**. The Psalmist unveils this in a breathtaking personification in Psalm 85:10: "*Steadfast love and faithfulness meet; righteousness and peace (*Shalom*) kiss each other.*"

This is one of the most theologically rich verses in all of Scripture regarding the nature of *Shalom*. It presents four divine attributes in relational motion. *Hesed*—the covenant loyalty, the relentless, merciful, steadfast love of God—moves toward *Emet*—faithfulness, truth, reliability. They "meet." They are in perfect concord. Simultaneously, *Tsedek*—righteousness, justice, the principle of moral rightness and equity—turns toward *Shalom*—the state of wholeness and flourishing. And they do not merely nod at each other from a distance; they "kiss." This is an image of intimate union, of inseparable connection.

The implication is revolutionary: *Shalom* cannot exist where righteousness and justice are absent. There can be no true, lasting peace without truth and justice. A community that ignores oppression, that tolerates economic exploitation, that turns a blind eye to the cry of the poor, may have a facade of quiet—a cold war, a tense truce—but it does not have *Shalom*. *Shalom* is not the absence of conflict; it is the active presence of right relationships, governed by *hesed* and *tsedek*. This is why the prophets, when they denounced Israel's sin, consistently linked the breakdown of *Shalom* with the abandonment of justice. They cried out against those who, while saying "Peace, peace," had no peace because they had forgotten *tsedek* (Jeremiah 6:14; 8:11).

Therefore, our pursuit of personal wholeness must never be divorced from a passion for God's righteousness to be manifest in our families, our churches, and our societies. To seek *Shalom* is to actively pursue justice, for the two are locked in a divine embrace.

Finally, we discover the pathway to this wholeness in the **Personification of Wisdom**. In Proverbs 3:17, Wisdom herself, who was with God at the beginning of creation (Proverbs 8:22-31), is described in this way: "*Her ways are ways of pleasantness, and all her paths are **shalom**.*"

This tells us that *Shalom* is not a mysterious, esoteric state that we stumble upon by accident. It is the inherent consequence of a life lived in alignment with the grain of the universe, which is the wisdom of God. The "ways" and "paths" of Wisdom are the created order, the moral fabric of reality, the divine design for how life is meant to be lived. When we walk according to this design—when our eating aligns with the nutritional wisdom built into creation, when our work follows the rhythm of labor and rest, when our relationships are governed by covenant faithfulness, when our minds are renewed by God's truth—the result is *Shalom*. The paths themselves *are Shalom*. The journey toward the destination is itself characterized by wholeness.

This is a profound insight for our Embodied Stewardship. We often think of health as a destination—a target weight, a blood pressure number, a state of mental calm we hope to achieve. But Proverbs 3:17 reframes it. The *process* of stewarding our bodies wisely—the daily choice of nourishing food, the consistent rhythm of exercise, the discipline of early sleep—is not a grim march toward a future goal. When done as an act of worship and in dependence on God's wisdom, these very paths *are* pleasantness and *are Shalom*. The disciplined life is not the opposite of the pleasant life; it is the very means of it. The chaos of gluttony, the anxiety of sloth, the fatigue of poor stewardship—these are the "paths" of folly, and they lead to disintegration. But the way of wisdom, even when it involves self-denial and effort, is a path of deepening harmony, integration, and peace, because it is a life in sync with the Creator's intent.

Thus, from these exegetical foundations, a magnificent picture emerges. *Shalom* is the covenantal gift of comprehensive well-being from a gracious God. It is a state of flourishing that is morally constituted by righteousness and justice. And it is the experiential reality of walking in the pleasant paths of God's created order. This is the vision that must captivate us—a vision far grander and more demanding than mere personal wellness, calling us into a holistic stewardship that encompasses our relationship with God, our inner life, our social obligations, and our interaction with the physical world.

3.3 The Four-Dimensional Matrix of *Shalom*

Beloved, having established the exegetical foundations of *Shalom* as covenantal wholeness, relational righteousness, and the way of wisdom, we must now map its magnificent architecture. *Shalom* is not a monolithic, undifferentiated state of bliss. It is a complex, dynamic, and multi-layered harmony that operates across four interdependent dimensions of existence. To understand the profound depth of biblical flourishing is to recognize that true *Shalom* requires right relationship in four distinct, yet inseparably connected, spheres: the vertical, the internal, the horizontal, and the environmental. A rupture in any one of these dimensions creates a tear in the entire fabric of *Shalom*, just as a single out-of-tune instrument can disrupt a grand symphony. Let us explore each of these dimensions in turn, understanding that our pursuit of holistic health is, in reality, the pursuit of harmony across this entire four-dimensional matrix.

First, and most foundationally, is ***Shalom* with God: The Vertical Dimension.** This is the primary axis upon which all other harmony depends. It is the state of being rightly related to our Creator, the source of all life and order. The Genesis narrative makes it devastatingly clear that the root of all cosmic disorder is the rupture of this primary relationship. When Adam and Eve chose autonomy over communion, they declared war on the divine order, and the consequence was immediate: they were cast out from the presence of God, the source of *Shalom*. This vertical rupture introduced dissonance into every other dimension of their existence. Their internal unity was shattered, leading to shame and fear (Genesis 3:7-10). Their horizontal relationship was fractured, leading to blame and domination (Genesis 3:12, 16). Their relationship with creation was cursed, leading to painful toil and ecological frustration (Genesis 3:17-19).

Therefore, the restoration of *Shalom* must begin here, at the point of the original breach. This is the glorious good news of the gospel. As the Apostle Paul triumphantly declares in **Romans 5:1**, "*Therefore, since we have been justified by faith, we have peace (*eirēnēn, *the Greek equivalent of Shalom) with God through our Lord Jesus Christ.*" Justification is not merely a legal declaration; it is the cosmic event of reconciliation. It is the ending of the hostility between a holy God and sinful humanity. Through the atoning sacrifice of Christ, the barrier of sin is removed, and we are brought back into a state of grace, into the shining presence of the God of peace. This vertical *Shalom* is the non-negotiable foundation. Without peace with God, any other peace we might experience is superficial, temporary, and ultimately illusory. It is the foundation upon which the entire structure of holistic human flourishing is built. You cannot have a whole life if you are at war with the source of life itself.

From this restored vertical axis flows the possibility of ***Shalom* with Self: The Internal Dimension.** This is the state of inner integrity where the heart, mind, and body are aligned under the lordship of Christ. The Fall created an internal civil war. The Apostle Paul describes this agonizing reality in **Galatians 5:17**: "*For the desires of the flesh are against the Spirit, and the desires of the Spirit are against the flesh, for these are opposed to each other, to keep you from doing the things you want to do.*" This is the experience of a person who has peace with God but has not yet experienced the full sanctifying work of that peace in their inner being. It is a state of disintegration: the spirit is willing, but the flesh is weak; the mind knows what is right, but the emotions rebel; the body craues what the soul despises.

Internal *Shalom* is the Holy Spirit's work of healing this fracture. It is the process of the renewed *pneuma* (spirit), now alive to God, gradually bringing the *psyche* (soul—mind, will, emotions) and the *soma* (body) into harmonious submission to Christ. This results in emotional stability that is rooted in God's character, not in circumstances. It produces psychological well-being that comes from a mind saturated with truth and a heart secure in God's love. It manifests as self-control, where physical appetites are disciplined servants rather than tyrannical masters. A person experiencing internal *Shalom* is not free from struggle, but they are free from the *dominion* of that struggle. They are integrated, whole, and directed toward a single, glorious purpose: the glory of God. This is why practices of embodied stewardship—caring for our physical and mental health—are so vital. They are the practical, daily outworking of pursuing internal harmony, of stilling the war within so that we can be effective peacemakers without.

The third dimension, which naturally extends from a whole self, is ***Shalom*** **with Others: The Horizontal Dimension.** The vertical peace with God and the internal peace within the self must inevitably spill over into our relationships. This dimension encompasses right relationships within the family, the church, the community, and the broader society. It is the practical outworking of the second greatest commandment: "*You shall love your neighbor as yourself*" (Matthew 22:39). Horizontal *Shalom* is the fruit of forgiveness, reconciliation, empathy, and sacrificial love. It is what Paul describes in Ephesians 2:14-16, where Christ Himself is our peace, breaking down the dividing wall of hostility between Jew and Gentile to create one new humanity, thus reconciling us all to God in one body.

This kind of *Shalom* creates the social environment where human flourishing becomes possible. It is the opposite of the isolation, competition, and violence that characterize a fallen world. It looks like a community where burdens are borne (Galatians 6:2), where there is no needy person among them (Acts 4:34), where people are quick to hear, slow to speak, and slow to anger (James 1:19). It requires immense energy, patience, and emotional resilience. This is a crucial point for our embodied stewardship: we cannot love our neighbor well if we are chronically exhausted, emotionally depleted, or physically incapacitated. Our pursuit of physical health and mental clarity is, in large part, so that we have the capacity to pursue horizontal *Shalom*—to be present, to listen, to serve, to forgive, and to build up.

Finally, and profoundly, is ***Shalom* with Creation: The Environmental Dimension.** Our modern concept of wellness is often tragically anthropocentric, but the biblical vision of *Shalom* is cosmically expansive. From the beginning, humanity was given a sacred vocation within the created order. In **Genesis 2:15**, "*The LORD God took the man and put him in the garden of Eden to work it and keep it.*" The Hebrew words are rich with meaning: *avad* means to work, serve, and worship; *shamar* means to keep, guard, and preserve. This was a call to priestly stewardship, to a harmonious relationship with the natural world where humanity would cultivate its potential and protect its integrity.

Environmental *Shalom* recognizes the natural world as God's good creation, worthy of respect and care, not merely a resource to be exploited or a backdrop for human drama. It understands that our own physical health is intimately connected to the health of the ecosystems of which we are a part. The food we eat comes from the soil, the water we drink from the cycles of evaporation and rain, the air we breathe from the photosynthesis of plants. To poison our rivers, to degrade our soil, to pollute our air is an act of violence against God's creation and, ultimately, against our own bodies. A theology of Embodied Stewardship must, therefore, extend to a theology of ecological stewardship. How we eat—choosing sustainable, locally grown foods when possible—is an act of environmental *Shalom*. How we conserve resources and reduce waste is an act of *shamar*, of guarding the garden. Our personal health and the planet's health are not separate concerns; they are different facets of the same divine harmony.

This four-dimensional matrix shows us that *Shalom* is the ultimate ecosystem of flourishing. We cannot have peace with God while harboring hatred toward our brother (1 John 4:20). We cannot have internal peace while living in unrepentant sin. We cannot experience social peace while exploiting the earth. It is all connected. Our calling as followers of Christ is to become agents of this comprehensive *Shalom*, pursuing harmony along every axis, starting with the vertical reconciliation we have in Jesus and allowing that peace to flow into every crack and crevice of our fractured world, until the knowledge of the Lord covers the earth as the waters cover the sea.

3.4 The Rupture of *Shalom*: Sin as Dis-integration

Beloved, having gazed upon the magnificent, four-dimensional harmony of *Shalom*, we must now, with sober hearts, turn to the catastrophic event that shattered this divine symphony. The vision of holistic flourishing is not our present reality because of a fundamental, cosmic rupture—the Fall, detailed in Genesis 3. This chapter is not a primitive myth to be demythologized; it is the definitive diagnosis of the human condition. It reveals that the root of all our pain, all our strife, and all our sickness is not merely imperfection or ignorance, but a willful rebellion that resulted in a comprehensive *dis-integration*. Sin is not just a list of moral infractions; it is a destructive force that tears apart the very fabric of *Shalom* at every level, introducing dissonance where there was harmony and fragmentation where there was wholeness. The disease, disorder, anxiety, and social strife that plague our existence are not random misfortunes; they are the systemic symptoms of this foundational collapse.

The rupture begins, as it must, in the **Vertical Dimension: The Breach with God.** Before the Fall, Adam and Eve walked with

God in the cool of the day in open, unashamed communion (Genesis 3:8). Their primary relationship was one of intimate trust and joyful submission. The serpent's temptation, however, was an invitation to distrust God's character and usurp His authority—to become "like God, knowing good and evil" (Genesis 3:5). The moment they acted on this temptation, the vertical axis of *Shalom* was severed. The immediate consequence was not a feeling of empowerment, but of terror and shame. They heard the sound of God walking, and they *hid* (Genesis 3:8). The communion was broken. The face-to-face relationship was replaced with fear and avoidance. This is the primal wound of humanity: a state of alienation from our Life-Source. We are, by nature, "alienated from the life of God" (Ephesians 4:18). Every human attempt to find meaning, purpose, and peace apart from God is a manifestation of this hiding, a futile effort to sew fig leaves together to cover our profound spiritual nakedness and shame before a Holy God. This vertical rupture is the taproot of all other forms of disintegration.

From this primary breach flows a torrent of disintegration into the **Internal Dimension: The Civil War Within.** The human person, created as an integrated *nephesh*, immediately experienced a terrifying internal fracture. The first emotion recorded after the Fall is *fear*: "I was afraid, because I was naked, and I hid myself" (Genesis 3:10). This is not a healthy reverence, but a paralyzing terror born of guilt and exposure. Along with fear comes *shame*, a profound sense of personal inadequacy and disgrace. Their unified self-image was shattered. Now, the body, which was good, becomes a source of shame. The mind, created to know God, now knows good and evil in a destructive, self-conscious way. The will, designed to freely obey, is now bent inward. This is the origin of the internal conflict described by

Paul in Romans 7, where he laments, "I do not understand my own actions. For I do not do what I want, but I do the very thing I hate" (Romans 7:15). The harmony between spirit, soul, and body was replaced by a state of internal civil war. The *psyche* is now a battlefield where truth and falsehood, love and hate, faith and fear wage a constant war for dominion. Our modern struggles with anxiety, depression, addiction, and self-loathing are not merely psychological disorders; they are the contemporary manifestations of this ancient, internal schism—the absence of internal *Shalom*.

This internal disintegration inevitably projects itself outward, rupturing the **Horizontal Dimension: The Blame Game and the Will to Power.** The first recorded human conversation after the Fall is not one of mutual comfort, but of blame and accusation. When God confronts Adam, he does not simply confess; he deflects: "The woman whom you gave to be with me, she gave me fruit of the tree, and I ate" (Genesis 3:12). In one sentence, he blames both Eve and God Himself. Eve, in turn, blames the serpent (Genesis 3:13). The relational harmony of "bone of my bones and flesh of my flesh" (Genesis 2:23) is instantly corrupted into a dynamic of self-justification and scapegoating. The partnership designed for mutual flourishing becomes a contest for dominance and self-protection. This is crystallized in the curse, where God tells Eve, "Your desire shall be contrary to your husband, but he shall rule over you" (Genesis 3:16). The relationship between the sexes, and by extension all human relationships, is now marred by a destructive power struggle—a desire to control and a tendency to dominate. All social strife—from marital conflict to ethnic cleansing, from office politics to international wars—finds its origin in this moment. Community is fractured by suspicion, competition, and violence, because the internal war within each person spills over into their relationships with others.

Finally, the rupture extends to the **Environmental Dimension: The Groaning Creation.** Humanity's rebellion did not occur in a vacuum; it had cosmic consequences. God's judgment pronounced a curse upon the very ground from which Adam was taken: "Cursed is the ground because of you; in pain you shall eat of it all the days of your life; thorns and thistles it shall bring forth for you... By the sweat of your face you shall eat bread" (Genesis 3:17-19). The creation, which was declared "very good" and entrusted to humanity's priestly care, now becomes resistant, frustrating, and dangerous. Work, which was meant to be joyful co-creation with God, becomes "painful toil." The harmonious relationship between humanity and nature is broken. Now, we must wrestle our sustenance from a recalcitrant earth. Natural disasters, disease, famine, and the entire phenomenon of natural evil are not part of God's original design but are manifestations of a creation that has been "subjected to futility" and now "groans" in its bondage to decay (Romans 8:20-22). Our ecological crisis—the pollution of our rivers, the erosion of our topsoil, the extinction of species—is not merely a problem of faulty technology or overpopulation. It is a direct result of humanity's failed stewardship, a consequence of the ruptured *Shalom* between us and the creation we were meant to "work and keep."

Therefore, when we look at the world and see cancer, mental illness, broken families, and a polluted planet, we are not looking at a series of unrelated, unfortunate events. We are looking at the symptoms of a single, deep-seated disease: the dis-integrating power of sin. The absence of *Shalom* is the presence of this four-dimensional fracture. A diagnosis, however, is only useful if it points to a cure. And this grim diagnosis of our disintegration makes the promise of a Redeemer, the one who will crush the head of the serpent (Genesis 3:15), not a peripheral religious idea, but the only possible hope for a world—and for hearts—that have been torn asunder. The gospel is the announcement that repair is possible, that reconciliation has been accomplished, and that the One who is Himself our *Shalom* (Ephesians 2:14) has come to make all things new.

3.5 Jesus Christ: The Prince of *Shalom* and Agent of Reconciliation

Beloved, having stood in the grim shadow of the Fall and witnessed the four-dimensional rupture of *Shalom*, we now turn to the glorious dawn of its restoration. The diagnosis of our disintegration would be utterly hopeless were it not for the divine intervention that pierces through the darkness. The entire Old Testament builds in a crescendo of longing, a prophetic ache for a day when the fractured pieces of God's good world would be gathered up and made whole again. This longing finds its stunning fulfillment in the person and work of Jesus of Nazareth. His ministry was not merely a series of religious teachings or miraculous exhibitions; it was the decisive, powerful inbreaking of God's *Shalom* into a world held captive by chaos and disintegration. He is the one prophesied by Isaiah, upon whose shoulders the government would rest, and whose name would be called, among other titles, ***Sar-Shalom***, "Prince of Peace" (Isaiah 9:6). In Him, the hope of covenantal wholeness, relational righteousness, and the way of wisdom becomes flesh and dwells among us.

To understand Jesus as the *Sar-Shalom* is to see His entire ministry through a new lens. His miracles were not arbitrary displays of power designed to prove His divinity. They were targeted, intentional acts of *Shalom*-restoration, strategic assaults on the kingdom of darkness, reversing the specific curses of the Fall and providing tangible foretastes of the coming Kingdom. Every healing, every exorcism, every act of power was a declaration that the reign of God—a reign of perfect harmony—was breaking into the present age.

Consider His works of healing as acts of restoring **Internal Shalom**. When Jesus healed the paralytic (Mark 2:1-12), the man with a withered hand (Mark 3:1-6), or the woman with the issue of blood (Mark 5:25-34), He was doing more than fixing broken biology. He was mending the internal fracture between the body and the soul. He was restoring physical integrity, freeing individuals from the shame, isolation, and pain that their conditions imposed. In these acts, He was confronting the symptom of the Fall that manifests as disease and bodily decay, demonstrating His authority to restore the human *nephesh* to wholeness. He was healing the *soma* to bring peace to the *psyche*.

But His restoration went deeper than the physical. In the very same story of the paralytic, Jesus first declares, "*Son, your sins are forgiven*" (Mark 2:5), before He heals the man's body. The religious teachers were correct in their silent objection that only God can forgive sins; they simply failed to recognize that God was standing in front of them in human flesh. In this profound moment, Jesus demonstrates the proper order of *Shalom*'s restoration. The most fundamental rupture is the vertical one. Therefore, His primary work is to address the root cause of all disintegration: sin and its resulting alienation from God. The healing of the body was a visible, tangible sign of the invisible, spiritual reality of forgiveness. By forgiving sins, Jesus was restoring **Vertical *Shalom***, bringing the individual out of hiding and shame and back into a state of grace and favor with the Father. He was re-establishing the foundational relationship upon which all other harmony depends.

Furthermore, Jesus actively worked to restore **Horizontal Shalom**. In a culture rigidly divided by purity laws and social hierarchies, Jesus consistently reached across those human-made barriers to reconcile outcasts to community. He touched lepers, who were forced to live in isolation, and made them clean, restoring them to their families and worshiping communities (Mark 1:40-42). He dined with tax collectors and sinners, welcoming them into fellowship and affirming their dignity (Luke 19:1-10). He spoke with the Samaritan woman at the well, shattering ethnic and gender barriers to offer her the water of life (John 4:1-42). In each of these encounters, Jesus was not merely being kind; He was actively dismantling the walls of hostility that sin had erected between people. He was modeling and enacting a new social order, the Kingdom of God, where the horizontal relationships of blame and domination are replaced by forgiveness, reconciliation, and mutual love.

Yet, all of these individual acts of *Shalom*-restoration during His ministry were localized and temporary. The paralytic would eventually die again. The forgiven sinner would need ongoing grace. The reconciled community would face new conflicts. The ultimate, cosmic, and permanent restoration of *Shalom* required a far more profound and costly action. It required the cross and the empty tomb.

The Apostle Paul unveils the cosmic scope of this work in **Colossians 1:19-20**: *"For in him all the fullness of God was pleased to dwell, and through him to reconcile to himself all things, whether on earth or in heaven, making peace by the blood of his cross."* Please, grasp the magnitude of this statement. The reconciliation achieved by Christ is not limited to human souls. It extends to "*all things*" (*ta panta*)—the entire cosmos. The four-dimensional rupture of *Shalom* required a four-dimensional reconciliation.

On the cross, Jesus, the *Sar-Shalom*, became the sin-bearer. He took upon Himself the full weight of the vertical rupture, enduring the Father's wrath and the agony of God-forsakenness so that we could be declared righteous and brought into a state of permanent peace with God. This is the ultimate fulfillment of the Aaronic blessing—the face of God now shines upon us in grace because of Christ.

On the cross, He bore our griefs and carried our sorrows (Isaiah 53:4). He entered into the depths of our internal disintegration—experencing anguish unto death, betrayal, and physical torment—in order to heal our fractured humanity from the inside out. By His stripes, we are healed (1 Peter 2:24).

On the cross, He " broke down in his flesh the dividing wall of hostility" (Ephesians 2:14), creating in Himself one new humanity, thus making horizontal *Shalom* a reality for all who are in Him, from every tribe, tongue, and nation.

And on the cross, the One through whom all things were created (Colossians 1:16) subjected Himself to the cursed ground, dying on a tree, to redeem the creation from its bondage to decay. His resurrection is the firstfruits of the new creation, the guarantee that the groaning of the earth will one day cease, and environmental *Shalom* will be fully realized in the New Heavens and New Earth.

Therefore, Jesus Christ is not merely a teacher of peace or an example of peace. He *is* our peace (Ephesians 2:14). He is the personal embodiment of the *Shalom* of God. In Him, the dis-integration of the Fall is met with the super-integration of redemption. All the fragmented pieces of God's good world—our relationship with God, our inner being, our social bonds, and our connection to creation—find their coherence, their reconciliation, and their ultimate flourishing in the person and work of the Prince of Peace.

3.6 The Role of the Church as a Community of *Shalom*

Beloved, the glorious work of the *Sar-Shalom*, Jesus Christ, does not end with His ascension. He has left behind a body, a community, an outpost of His kingdom in the midst of a world still groaning under the weight of disintegration. This community, the Church, is not a social club or a voluntary association for religious people. It is the chosen instrument of God, the living organism through which the reality of Christ's accomplished *Shalom* is to be manifested, demonstrated, and proclaimed to the principalities and powers in the heavenly places (Ephesians 3:10). The Church is called to be nothing less than a living, breathing **embassy of the coming Kingdom of *Shalom***. An embassy is a sovereign territory of a foreign nation located within a host country. Its staff lives by the laws, customs, and culture of their homeland, and they offer a place of refuge and a foretaste of home for their citizens abroad. This is our identity. Our homeland is the New Creation, the Kingdom of God, where *Shalom* is all in all. We are stationed here, in the present evil age, to live according to the laws and culture of our true homeland, offering the world a tangible, compelling foretaste of the wholeness that is to come.

This means the local church is to be a laboratory of *Shalom*, a place where the four-dimensional harmony restored by Christ is actively practiced and experienced. It is a community where the sick are not merely referred to doctors, but where **the sick are prayed for and cared for.** The apostle James gives us a profound template for this in James 5:14-16: "*Is anyone among you sick? Let him call for the elders of the church, and let them pray over him, anointing him with oil in the name of the Lord. And the prayer of faith will save the one who is sick, and the Lord will raise him up. And if he has committed sins, he will be forgiven. Therefore, confess your sins to one another and pray for one another, that you may be healed.*"

Notice the holistic, *Shalom*-oriented nature of this instruction. It is not a prescription for a "faith healing" service divorced from reality. The elders are called to the sick person's bedside. They pray *and* they anoint with oil—a symbol of the Holy Spirit's presence and, in the ancient world, a common medicinal practice. This act beautifully integrates the spiritual and the physical. It acknowledges that healing is from the Lord, while also honoring the means of healing He provides in His creation. Furthermore, James immediately connects physical healing with the confession of sins and mutual prayer. He understands that sickness can be a symptom of the internal and vertical ruptures of *Shalom*. The church, as a community of *Shalom*, is to address the whole person—their spiritual, emotional, and physical state—in an atmosphere of faith, love, and vulnerability. This is a far cry from a congregation that ignores physical suffering or, conversely, one that medicalizes all pain without attending to the state of the soul.

Furthermore, the church as an embassy of *Shalom* is a community where **the brokenhearted are comforted.** The world offers platitudes, distractions, or toxic positivity in the face of grief, loss, and deep emotional pain. But the church operates with a different currency. Paul, in 2 Corinthians 1:3-4, reveals the divine economy of comfort: "*Blessed be the God and Father of our Lord Jesus Christ, the Father of mercies and God of all comfort, who comforts us in all our affliction, so that we may be able to comfort those who are in any affliction, with the comfort with which we ourselves are comforted by God.*"

The comfort we offer is not a shallow, "There, there, it will be okay." It is the profound, strengthening, and hope-infusing comfort that flows from the God of all comfort, who Himself entered into our affliction in the person of His Son. This comfort is born of shared suffering and a shared hope. It is the ministry of "sitting shiva" with those who mourn, of weeping with those who weep (Romans 12:15). It is the practical, tangible love that provides meals, listens without judgment, and simply abides in the painful silence with a brother or sister. In a world that prizes strength, success, and the curated life, the church is to be a sanctuary for the broken, a place where internal *Shalom* begins to be restored not through denial, but through the healing balm of compassionate presence and the hope of the resurrection.

As an embassy of the Kingdom, the church must also be a place where **reconciliation is practiced as a spiritual discipline.** Horizontal *Shalom* does not happen by accident in a fallen world; it must be intentionally pursued. Jesus provided a clear, step-by-step protocol for this in Matthew 18:15-17. It begins with private, humble confrontation, moves to a small group for accountability, and, if necessary, involves the wider church community. The goal at every stage is not to punish or ostracize, but to "*gain your brother*" (Matthew 18:15). The goal is restoration, the mending of the torn social fabric. This process stands in stark contrast to the world's patterns of gossip, bitterness, and relational cut-off. It requires immense humility, courage, and a commitment to the unity of the body of Christ over personal pride or preference. A church that actively and lovingly practices biblical discipline and reconciliation is a powerful sign to a fractured world that there is a way through conflict that leads to deeper, more authentic *Shalom*, rather than to further disintegration.

Finally, and most comprehensively, the church as an embassy of *Shalom* is called to **model the integrated wholeness that God intends** by bringing all aspects of life under the Lordship of Christ. This is where our theology of Embodied Stewardship finds its natural home. The church should be a place where it is normal and encouraged to talk about how our faith informs our eating habits, our exercise routines, our work-life balance, our financial decisions, our marital intimacy, and our care for the environment. We are to be a people who demonstrate that the gospel is not a separate, "spiritual" compartment of life, but the integrating principle that brings coherence to all of it.

When a church small group studies Scripture *and* shares healthy recipes, it is modeling integrated wholeness. When a pastor preaches on the fruit of the Spirit of self-control *and* the congregation supports a weight-loss support group, it is tearing down the sacred-secular divide. When a church creates a community garden, it is enacting environmental *Shalom* and providing nutritious food, all while fostering community. In these practical ways, the church becomes a living exhibit of what it means to be a fully human, fully redeemed people. We are to be a preview of the New Jerusalem, a city where the healing of the nations takes place (Revelation 22:2), and where the glory of God illuminates every aspect of a life fully alive. This is our high calling: to be so saturated with the *Shalom* of Christ that our very life together becomes an irresistible invitation to a weary world to be reconciled to God.

3.7 Eschatological *Shalom*: The Hope of Complete Restoration

Beloved, as we have surveyed the biblical landscape of Shalom—from its creational design to its catastrophic rupture and its glorious inauguration in Christ—we must now fix our gaze on the far horizon. The full, unadulterated, and permanent realization of Shalom is, in its ultimate expression, eschatological. It belongs to the eschaton, the final culmination of all things in Christ. The partial healing we experience now, the fleeting moments of harmony, the temporary mending of relationships, and the fragile health we steward in these mortal bodies—all of these are but shadows and foretastes. They are down payments on a future reality so magnificent, so comprehensive in its wholeness, that it defies our present imagination. This hope is crystallized for us in the climactic vision of the Apostle John in Revelation 21:1-5, where he beholds "*a new heaven and a new earth,*" and hears a loud voice from the throne proclaiming the final state of *Shalom*: "*Behold, the dwelling place of God is with man. He will dwell with them, and they will be his people, and God himself will be with them as their God. He will wipe away every tear from their eyes, and death shall be no more, neither shall there be mourning, nor crying, nor pain anymore, for the former things have passed away.*" (Revelation 21:3-4).

This vision is the antithesis of every form of Gnostic escapism that has plagued the church. Our ultimate hope is **not an escape *from* the physical world, but the final redemption *of* the physical world.** The promise is not that we will be disembodied souls floating in a ethereal, non-material realm, but that we will be resurrected, glorified beings inhabiting a resurrected, glorified creation. The "new earth" is the direct descendant and transformation of this earth, just as our resurrection bodies will be the direct descendant and transformation of these bodies. The curse of Genesis 3 is utterly reversed. The thorns and thistles give way to the tree of life, whose leaves are "for the healing of the nations" (Revelation 22:2). The painful toil is transformed into purposeful, joyful, and effortless cultivation. The rupture between humanity and creation is fully healed, and we will once again exercise a perfectly righteous and loving dominion as the image-bearers of God. This is the full flowering of Environmental *Shalom*.

In this consummated state, the four-dimensional matrix of Shalom reaches its perfect, eternal integration. Vertical Shalom is absolute and immediate: we will see God's face, and His name will be on our foreheads (Revelation 22:4). There will be no more sin, no more separation, no more veil. We will know even as we are fully known (1 Corinthians 13:12). **Internal *Shalom*** will be complete: the civil war between the flesh and the spirit will be over. Our minds, wills, emotions, and bodies will be in perfect, seamless harmony, all joyfully aligned with the will of God. There will be no more internal conflict, no more psychological distress, no more shame or fear. **Horizontal *Shalom*** will be universal: the nations will be healed, and the people of God from every tribe, tongue, and nation will dwell together in perfect unity, love, and mutual delight. There will be no more injustice, no more conflict, no more betrayal, and no more loneliness.

This glorious, future certainty is not meant to be a mere comfort for the distant future, a pie-in-the-sky fantasy that helps us endure present misery. No, this eschatological hope is a dynamo of power for the present. It is the engine that drives and empowers faithful action here and now. The sure and certain hope of the New Creation provides the ultimate rationale and motivation for our present pursuit of Embodied Stewardship and our work as agents of *Shalom*. Why should we care for these bodies that are wasting away? Because they are the seeds of our resurrection bodies (1 Corinthians 15:42-44). Our present stewardship is an act of faith in their future glorification. We treat them with reverence now because they have an eternal destiny. Why should we work to alleviate suffering, to heal the sick, to comfort the brokenhearted, and to pursue justice? Because these actions are not in vain. They are tangible, provisional manifestations of the coming reality. They are signposts pointing toward the day when God Himself will wipe away every tear. They are acts of "pulling the future into the present."

This hope infuses our daily, often mundane, acts of stewardship with cosmic significance. When you choose to eat a meal that nourishes your body, you are not just managing a biological machine. You are honoring a future vessel of glory. You are making a statement of faith that this body matters to God, not just for the few decades of this life, but for all eternity. When you engage in physical exercise, you are not merely pursuing vanity or even just present-day health; you are cultivating strength and discipline in a body that will one day be raised in power. When you work to reconcile a broken relationship, to forgive a deep hurt, or to serve the poor, you are not just engaging in social work. You are participating in the inbreaking of the Kingdom of God. You are creating a little pocket of the New Creation in the midst of the old. You are, in the power of the Spirit, making the future *Shalom* audibly and visibly present in a world that desperately needs to see it.

Therefore, the hope of eschatological *Shalom* saves us from both presumption and despair. It saves us from the presumption of thinking we can build a utopia here and now through our own efforts—a theology of glory that is inevitably crushed by the persistent reality of sin and death. But it also saves us from the despair of thinking that our present struggles and labors are meaningless because the world is beyond repair. We live in the tension of the "already but not yet." We already possess the firstfruits of the Spirit—the down payment of *Shalom* in our reconciled relationship with God and the transformative work within us. But we have not yet received the full harvest. So we labor, we steward, we heal, we reconcile, and we care for creation, not with the illusion that we will complete the task, but with the confident hope that our labor in the Lord is not in vain (1 Corinthians 15:58). It is all taken up into God's great redemptive plan and will find its fulfillment in the day when the knowledge of the Lord covers the earth as the waters cover the sea, and *Shalom* is all in all.

3.8 Conclusion: Health as a Foretaste of the Kingdom

Beloved, we have journeyed to the heights and depths of the biblical concept of *Shalom*—from its original harmony to its catastrophic rupture, from its glorious inauguration in Christ to its ultimate consummation in the New Creation. We now arrive at the powerful, practical synthesis that must govern our daily lives. A biblically informed pursuit of health—of holistic, embodied well-being—is far more than personal discipline or prudent self-interest. It is, at its core, a profound and active **participation in God's cosmic mission of *Shalom***. Every conscious choice we make to steward the integrated unity of our body, soul, and spirit is a deliberate strike against the kingdom of darkness and a tangible alignment with the inbreaking Kingdom of God. It is a declarative act that proclaims, in the flesh-and-blood theater of our own existence, that the reign of Christ is a reality that has implications for every facet of creation, including our very metabolism, our neural pathways, and our emotional resilience.

To grasp this is to be liberated from the petty and ultimately futile motivations of vanity or performance. When you choose to **eat well**—to select foods that are nourishing, life-giving, and ethically sourced—you are not merely following a diet. You are engaging in a theological act. You are acknowledging that your body is a temple of the Holy Spirit, and you are refusing to defile it with that which degrades and corrupts. You are participating in the original creational design where food was given as a good gift for sustenance and pleasure. You are also, by your choices, participating in environmental *Shalom*, supporting agricultural systems that honor the earth rather than exploit it. And you are cultivating the physical vitality necessary to be an effective agent of horizontal *Shalom* in your family and community. A meal becomes a sacrament of stewardship, a daily opportunity to choose life over the slow decay that is the legacy of the Fall.

When you diligently **manage stress** through prayer, Scripture meditation, Sabbath rest, and healthy boundaries, you are doing something far more significant than practicing self-care. You are actively combatting the internal disintegration that sin introduced into the human psyche. You are declaring that you will not be governed by the anxiety and hurry that characterize a fallen world alienated from its Creator. By entrusting your burdens to God in prayer, you are reinforcing your vertical *Shalom*, acknowledging your dependence on Him. By stilling your soul before Him, you are allowing the peace of Christ to rule in your heart, which is the very essence of internal *Shalom* (Colossians 3:15). This cultivated inner tranquility then becomes a wellspring from which you can offer peace to others, rather than projecting your own anxiety onto them.

When you consistently **exercise** and strengthen your body, you are not worshipping at the altar of physical appearance or athletic prowess. You are honoring the *soma* as an essential part of your God-given identity, destined for resurrection. You are preparing a fit instrument for service, increasing your capacity for the "good works, which God prepared beforehand, that we should walk in them" (Ephesians 2:10). The strength in your muscles and the stamina in your cardiovascular system are resources for loving your neighbor—for helping a friend move, for playing with your children, for serving on a mission trip, for enduring long days of fruitful labor. Physical discipline is a form of training in godliness (1 Timothy 4:7-8), teaching perseverance, self-control, and the ability to push through present discomfort for a future good—a spiritual lesson embodied in a physical practice.

And when you intentionally **care for your mental state**—guarding your thought life, renewing your mind with truth, seeking healing for past trauma, and fostering emotional health—you are tending to the garden of your *psyche*. You are pulling down "strongholds" and taking "every thought captive to obey Christ" (2 Corinthians 10:4-5). You are recognizing that a healthy mind is not a luxury but a crucial component of your ability to discern the will of God, to resist the lies of the enemy, and to bear the fruit of the Spirit. This is the ongoing sanctification of the soul, the renewal that is essential for a life that truly glorifies God.

In all these ways, the faithful stewardship of your health becomes a **tangible way to align your personal existence with the harmony of God's ultimate will.** It is a life lived in sync with the grain of the universe, which is the wisdom and order of its Creator. It is a proactive rejection of the chaos and disintegration that entered the world through sin. You are, in a very real sense, "working out your own salvation" (Philippians 2:12) in the physical and psychological realm, cooperating with the Holy Spirit who is at work within you to will and to work for His good pleasure.

Therefore, your body, your health, your wholeness, becomes a **signpost.** In a world that treats the body as either a god to be worshipped or a machine to be used and discarded, your reverent, disciplined, and joyful stewardship points beyond itself. It points to a comprehensive restoration that is not merely physical, but spiritual, relational, and cosmic. It points to a Savior, Jesus Christ, who took on flesh to redeem flesh, who heals the brokenhearted and binds up their wounds (Psalm 147:3), and who is even now making all things new. Your choice for wholeness, however imperfect, is a testimony to the world that the gospel is true, that it is powerful, and that it has implications for the whole person. It is a foretaste of the Kingdom, a living, breathing preview of the day when death will be no more, when mourning and crying and pain will have passed away, and when the *Shalom* of God will be the very air we breathe. Let us then pursue health not as an end in itself, but as an act of worship, a weapon of warfare, and a witness to the world—a daily, embodied proclamation that Jesus Christ is Lord, to the glory of God the Father.

CHAPTER 04

The Fall and its Impact on Human Health: A Theological Perspective on Disease and Disorder

4.1 Introduction: The Problem of Evil in the Temple

Beloved, we now arrive at the most pastorally urgent and intellectually formidable question in our entire study of Embodied Stewardship. We have established with exegetical and theological force that the human body is a sacred temple, a *naos* of the Holy Spirit, fearfully and wonderfully made for divine glory and eternal purpose. We have contemplated the majestic vision of *Shalom*, the harmonious flourishing for which we were created. Yet, we are confronted daily by a reality that seems to mock these lofty truths. We live in a world convulsed by disease, a world where bodies—these supposed temples—are ravaged by cancer, crippled by genetic disorders, and slowly dismantled by decay. We witness the anguish of chronic pain, the shadow of mental illness, and the relentless, universal march toward death. If our theology is to be more than a beautiful but irrelevant fantasy, it must stare unflinchingly into this abyss of suffering and provide a framework that does not collapse under the weight of human agony.

This is the ancient problem of theodicy, applied with piercing specificity to the realm of human health. **The Problem of Evil in the Temple** can be stated with stark simplicity: If the body is God's holy dwelling place, why is it so profaned by sickness? If *Shalom* is God's will, why does such profound *dis-integration* characterize our physical existence? How can we proclaim a God of love and power who presides over a creation groaning with tumors, infections, and fractured minds? This is not an abstract philosophical puzzle; it is the cry of the parent watching their child suffer, the silent scream of the one receiving a terminal diagnosis, the weary sigh of the saint battling decades of chronic pain. To offer glib answers is to commit pastoral malpractice. To ignore the question is to abandon the faithful to confusion and despair.

We must, therefore, confront this theodicy directly. And the only biblically faithful starting point is to trace the origin of bodily affliction not to the original design of God, but to the cosmic catastrophe of the **Fall**, as recorded in Genesis 3. The pervasive reality of disease, disability, decay, and death is not part of the "very good" creation. It is an intruder, a violent disruption of the created order, a direct consequence of humanity's catastrophic rebellion against its Creator. The Fall was not a minor misstep; it was an ontological earthquake that shattered the foundations of *Shalom* at every level, and its seismic shockwaves continue to ripple through our cellular biology, our neurochemistry, and our very genetic code.

To understand the Fall's impact on health, we must first reject the simplistic and deeply harmful notion that all sickness is the direct, immediate result of an individual's personal sin. This was the error of Job's friends, whom God Himself condemns for speaking falsely (Job 42:7). While Scripture does acknowledge that some illnesses can be a direct consequence of specific sins (e.g., 1 Corinthians 11:29-30), to universalize this principle is to heap condemnation upon the suffering and to fundamentally misread the biblical narrative. The Fall introduces a systemic, corporate, and cosmic dimension to brokenness that transcends individual culpability. We are born into a world already broken, a world whose very systems—biological, ecological, social—are bent toward disorder and death as a result of humanity's collective rebellion.

This chapter will, therefore, explore the multifaceted consequences of the Fall for human health. We will delve into the four channels through which affliction enters our lives, recognizing that they are often intertwined in complex and mysterious ways. We will examine how the Fall corrupted the very physical structures of creation, turning a world of life-giving order into a theater of entropy and decay. We will consider how our own personal choices, our participation in sinful patterns, can have direct and devastating physiological consequences. We will acknowledge, with biblical sobriety, the reality of demonic activity that can manifest in physical and psychological torment. And we will wrestle with the mysterious reality that God, in His sovereign purposes, sometimes permits suffering for reasons that transcend our finite understanding, as in the case of Paul's thorn in the flesh (2 Corinthians 12:7-9).

Our goal is to develop a pastoral theology of suffering that is both honest and hopeful. It must be honest enough to name the horror of cancer as an evil, a violation of God's good design, and not somehow secretly "good" in itself. It must be hopeful enough to affirm that even in the midst of the temple's ruin, the Divine Resident has not abandoned it, and that the Cross and Resurrection of Jesus Christ are the definitive divine responses to this cosmic tragedy. We are called to be stewards of these fragile, fallen temples, not in a naive denial of their fragility, but in a hopeful defiance of the decay that assails them, knowing that our present sufferings are not worth comparing with the glory that will be revealed in us, and that the redemption of our bodies is our sure and certain hope (Romans 8:18, 23). Let us then, with courage and compassion, explore the difficult terrain of disease and disorder, seeking a wisdom that can only be found at the foot of the cross.

4.2 Exegesis of Genesis 3: The Catastrophic Pivot

Beloved, to understand the world of disease and disorder in which we live, we must return to the moment the universe fractured. The narrative of the Fall in Genesis 3 is not a simple allegory about disobedience; it is the sober, historical account of a cosmic unraveling, a catastrophic pivot in the relationship between God, humanity, and all creation. Every pathology, every malignancy, every anxious thought, and every grieving heart finds its origin in the events of this chapter. We must approach this text not as a distant myth, but as the diagnosis for our terminal condition, the explanation for the profound dissonance between the temple we are meant to be and the crumbling ruins we often experience.

The unraveling begins with what we must term **The Spiritual Rupture: The Primacy of Alienation.** Before any physical consequence is felt, the immediate and most devastating result of Adam and Eve's sin is a fundamental breach in their relationship with God. Genesis 3:8-10 depicts this with heartbreaking clarity: "*And they heard the sound of the LORD God walking in the garden in the cool of the day, and the man and his wife hid themselves from the presence of the LORD God among the trees of the garden. But the LORD God called to the man and said to him, 'Where are you?' And he said, 'I heard the sound of you in the garden, and I was afraid, because I was naked, and I hid myself.*'"

Consider the staggering shift. The couple created for open-faced, intimate communion with their Creator now flees from the sound of His approach. The relational *Shalom*—the joyful, trusting fellowship—is instantly replaced by terror, shame, and hiding. The question, "Where are you?" is not a request for geographical data; it is the poignant cry of a grieving Father to His estranged children. This is spiritual death—not annihilation, but separation. It is the severing of the soul from its life-source. This primary, vertical alienation is the root of all other disharmony. When the human spirit is cut off from the Spirit of God, the entire psychosomatic system is thrown into chaos. The mind, no longer illuminated by divine truth, becomes a factory of fear and rationalization. The emotions, untethered from the love of God, spiral into shame and anxiety. The body, divorced from the sustaining power of its Maker, becomes vulnerable to the entropy and corruption that will now define a fallen creation. All physical death begins with this spiritual death. All sickness is, at its deepest level, a symptom of this foundational separation. The disintegration of the body mirrors the prior disintegration of the relationship.

From this primary spiritual rupture flows the divine pronouncement of judgment, which details the specific ways in which *Shalom* is systematically shattered across the four dimensions of existence. While the consequences for the woman (pain in childbearing and relational strife) and the serpent are profound, of particular relevance to our focus on embodied stewardship is **The Pronouncement of Judgment upon Adam and the Ground.** God declares to Adam in Genesis 3:17-19:

"*Cursed is the ground because of you; in pain you shall eat of it all the days of your life; thorns and thistles it shall bring forth for you; and you shall eat the plants of the field. By the sweat of your face you shall eat bread, till you return to the ground, for out of it you were taken; for you are dust, and to dust you shall return.*"

Let us unpack the monumental implications of this curse, which establishes a direct, causal link between human sin and a corrupted creation that now actively resists humanity's God-given stewardship, a resistance that culminates in physical death.

First, God pronounces a curse upon the **ground** (haadamah). This is profoundly significant. The very material from which Adam (haadam) was formed—the "ground" that was his source and his charge to cultivate—is now cursed *because of him*. The creation, which was declared "very good" and was designed to respond willingly and fruitfully to humanity's priestly care, now becomes antagonistic. It will now produce "thorns and thistles"—useless, painful, and obstructive growth—alongside the nourishing plants. This is the origin of what we might call "Natural Evil" or systemic corruption within the created order. The soil becomes less fertile, the weather becomes hostile, the plants develop defenses, and the entire ecosystem is thrown out of balance. This is not merely a agricultural difficulty; it is a cosmic sign that the harmony between humanity and creation has been broken. The environment itself becomes a source of frustration, toil, and danger. This corrupted creation is the environment in which our bodies now exist, an environment filled with pathogens, natural disasters, and a general tendency toward disorder rather than sustaining order.

Second, humanity's **vocation** is corrupted. The joyful, co-creative work of "working and keeping" the garden (Genesis 2:15) is now transformed into "painful toil" and eating bread "by the sweat of your face." Work itself, which was meant to be a source of fulfillment and a channel for imaging God's creative power, becomes burdensome, exhausting, and fraught with frustration. This has direct implications for our physical health. The chronic stress of futile labor, the bodily wear and tear of struggling against a resistant creation, and the mental anguish of financial insecurity and vocational meaninglessness are all fruits of this aspect of the curse. Our bodies break down under the strain of a struggle that was not part of the original design.

Finally, and most definitively, the judgment culminates in the pronouncement of **physical death**. "For you are dust, and to dust you shall return." This is the ultimate dis-integration. The psychosomatic unity of the *nephesh chayyah*, the living being, is violently torn apart. The body, formed from the dust, returns to the dust. The breath of life (*nishmat chayyim*) returns to God who gave it. This is the final enemy (1 Corinthians 15:26). The curse establishes a direct, causal chain: human sin leads to a cursed ground, which leads to a life of painful toil and struggle, which culminates in the body's return to that same cursed ground. Death is not natural. It is an intruder, a judicial sentence, the final and most visible signature of sin upon the physical creation. Every disease, every disability, every ache and pain is a precursor, a herald of this ultimate return to dust. The pathology in our cells, the genetic mutations, the failing organs—all are participating in this long, slow, or sometimes terrifyingly swift, process of returning to the dust.

Therefore, this exegesis of Genesis 3 provides the only adequate foundation for a theology of health and sickness. It tells us that our bodies are not failing because God designed them poorly. They are failing because we, as a race, rebelled against the Designer, and the entire system of creation was consequently subjected to futility and decay (Romans 8:20). The problem of evil in the temple begins here, in a choice that shattered the relationship with the Temple's divine Architect, resulting in a curse that extends to the very materials from which the temple is built and the environment in which it stands.

4.3 The Four Channels of Affliction

Beloved, having established the cosmic catastrophe of the Fall as the origin point of all disorder, we must now navigate the complex and often painful question of how this general curse manifests in our individual lives. Why does one person struggle with a genetic illness from birth, while another develops heart disease from decades of poor choices? Why do some face sudden, "random" tragedies, while others endure persistent, unexplained suffering? A simplistic theology that attributes all affliction to a single cause will inevitably wound the suffering and misrepresent the character of God. Scripture reveals a more nuanced, multi-faceted reality. The effects of the Fall on human health flow through at least four distinct, yet often tragically intertwined, channels. A wise and compassionate stewardship, both of our own health and in ministering to others, requires that we learn to discern these different streams.

The first channel is the most direct and, in some ways, the most understandable: **The Direct Consequence of Personal Sin.** The Apostle Paul provides a sobering and explicit example of this in his first letter to the Corinthians. Addressing their sacrilegious conduct during the Lord's Supper, he declares, "*For anyone who eats and drinks without discerning the body eats and drinks judgment on himself. That is why many of you are weak and ill, and some have died.*" (1 Corinthians 11:29-30). Here, a specific spiritual failure—the unworthy participation in a holy sacrament—results directly in physical weakness, sickness, and even death. This is not God capriciously zapping people from heaven; it is the built-in moral and physiological fabric of reality asserting itself. When we violate the created order, there are consequences.

This principle extends far beyond this specific context. Diseases linked to gluttony, such as type 2 diabetes and hypertension, are not arbitrary punishments. They are the natural, physiological outcome of consistently overloading the body's God-designed systems. The liver, pancreas, and cardiovascular system were created to function within certain parameters; to chronically violate those parameters is to invite dysfunction. Similarly, substance abuse directly damages the brain, liver, and other organs. The ravages of sexually transmitted diseases are a direct consequence of violating the "one-flesh" union for which sexuality was designed. This is not to heap shame upon the sick, but to acknowledge a foundational biblical truth: we live in a moral universe where our choices have real, physical effects. This channel calls us to personal responsibility and repentance, reminding us that part of stewarding the temple is to flee from sin, which so often wages war not only against our soul but against our very body (1 Peter 2:11).

However—and this is a crucial pastoral distinction—we must never universalize this principle. This leads us to the second, and far more common, channel of affliction: **The General Brokenness of a Fallen World (Natural Evil).** The vast majority of human suffering is not the direct result of an individual's specific sin, but is a consequence of living in a creation that has been "subjected to futility" and now exists in "bondage to decay" (Romans 8:20-21). We are all born into a world system that is fundamentally broken at a cosmic level.

This channel encompasses a wide range of afflictions. **Genetic disorders** like cystic fibrosis or Down syndrome are the result of corrupted genetic information, mutations that accumulate and are passed down in a world groaning under the curse. **Viruses and bacteria**, which can cause everything from the common cold to devastating pandemics, are part of a biological world no longer in perfect harmony with humanity. **Natural disasters**—earthquakes, tornadoes, famines—are the result of a physical creation whose systems are unstable and violent. "Random" accidents, like a tree falling on a hiker or a child being born with a birth defect due to a prenatal infection, fall into this category. These are not acts of a vengeful God targeting individuals; they are the general, systemic conditions of a fallen planet.

Our Lord Jesus Christ Himself explicitly refuted the simplistic idea that all suffering is tied to personal sin. In John 9, His disciples, seeing a man blind from birth, ask, "*Rabbi, who sinned, this man or his parents, that he was born blind?*" (John 9:2). This question reflects the very theological error we are addressing. Jesus' answer is definitive and liberating: "*It was not that this man sinned, or his parents, but that the works of God might be displayed in him.*" (John 9:3). He redirects their focus from a backward-looking search for blame to a forward-looking anticipation of God's redemptive power. The man's blindness was a result of the general brokenness of the fallen world, but it became a platform for a divine revelation of healing and grace. This channel calls us away from judgment and into compassion, recognizing that much suffering is simply part of the shared human condition in a creation that desperately needs redemption.

The third channel, which the modern Western mind often struggles to accept, is that of **Demonic Affliction.** The New Testament unambiguously acknowledges a category of illness that is directly linked to the activity of demonic spirits. This is not a primitive superstition but a sober recognition of the ongoing spiritual war against the kingdom of darkness. We see this in passages like Matthew 9:32-33, where a demon-oppressed man who was mute is brought to Jesus, and when the demon is cast out, the man speaks. Similarly, in Luke 13:11-16, Jesus heals a woman who had "a disabling spirit" for eighteen years, whom He explicitly describes as one "whom Satan bound for eighteen years."

It is critically important to state that *not all disease is demonic.* To see a demon behind every illness is a form of spiritual paranoia that can lead to great harm. However, to dismiss the possibility entirely is to ignore a clear strand of the biblical witness. Demonic affliction seems to often manifest in specific kinds of disorders, particularly those affecting the mind, speech, and musculoskeletal system (e.g., the epileptic boy in Matthew 17:14-18). This channel reminds us that our struggle is not merely against flesh and blood, but against spiritual forces of evil (Ephesians 6:12), and that some forms of brokenness require not only medical or psychological intervention but spiritual authority and deliverance through the powerful name of Jesus.

Finally, we come to the most mysterious and difficult channel to comprehend: **The Sovereign Purpose of God.** In rare but significant cases, Scripture shows us that God, in His inscrutable wisdom, permits or even appoints suffering for a greater purpose that transcends our immediate understanding. We have already seen one example in John 9, where the man's blindness from birth was ordained as an occasion for the works of God to be displayed.

The paradigmatic example for the believer, however, is the Apostle Paul's "thorn in the flesh" in 2 Corinthians 12:7-10. Paul pleads with the Lord three times for this affliction—which many scholars believe was a chronic, debilitating physical condition—to be removed. God's answer is not healing, but a promise: "*My grace is sufficient for you, for my power is made perfect in weakness.*" (2 Corinthians 12:9). Paul comes to understand that this "messenger of Satan" was given to him *to keep him from becoming conceited* because of the surpassing greatness of the revelations he had received. The affliction had a sanctifying purpose: to cultivate humility and a deeper dependence on Christ. In such cases, the suffering is reframed from a meaningless tragedy to a redemptive experience within the sovereign care of a loving Father. It is not that God is the author of the evil, but that He sovereignly harnesses even the attacks of the enemy and the brokenness of the world to accomplish His good and perfect purposes in the lives of His children, conforming them to the image of Christ who learned obedience through what He suffered (Hebrews 5:8). This channel calls us to a posture of profound trust, even when we cannot see the reason for our pain, believing that our loving Father is at work in the midst of it.

4.4 The "Already but Not Yet" Tension of Redemption

Beloved, as we grapple with the grim reality of the four channels of affliction, we now arrive at the critical, dynamic tension that defines the Christian life in this present age. The work of Christ on the cross and in His resurrection was a decisive, finished, and cosmically victorious act. He truly and utterly defeated sin and death, disarming the principalities and powers and making a public spectacle of them (Colossians 2:15). And yet, we look around and see that sin and death appear to be very much alive and active. The resolution to this apparent contradiction lies in understanding the biblical timeline of redemption. We live in the era between the *inauguration* of Christ's kingdom and its final *consummation*. This places every believer in a state of profound paradox, a dynamic and often painful tension between the "Already" and the "Not Yet." Our experience of health, healing, and suffering is utterly framed by this reality.

Let us first contemplate the glorious reality of the **"ALREADY."** Through faith in Jesus Christ, we have been transferred from the kingdom of darkness into the kingdom of God's beloved Son (Colossians 1:13). We are new creations; the old has passed away, behold, the new has come (2 Corinthians 5:17). This is not merely a future hope but a present-tense reality. Crucially, we have received the Holy Spirit as a down payment, the "firstfruits" of our full inheritance (Romans 8:23). The same divine power that raised Jesus from the dead now dwells within us (Romans 8:11). This indwelling presence of the Spirit is the engine of the "Already."

Because of this, we can and do experience real, tangible foretastes of the Kingdom's power *now*. We experience **healing**. Throughout the New Testament and in the life of the church today, God, in His sovereign mercy, graciously grants miracles of physical and emotional restoration. These are not illusions; they are genuine inbreakings of the life of the age to come into the present evil age. They are signposts pointing to the day when every tear will be wiped away. We experience strength that surpasses our natural capacity—the strength to endure suffering, to resist temptation, and to serve tirelessly. This is the "power of Christ" resting upon us and being perfected in our weakness (2 Corinthians 12:9). We experience **victory over sinful habits**. The chains of addiction, the patterns of bitterness, and the strongholds of lust can be broken by the Spirit's power. The Kingdom has truly broken in. We are not merely waiting for salvation; we are actively being saved, being sanctified, and being renewed day by day (2 Corinthians 4:16). This is the foundation for our faith-filled prayers for healing and our confident warfare against every form of affliction. We pray with expectation because we know our God is a God who heals and who delivers.

However, this "Already" exists in constant, sometimes agonizing, tension with the **"NOT YET."** While the Spirit within us is life, our bodies are still subject to the consequences of the Fall. As Paul states with stark honesty, "*So we do not lose heart. Though our outer self is wasting away, our inner self is being renewed day by day.*" (2 Corinthians 4:16). The Greek word for "wasting away" (*diaphtheirō*) is strong; it means to decay, to corrupt, to destroy. This is the present reality of our *soma*. We still inhabit bodies that are susceptible to viral infection, genetic disorders, and cellular mutation. We still get the flu. We still develop cancer. We still age, our muscles atrophy, our memories fade. We are still destined for physical death, barring the Lord's return. The full and final redemption of our bodies is a future hope. Paul makes this explicit in Romans 8:23: "*And not only the creation, but we ourselves, who have the firstfruits of the Spirit, groan inwardly as we wait eagerly for adoption as sons, the redemption of our bodies.*"

This "Not Yet" is the reason why the most faithful saint can still die of a brain tumor. It is the reason why a prayer for healing, offered in fervent faith and full alignment with God's will, may not result in physical restoration in this life. It is the reason why we must carry our cross daily, participating in the sufferings of Christ in these mortal bodies.

Therefore, this "Already but Not Yet" tension demands a corresponding tension in our pastoral practice and personal faith. **We pray for healing with faith, yet we accept that God's sufficient grace is often perfected in our weakness.** This is the perfect balance modeled by the Apostle Paul in 2 Corinthians 12. He prayed in faith for his thorn to be removed—three times. He believed in the "Already" power of God to heal. But when the healing did not come in the way he requested, he did not descend into despair or self-recrimination. He received a revelation of the "Not Yet" purpose of God: that Christ's power is made manifest not in the absence of weakness, but in its very presence. He learned to boast in his weaknesses, so that the power of Christ might rest upon him.

The absence of healing in the present, then, **does not necessarily signify a lack of faith.** To teach otherwise is to inflict terrible pastoral harm on those who are suffering. It is to ignore the clear testimony of Scripture that some of God's most faithful servants—from Paul to Timothy with his frequent ailments (1 Timothy 5:23)—endured chronic physical suffering. It is a failure to understand the "Not Yet" dimension of our existence. We live in the time between the D-Day of the cross—the decisive victory—and the V-Day of the Second Coming—the final mopping-up operation. Battles still rage, and casualties are still taken, even though the war's outcome is certain.

This tension is the key to a resilient, hopeful, and realistic Christian life. It allows us to pray with bold faith for miracles, believing God can and does act now. Simultaneously, it allows us to endure prolonged suffering without our faith shattering, because our hope is not anchored in our present physical comfort, but in the future resurrection of our bodies. We steward our health diligently, fighting the "wasting away" with every God-honoring means at our disposal, because our bodies are temples of the Spirit. Yet, we do so with the peaceful acknowledgment that our best efforts are but a holding action against the inevitable tide of mortality, a tide that will only be finally turned when the trumpet sounds and the dead in Christ are raised imperishable (1 Corinthians 15:52). We live in the paradox, held by the grace that is sufficient for today, and looking with eager longing for the grace that will be revealed in the redemption of these very bodies.

4.5 A Pastoral Theology of Suffering and Care

Beloved, the complex theological framework we have built—comprehending the Fall's curse and the four channels of affliction within the "Already but Not Yet" tension—is not meant for abstract speculation. It is meant to be applied with tenderness and wisdom at the bedside of the sick, in the counseling room with the despairing, and in the quiet hearts of those who suffer. This framework provides the church with a compassionate, realistic, and profoundly hopeful approach to ministry that can withstand the brutal realities of a broken world. It equips us to be true physicians of the soul and companions in suffering, rather than dispensing simplistic platitudes that shatter upon impact with genuine pain.

First and foremost, this framework **removes the crushing burden of guilt from those suffering from non-moral causes of illness.** For the parent of a child born with a severe genetic disorder, for the faithful saint diagnosed with aggressive leukemia, for the victim of a random accident or a natural disaster, the most common and toxic spiritual question that arises is, "What did I do to deserve this?" This is the echo of the disciples' question to Jesus in John 9: "Who sinned?" When the church, wittingly or unwittingly, promotes a theology that directly or indirectly links all suffering to personal sin, it becomes an instrument of torture rather than a haven of grace. It compounds physical agony with spiritual condemnation. But our framework, following Jesus' own teaching, liberates the sufferer. It clearly distinguishes the channels of affliction. It affirms that a vast amount of human suffering falls under Channel 2—the general brokenness of a fallen world. It declares that a child's disability is a result of a cosmos groaning under the curse of Genesis 3, not a specific failure of the parents. It tells the cancer patient that their disease is a manifestation of cellular corruption in a creation subjected to futility (Romans 8:20), not a punishment from God. This is not a cold, clinical diagnosis; it is a pastoral balm. It lifts the weight of false responsibility and allows the sufferer to direct their energy away from fruitless self-recrimination and toward receiving grace and comfort from the God who Himself enters into our suffering.

Secondly, this framework provides balanced guidance for life, for it **encourages responsible stewardship while simultaneously acknowledging the limits of our control.** It calls us to take full responsibility for Channel 1—the direct consequences of personal sin. This is a vital part of discipleship and health. We are to preach, teach, and model the truth that our choices matter. We are to call people to repent of gluttony, sloth, substance abuse, and sexual immorality, not merely as spiritual offenses, but as acts that physically defile the temple of the Holy Spirit and lead to predictable paths of destruction. This is a prophetic and loving ministry. A church that remains silent on these issues is not being "gracious"; it is being negligent.

However, this call to stewardship is held in tension with a humble acknowledgment of Channels 2 and 4. We must acknowledge the limits of our control. We cannot through sheer willpower or perfect behavior inoculate ourselves against a random virus, a genetic predisposition, or the sovereign purposes of God that may include a "thorn in the flesh." This prevents a health-and-wealth gospel that promises perfect health as a reward for faith and inevitably blames the sick for their lack of it. It also prevents a neurotic, anxious pursuit of wellness where every minor ailment is seen as a personal failure. We are called to be faithful stewards of what we can control—our choices, our habits, our disciplines—while simultaneously entrusting to our sovereign Father all that we cannot control, resting in the truth that even the things that are outside our dominion are still inside His.

Thirdly, this framework **provides a robust theodicy—a defense of God's justice and goodness in the face of evil.** The problem of evil is the greatest stumbling block to faith for many. A weak theodicy either minimizes the reality of evil or makes

God its author. Our framework does neither. It acknowledges the full, horrifying reality of evil—cancer is evil, dementia is evil, childhood leukemia is a monstrous evil. It does not call it "good" or pretend it is not there. It rightly identifies the origin of this evil not in God, but in the cosmic rebellion of humanity and the subsequent curse upon creation. God is not the author of evil; He is its ultimate conqueror.

Yet, at the same time, this theodicy affirms God's ultimate sovereignty. He is not a passive bystander wringing His hands in heaven. Even in the midst of the evil that flows from Channels 1, 2, and 3, He is sovereign. He sets limits on suffering (Job 1:12; 2:6). And, mysteriously and wonderfully, He can sovereignly harness even these evil things and weave them into His redemptive plan for our good and His glory (Channel 4), as He did with Joseph's betrayal (Genesis 50:20) and most supremely with the cross of Christ. This theodicy allows us to weep with those who weep, to name evil as evil, and yet to still confess through our tears, "I believe in God the Father Almighty."

Finally, and most importantly, this framework **directs the sufferer to the certain and glorious hope of the resurrection.** All pastoral care that stops at the grave is ultimately bankrupt. Our comfort is not that we might be healed in this life—though we pray for that fervently. Our ultimate comfort is that, healed or not, these perishable bodies will one day put on imperishability, and these mortal bodies will put on immortality (1 Corinthians 15:53). The resurrection of the body is the Christian answer to the problem of suffering. It is the divine guarantee that the story of every believer does not end with the slow decay of the body or the sudden violence of death. It ends with restoration, with wholeness, with a body like Christ's glorious body (Philippians 3:21), forever free from the four channels of affliction.

This hope is not a spiritualized fantasy; it is a physical reality. The same power that raised Jesus from the dead will raise us. This means that the suffering of the present, however long and deep, is momentary and light compared to the eternal weight of glory that is being prepared for us (2 Corinthians 4:17). This hope allows a dying saint to face death not with terror, but with defiance. It allows the chronically ill to endure another day of pain, knowing it is not the final word on their body. It is the solid rock upon which we can stand when everything else is giving way. Our pastoral care, therefore, must always point beyond the sickbed, beyond the hospital room, beyond the grave, to the empty tomb of Jesus and the promise of our own resurrection. In this hope, we find the strength to suffer well, to care faithfully, and to wait with patience for the redemption of our bodies.

4.6 Conclusion: Groaning in Hope

Beloved, as we draw this profound and sobering chapter to a close, we are left standing at the intersection of two monumental truths. On one hand, the impact of the Fall upon human health is **profound and inescapable.** It is the universal human experience, the foundational reality of our biological existence. We have traced its origins to the catastrophic pivot in Eden, where spiritual rupture unleashed a cascade of disintegration into every dimension of our being. We have seen its multifaceted expression through the four channels of affliction—the direct consequences of our own sin, the general brokenness of a fallen world, the malicious activity of demonic forces, and the mysterious, sovereign purposes of God. This reality explains the universality of suffering—why no one, from the most pious saint to the most hardened atheist, is exempt from sickness and pain. It explains the inevitability of death—the final, grim signature of sin upon our physical frames, the return to dust from which we were taken. To deny this is to be deluded. To be unaware of it is to be unprepared for life in a world under curse.

And yet—and this is the glorious, resounding "yet" of the gospel—**the Christian does not groan without hope.** Our groaning is not the hopeless wail of despair of those who have no future. It is a different kind of groaning altogether. The Apostle Paul, in his magnificent treatise in Romans 8, masterfully connects our personal suffering to the cosmic drama of redemption. He acknowledges the reality of our pain: "*For we know that the whole creation has been groaning together in the pains of childbirth until now.*" (Romans 8:22). The entire cosmos is in a state of agonized longing, like a woman in labor, yearning for deliverance. And then he includes us in this cosmic sigh: "*And not only the creation, but we ourselves, who have the firstfruits of the Spirit, groan inwardly as we wait eagerly for adoption as sons, the redemption of our bodies.*" (Romans 8:23).

Do you see it? Our groaning—the ache in our bones, the fatigue in our bodies, the anguish of a diagnosis, the slow decline of age—is not meaningless. It is a participation. It is our personal, embodied echo of the creation's own eager longing for final redemption. When your body groans with illness, it is joining the mountains, the forests, and the oceans in their collective cry for liberation from the bondage to decay. This groaning is, paradoxically, a sign of the Spirit's work within us, for it is the Spirit who creates in us this eager longing for a reality we do not yet see in full. The person who is perfectly content with a decaying body is a person who has not yet grasped the hope of glory. Our discontent with sickness, our rage against the dying of the light, is a holy impulse, a Spirit-inspired recognition that this is not the way things are supposed to be.

This is why the gospel does not promise us a trouble-free life now. Such a promise would be a lie, and it would make heaven irrelevant. Instead, it assures us of something far more substantial and enduring: "*For I consider that the sufferings of this present time are not worth comparing with the glory that is to be revealed to us.*" (Romans 8:18). The glory that awaits us so infinitely outweighs the suffering we endure now that they cannot even be placed on the same scale. The momentary, light affliction of a lifetime of cancer or chronic pain is producing for us an eternal weight of glory beyond all comparison (2 Corinthians 4:17). This is not a call to stoic resignation, but to hopeful endurance. We are not merely waiting for the pain to stop; we are waiting for a glory so magnificent that the memory of our suffering will be swallowed up in its radiance.

Therefore, our bodies, though subject to decay, are still temples of the Holy Spirit. Even in their weakened, groaning state, they are sacred. The divine Resident has not evacuated the premises because the roof is leaking and the walls are crumbling. He remains, a present help in trouble, the source of our strength in weakness, the guarantee of our future redemption. This truth sanctifies our present suffering and transforms our daily stewardship.

Our stewardship, then—the careful, disciplined, loving care of these physical bodies—is ultimately **an act of hope.** It is a defiant declaration of faith in the future. When we choose to eat nourishing food, we are not just feeding a dying body; we are honoring a future vessel of glory. When we engage in physical exercise, we are not just building muscle that will one day atrophy; we are cultivating strength and discipline in a body that will be raised in power. When we pursue rest and manage stress, we are not just optimizing a biological machine; we are maintaining the temple for the Spirit's work and bearing witness to a rhythm of grace in a frantic world. We are caring for these "jars of clay" (2 Corinthians 4:7)—these fragile, ordinary, cracked pots—in the sure and certain hope that the transcendent power within them belongs to God and not to us, and that the same power will one day transform the jar itself into a flawless vessel of unimaginable beauty and strength.

We groan, yes. But we groan *in hope*. We steward these bodies not with the despair of those who are maintaining a sinking ship, but with the hopeful anticipation of gardeners tending seeds that will one day explode into glorious, eternal life. We look forward with eager longing, not for an escape from our bodies, but for their redemption. We await the day when the groaning will cease, not in silence, but in the triumphant shout of resurrection, when the perishable puts on the imperishable, and death is swallowed up in victory. Until that day, we steward, we groan, and we hope, sustained by the promise that the one who began this good work in us will be faithful to complete it on the day of Christ Jesus.

PART II

NUTRITIONAL STEWARDSHIP: NOURISHING THE TEMPLE

CHAPTER 05

Divine Provision: A Theological Analysis of Food in Scripture

5.1 Introduction: From Fuel to Sacrament

Beloved, we now turn our attention to one of the most fundamental, daily, and yet profoundly misunderstood acts of our embodied existence: the act of eating. In our modern, disenchanted age, food has been largely reduced to its biochemical constituents—macronutrients, calories, vitamins, and minerals. It has become "fuel," a commodity to be optimized for performance, a variable in a weight management equation, or a source of fleeting sensory pleasure. This **functional nutrition** perspective, while containing elements of truth from General Revelation, represents a catastrophic flattening of a reality that Scripture reveals to be deep, wide, and shot through with theological significance. It is a view from the laboratory that is blind to the view from the altar.

A robust theological vision, however, restores to food its God-ordained majesty and meaning. It calls us to see beyond the plate to the Provider, beyond the metabolism to the mystery. This chapter will argue a singular, transformative thesis: **Eating is a theological act.** It is never merely a biological transaction. Every meal, from the simplest snack to the most elaborate feast, is a daily participation in the Creator's sustaining goodness, a tangible experience of His covenant faithfulness, a locus for the formation of community, and a sacred channel of His grace. Furthermore, our earthly eating is a profound foreshadowing, a daily rehearsal, for the great eschatological feast of the Lamb. To eat with theological awareness is to transform the dining table into a sanctuary and the act of consumption into an act of communion.

We must first recognize that in the biblical worldview, food is, first and foremost, a **primary means of God's provision.** From the very beginning, the Creator's care for His creatures is expressed through the gift of food. In the pristine goodness of Eden, God does not merely give Adam and Eve abstract sustenance; He gives them specific, good things to eat: "*And God said, 'Behold, I have given you every plant yielding seed that is on the face of all the earth, and every tree with seed in its fruit. You shall have them for food.'*" (Genesis 1:29). Food is the original gift, a tangible expression of divine generosity and a central component of the *Shalom* for which we were created. This establishes a pattern that runs throughout Scripture: God is the one who feeds His people. He provides manna in the wilderness (Exodus 16), water from the rock (Exodus 17:6), and quail in the camp (Numbers 11). The Psalmist declares, "*The eyes of all look to you, and you give them their food in due season. You open your hand; you satisfy the desire of every living thing.*" (Psalm 145:15-16). Jesus Himself teaches us to pray for "our daily bread"

(Matthew 6:11), grounding our most basic physical need in a posture of radical dependence on our Heavenly Father. Therefore, when we eat, we are not just consuming calories; we are receiving a gift. We are participating in the ongoing, creational providence of God. This transforms our eating from an act of autonomous consumption to an act of receptive gratitude.

Secondly, food is a powerful **locus of community and covenant.** In the ancient Near Eastern world, and throughout the Bible, to share a meal was to establish a bond of fellowship, trust, and peace. It was a covenant-making activity. When Abimelech and Isaac made a treaty, they sealed it with a feast (Genesis 26:30). The entire Levitical system of sacrifices, while dealing with atonement, often culminated in a communal meal where the worshipper and his family would eat a portion of the sacrifice in God's presence (Deuteronomy 12:17-18). This was a powerful act of communion with God and with one another. Jesus' ministry was constantly criticized precisely because He ate with "tax collectors and sinners" (Matthew 9:11). In doing so, He was not merely being sociable; He was demonstratively enacting the inclusive grace of the Kingdom, welcoming outcasts into covenant fellowship. The table is where relationships are built, where stories are shared, where the body of Christ is knit together. The early church devoted itself to "the breaking of bread" (Acts 2:42), recognizing that their shared life in Christ was nurtured around a common table. To eat alone, habitually and by choice, is to miss a fundamental dimension of what food is for. It is designed to draw us into community, to break down barriers, and to strengthen the bonds of *Shalom*.

Finally, and most gloriously, food functions as a **channel of grace and a foreshadowing of the eschatological feast.** God uses physical food to convey spiritual realities. The manna in the wilderness was not merely caloric sustenance; it was a "test" of Israel's obedience and a lesson in daily dependence, and Jesus later identifies it as a type of His own person, the true "bread from heaven" (John 6:32-35). But the supreme example is the Lord's Supper, the Eucharist. In this sacrament, God takes the most basic elements of food and drink—bread and wine—and makes them the vehicles of the most profound spiritual reality. We do not merely *think* about Christ's sacrifice; we physically partake of it. "*Take, eat; this is my body...*" (Matthew 26:26). In the Eucharist, the theological nature of all eating is revealed in its fullest clarity: the physical nourishes the spiritual; God's grace comes to us through material means; and our daily bread points to the True Bread that gives eternal life.

This sacred meal, in turn, points forward. It is an "anticipatory sign" of the Marriage Supper of the Lamb (Revelation 19:9). Our daily meals, our church potlucks, our family dinners—all are small, imperfect foretastes of that great and final banquet when people from every nation will sit down at the table of the King in the New Creation. Every time we eat with gratitude, in community, and in remembrance of God's provision, we are rehearsing for eternity. We are proclaiming that our ultimate hunger and thirst will be satisfied not by a meal that perishes, but by the presence of God Himself.

Therefore, to approach food merely as fuel is to live in a state of profound spiritual poverty. It is to be like Esau, who saw only the lentil stew and was blind to the birthright (Genesis 25:29-34). But to approach food theologically is to open our eyes to the divine drama in which every meal is a scene. It is to see our daily bread as a gift from our Father's hand, our shared tables as a foretaste of heavenly fellowship, and our hunger as a God-given pointer to our ultimate satisfaction in Christ. Let us then journey through the biblical narrative of food, from Eden to the New Jerusalem, and learn once again how to eat to the glory of God.

5.2 The Creational Menu: Food in the Pre-Lapsarian World (Genesis 1-2)

Beloved, to understand the deep theology of food, we must return to the beginning, to the pristine state of creation as God intended it, before the rupture of sin introduced violence, toil, and death into the world. The original dietary design, revealed in the opening chapters of Genesis, is not a primitive nutritional footnote. It is a profound theological revelation, a blueprint for the harmonious relationship between humanity, creation, and Creator. It reveals God's intention for a perfect *Shalom* in which our most basic act of sustenance—eating—would be an act of worship, communion, and joyful participation in a life-giving order.

The foundational text for this creational menu is **Genesis 1:29-30**. Here, God articulates His original provision for humanity and, indeed, for all creatures: "*And God said, 'Behold, I have given you every plant yielding seed that is on the face of all the earth, and every tree with seed in its fruit. You shall have them for food. And to every beast of the earth and to every bird of the heavens and to everything that creeps on the earth, everything that has the breath of life, I have given every green plant for food.'*"

This establishes what we must term the **Plant-Based Paradigm**. In the pre-lapsarian world, the entire system of nourishment was founded on plants—specifically, seed-bearing plants and fruit-bearing trees. This is a vision of staggering theological significance. First and foremost, it establishes a **non-violent system of nourishment.** In the original *Shalom* of Eden, there was no death. The taking of life, whether animal or human, was utterly foreign to God's perfect design. The human consumption of food did not require the death of another creature. Humanity's dominion over the animal kingdom, therefore, was not predatory; it was **priestly**. Adam's role was to "work and keep" the garden (Genesis 2:15)—to cultivate, protect, and oversee this vibrant, life-filled ecosystem. He was to be a steward and a shepherd, not a hunter or a slaughterer. The food system itself reflected this harmonious relationship: both humanity and the animals were sustained by the same life-giving vegetation, all provided directly from the hand of the Creator. This original menu stands as an eternal testament to God's desire for a world without violence, a world where life is sustained by life that freely gives itself in the form of fruit and grain, not by life that is taken by force. It points forward to the prophetic vision of the messianic kingdom, where "the wolf shall dwell with the lamb... and the lion shall eat straw like the ox" (Isaiah 11:6-7), and finds its ultimate fulfillment in the New Creation where death will be no more.

Furthermore, this creational menu reveals that God's provision is inherently **sustainable and regenerative.** The emphasis on plants "yielding seed" and trees with "seed in its fruit" is crucial. This was not a system of extraction and depletion. It was a system designed for ongoing life, for perpetual fruitfulness. The very act of eating involved participating in a cycle of life that would ensure future provision. The seeds within the food guaranteed the next harvest. This reflects the nature of God's Kingdom, which is a kingdom of abundance and multiplication, not of scarcity and hoarding. Our modern industrial food systems, which often degrade the soil, rely on synthetic inputs, and produce immense waste, stand in stark contrast to this creational model of sustainable, regenerative nourishment that honors the cycles of life God embedded in His world.

But God's provision was not merely functional; it was also beautiful. **Genesis 2:9** offers another dimension of the creational menu that is often overlooked: *"And out of the ground the LORD God made to spring up every tree that is pleasant to the sight and good for food."* Here we see the **Aesthetic and Functional** unity of God's design. The trees of the garden were not merely caloric fuel depots. They were "pleasant to the sight"—they were beautiful, appealing, and delightful to behold. God designed our sustenance to engage the whole person. The vibrant color of a ripe fruit, the intricate pattern on a vegetable, the fragrant aroma of an herb—all of these were part of the original eating experience. God could have created bland, gray, nutrient-dense cubes to meet our biological needs. Instead, He created a cornucopia of sensory delights. This tells us that God is not only concerned with our survival but with our *flourishing*. He created us as integrated beings whose senses, intellect, and spirit are all to be engaged in the simple act of receiving His gifts. The pleasure of taste, the joy of a beautiful meal, the satisfaction of a shared feast—these are not sinful indulgences but creational goods, designed by God to draw us into a deeper appreciation of His goodness and generosity. To eat without noticing, without gratitude, without savoring the beauty and variety of God's provision, is to miss a fundamental aspect of why He made food the way He did.

Finally, we encounter the profound theological significance of **The Prohibitive Tree.** Amidst the abundant and unrestricted provision of the garden, God placed a single, crucial boundary: *"And the LORD God commanded the man, saying,*

'You may surely eat of every tree of the garden, but of the tree of the knowledge of good and evil you shall not eat, for in the day that you eat of it you shall surely die.'" (Genesis 2:16-17).

This single prohibition transformed the entire landscape of eating. It introduced the concept of **dietary restraint as an act of trust and obedience.** In a world of limitless permission, one limit was set. Food became a test, a boundary that defined the relationship between the creature and the Creator. The question posed by the forbidden tree was not primarily about nutrition, but about authority and trust: Would humanity trust that God's "no" was for their ultimate good? Would they be content to live within the bounds of His wisdom, or would they seize autonomy, determining for themselves what was good and evil? The act of eating, therefore, from the very beginning, was laden with moral and spiritual significance. It was the primary arena in which faith and obedience were to be exercised. To abstain from that one tree was an act of worship, a tangible declaration that "man does not live by bread alone, but by every word that comes from the mouth of the LORD" (Deuteronomy 8:3). The Fall itself was triggered by a dietary choice—a decision to transgress a God-ordained food boundary, driven by distrust of God's word and a desire for self-determination. This foundational story teaches us that our relationship with food is always, at its heart, a spiritual issue. It is about whether we will receive food as a gift from God with gratitude and within His limits, or whether we will grasp for it as a right, using it to satisfy our own desires for control, pleasure, and autonomy, apart from Him. The creational menu, therefore, sets the stage for all that follows: food is God's good gift, meant for our pleasure and sustenance within the context of a trusting, obedient relationship with Him.

5.3 The Post-Diluvian Concession: Meat-Eating in a Fallen World (Genesis 9:1-4)

Beloved, the pristine harmony of Eden's plant-based paradigm was shattered by the cataclysm of the Fall. The world that emerged from the Great Flood was not a restored Eden, but a world purged yet still fundamentally scarred by sin. It is in this new, post-diluvian reality that we encounter a profound and sobering shift in the divine dietary ordinance. In Genesis 9:1-4, God establishes His covenant with Noah and his descendants, and in doing so, He formally alters the creational menu: "*And God blessed Noah and his sons and said to them, 'Be fruitful and multiply and fill the earth. The fear of you and the dread of you shall be upon every beast of the earth and upon every bird of the heavens, upon everything that creeps on the ground and all the fish of the sea. Into your hand they are delivered. Every moving thing that lives shall be food for you. And as I gave you the green plants, I give you everything. But you shall not eat flesh with its life, that is, its blood.*'"

This passage marks a monumental theological pivot. The permission to eat animal flesh represents a dramatic departure from the non-violent, priestly dominion of Genesis 1. We must understand this not as a new ideal, but as a **Concession, Not a Command.** This is a crucial distinction. God is not now declaring that eating meat is inherently superior or more aligned with His ultimate will than the original plant-based design. Rather, this is a divine accommodation to a new, harsh, and violent reality. The original *Shalom* is irrevocably fractured. The world after the Flood is one where "the intention of man's heart is evil from his youth" (Genesis 8:21). It is a world now characterized by fear and dread between humanity and the animal kingdom. The harmonious relationship is broken, replaced by a dynamic of terror and domination.

This concession, therefore, is a tangible acknowledgment of the full implications of the Fall. Death has entered the world not just as a spiritual reality, but as a physical, systemic one. The taking of life for sustenance is now permitted, but it is framed within this new context of brokenness. It is a provision for survival in a world where the perfect, self-perpetuating abundance of Eden is no longer the operating principle. This divine allowance carries a tone of solemnity, even tragedy. It is God providing for humanity in their fallen state, meeting them where they are, yet it forever memorializes the loss of the original peaceable kingdom. Every time an animal is slaughtered for food, it should serve as a silent, sobering sermon on the devastating consequences of human sin—a consequence that ripples out to encompass the entire created order, forcing the taking of life to sustain life.

Yet, even in this concession, God immediately establishes a crucial, non-negotiable boundary that infuses this new, violent reality with sacred meaning. This is the law of **The Sanctity of Blood.** God declares, "*But you shall not eat flesh with its life, that is, its blood.*" This prohibition is not an arbitrary dietary restriction; it is dense with theological significance. In the Hebrew worldview, blood is not merely a biological fluid; it is the seat of life, the *nephesh*. As God will later articulate to Moses in Leviticus 17:11, "*For the life of the flesh is in the blood, and I have given it for you on the altar to make atonement for your souls, for it is the blood that makes atonement by the life.*"

This prohibition, therefore, serves several profound purposes. First, it **instills a sacred reverence for life, even in the act of**

taking it. By forbidding the consumption of blood, God is drawing a stark line. He is saying, "I am giving you the animal's flesh for your sustenance, but its *life* remains mine. You may use the body, but you must acknowledge that the life-principle belongs to Me alone." The act of slaughter, therefore, could not become a casual, desensitized, or bloodthirsty affair. It had to be done in a way that ritually acknowledged the gravity of taking a life. The blood, representing the God-given life, was to be drained out and, in later Mosaic law, returned to God by being poured out on the ground or sprinkled on the altar. This practice was a tangible confession that God is the sole author and owner of life.

Second, this law **serves as a constant reminder of the cost of sin.** In a world without death, no blood needed to be shed. But in a fallen world, the sustaining of human life now, in this concessionary diet, required the death of another creature. The sight of blood, spilled out and offered to God, was a visceral, daily reminder that sin has a terrible price. It pointed to the fundamental brokenness of the world, where one life must be given for another to continue.

Finally, and most significantly, the sanctity of blood **points forward to the ultimate need for atonement.** The life-in-the-blood that was forbidden for consumption was the very thing that God would later designate for use on the altar for sacrifice. The blood of bulls and goats could never truly take away sin (Hebrews 10:4), but it was a God-appointed symbol, a placeholder, pointing toward the one, final, sufficient sacrifice. It all pointed to the day when the Lamb of God would take away the sin of the world (John 1:29). The blood of Jesus Christ, shed on the cross, was the ultimate and perfect life given as a ransom for many. The prohibition against consuming blood in Genesis

9, therefore, sets the stage for the entire theology of sacrifice and atonement that unfolds in Scripture. It reserves the significance of blood for God's redemptive purposes, teaching humanity that the problem of sin is so grave that it can only be addressed by a life given up—a lesson that finds its ultimate fulfillment on Calvary.

Thus, the post-diluvian concession to eat meat is a complex, multi-layered divine action. It is an accommodation to a fallen reality, a perpetual reminder of the loss of *Shalom*, a call to reverence for God's gift of life, and a profound prophetic pointer to the gospel of Jesus Christ. It teaches us that our eating is never divorced from the grand narrative of creation, fall, and redemption.

5.4 Manna in the Wilderness: A Paradigm of Dependence (Exodus 16)

Beloved, we now journey from the broad creational and post-diluvian frameworks into a specific, miraculous, and deeply instructive episode in Israel's history: the provision of manna in the wilderness. The story found in Exodus 16 is far more than a record of supernatural catering; it is a masterclass in nutritional theology. Here, God uses the most basic human need—daily bread—to teach His people fundamental spiritual truths about His character, their dependence, and the proper posture for receiving all good gifts. In the barren, lifeless desert, God establishes a school of faith, and the curriculum is food.

At the heart of this divine pedagogy is the principle of **Daily Dependence.** The instructions for gathering the manna were precise and non-negotiable. Exodus 16:4 states, "*Then the LORD* *said to Moses, 'Behold, I am about to rain bread from heaven for you, and the people shall go out and gather a day's portion every day, that I may test them, whether they will walk in my law or not.'"* The people were to gather only what they needed for that single day. If they tried to hoard it out of anxiety for the future, the leftover manna would breed worms and stink (Exodus 16:20). This was a direct assault on the human tendency toward self-reliance, anxiety, and hoarding. In the desert, there were no grain silos, no backup plans, no 401(k) retirement accounts. There was only God's promise and His daily, faithful provision.

This discipline of daily gathering was a tangible, physical rehearsal of the trust Jesus would later teach us to pray: "*Give us this day our daily bread*" (Matthew 6:11). It forced Israel to live in the present, to trust that the same God who provided today would be just as faithful tomorrow. It was a detox from the Egyptian mindset of accumulation and security through human systems. Every morning, as they walked out of their tents to find the ground covered with God's grace, they were being schooled in the truth that life is not sustained by bread alone, but by every word that proceeds from the mouth of the Lord (Deuteronomy 8:3). Their stomachs, and thus their entire beings, were being trained in the posture of receptive gratitude, one day at a time. This stands as a permanent critique of our modern culture of excess, food waste, and the frantic stockpiling of resources driven by a deep-seated fear of scarcity, a fear that fundamentally doubts the providence of a good Father.

Furthermore, God wove His creational rhythm directly into this system of provision, creating a **Sabbath Rhythm.** The instructions included a profound exception: "*On the sixth day, when they prepare what they bring in, it will be twice as much as they gather daily.*" (Exodus 16:5). On the day before the Sabbath, the manna would not spoil, providing sustenance for the day of rest. This was a miraculous suspension of the normal rules, a divine endorsement of the Sabbath principle established at creation. God was teaching them that His provision includes rest. The rhythm of work and cessation from work was not an afterthought; it was built into the very metabolism of their existence. They did not need to anxiously gather on the Sabbath, violating God's command for rest, because He had already provided.

This teaches us a vital lesson for our own embodied stewardship. Our relationship with food and work is not meant to be one of constant, anxious striving. The Sabbath principle, modeled in the manna, tells us that God's economy is one of grace and sufficiency. It calls us to a rhythm where we work diligently during six days, trusting God for the yield, and then we cease, recognizing that our ultimate security and sustenance come from Him, not from our relentless labor. To ignore this rhythm is to fall back into the Egyptian bondage of endless production, a state that is physically, mentally, and spiritually destructive. The manna on the sixth day was a gift of time, a gift of peace, a declaration that our worth is not in our productivity but in our identity as God's dependent children.

Yet, despite this perfect, miraculous provision, the human heart revealed its corruption. We see the tragedy of **Rejecting Monotony and Discontent.** The manna is described as being like coriander seed, white, and tasting like wafers made with honey (Exodus 16:31). It was a perfectly designed, nutritionally complete food, provided without cost or toil, directly from the hand of God. But in Numbers 11:4-6, the narrative takes a dark turn: "*The rabble that was among them had a strong craving. And the people of Israel also wept again and said, 'Oh that we had* *meat to eat! We remember the fish we ate in Egypt that cost nothing, the cucumbers, the melons, the leeks, the onions, and the garlic. But now our strength is dried up, and there is nothing at all but this manna to look at.*'"

This is a stunning indictment. The very perfection of the manna—its consistent, reliable, sufficient nature—became the object of their contempt. They romanticized their past slavery in Egypt, focusing only on the variety and intensity of flavors, while willfully forgetting the whips and the bondage. Their desire for culinary variety metastasized into a rejection of God's sufficiency. They allowed their palates to dictate their theology, and their cravings to corrupt their memory. This illustrates a profound spiritual danger: our sinful desires can corrupt God's good provision and lead us to reject Him. The manna was good, but their hearts were not. They preferred the stimulating, varied, yet ultimately enslaving foods of Egypt over the simple, sustaining, and freeing bread of heaven.

This speaks directly to our modern food culture, saturated with hyper-palatable, artificially flavored, and marketing-driven food products designed to exploit our natural desire for variety and intensity. Like Israel, we can easily become discontent with simple, wholesome, God-given foods, craving instead the "onions and garlic" of a world system that, while offering fleeting sensory pleasure, ultimately leads to bondage—bondage to unhealthy cravings, to poor health, and to a spirit of ingratitude. The manna story calls us to examine our hearts: Do we receive God's good provision with gratitude, or do we grumble because it lacks the exciting variety and intensity the world promises? Do we trust that what God provides is truly sufficient, or do we secretly long for the "cuisine of Egypt"? The test in the wilderness was not merely about gathering food; it was about the state of the heart that receives it.

5.5 The Dietary Laws of Leviticus: Holiness Embodied

Beloved, we now arrive at one of the most distinctive and often misunderstood aspects of Israel's identity: the dietary laws, known as the *kashrut* laws, detailed primarily in Leviticus 11 and Deuteronomy 14. In our modern, scientifically-oriented age, there is a strong temptation to read these texts through a purely hygienic or medical lens, searching for the hidden health benefits that would explain God's seemingly arbitrary choices. While it is true that some of these laws, such as the prohibition of pork, likely had the secondary benefit of protecting Israel from diseases like trichinosis, to view this as their primary purpose is to miss their profound theological heart. The *kashrut* laws were not fundamentally about physical health; they were about **holiness embodied**. They were a divine curriculum designed to teach a visceral, daily lesson about what it means to be *qadosh*—set apart, holy, belonging exclusively to Yahweh.

The core purpose of these laws was to function as a **Pedagogy of Separation.** In a world populated by nations with their own gods, customs, and cuisines, Israel was called to be a unique treasure, a kingdom of priests, a holy nation (Exodus 19:5-6). This identity could not remain an abstract theological concept; it had to be woven into the very fabric of their daily existence. What could be more daily than eating? By dividing the animal kingdom into "clean" and "unclean" categories, God created a tangible, inescapable system that constantly reinforced their distinct identity. Every single meal—from a simple family supper to a great communal feast—became a theological statement. To choose a clean animal over an unclean one was to declare, "I am not an Egyptian, a Canaanite, or an Assyrian. I belong to Yahweh." The act of chewing and swallowing became a physical rehearsal of their covenant identity.

This separation was not rooted in a concept of intrinsic evil within the material creation. The unclean animals were still part of God's "very good" creation. Rather, their designated status as unclean for Israel's consumption was a symbolic boundary marker. It taught them that holiness requires distinction. It required them to exercise discernment in the most mundane areas of life. They could not simply eat whatever their neighbors ate. Their palates, their appetites, and their dinner tables were to be consecrated to God. This daily discipline of saying "no" to certain foods was a training ground for the much larger task of saying "no" to pagan idolatry, immoral practices, and the spiritual syncretism that constantly threatened to engulf them. Their diet was a fence around their identity, protecting them from assimilation and reminding them that they were a people set apart for a special purpose and relationship.

Beyond this overarching theme of separation, the laws were built upon deep **Symbolic Foundations** that taught moral and spiritual truths through physical categories. The system was a divinely instituted language of symbols, where the physical characteristics of animals represented spiritual realities.

The criteria for clean land animals, for instance, were that they must both chew the cud and have a cloven hoof (Leviticus 11:3). These are not random biological traits. **Chewing the cud** (*ma'aleh gerah*) is a powerful picture of meditation, of patiently and repeatedly processing what one has taken in. It symbolizes a life that ruminates on the Word of God, that does not merely hear it but inwardly digests it, extracting its full nutritional value for the soul. The **cloven hoof** (*mafreset parsah v'shosa'at shesa parsin*), a hoof completely divided, symbolizes a clear and distinct walk. It represents a life that is separated from the world, that walks on a distinct path, whose steps are clearly defined by God's law and not blurred by compromise. An animal that had one trait but not the other was unclean. This taught that true holiness requires both internal reflection on God's truth *and* an external lifestyle that is clearly distinct from the world. One without the other is incomplete and ultimately defiling.

Furthermore, the prohibition of certain creatures carried profound symbolic weight. **Predatory birds**—the eagle, the vulture, the hawk—were forbidden (Leviticus 11:13-19). These are birds of prey that live by violence and scavenging, that seize and tear. Their exclusion from Israel's diet symbolized a rejection of a predatory lifestyle, of gaining wealth or power through violence and exploitation of the weak. **Swarming creatures** and those that crawl on the earth were also largely forbidden (Leviticus 11:29-31, 41-44). These creatures often operated in the hidden, dark, and dusty places, symbolizing that which is secret, insidious, and low. God calls His people to a higher, more open way of living. Most famously, the **pig** was declared unclean (Leviticus 11:7), despite having a cloven hoof, because it does not chew the cud. The pig, in the ancient Near East, was also heavily associated with the religious rituals of Canaanite fertility cults. To abstain from pork was not only to avoid potential disease but to make a clear break from the idolatrous practices of the surrounding nations. It was a rejection of chaos, of spiritual promiscuity, and of that which appears righteous on the outside (the divided hoof) but lacks the internal meditation and transformation (chewing the cud).

Thus, the Levitical dietary code was a comprehensive spiritual training system. It taught discernment: just as they were to distinguish between the clean and the unclean animal, so they were to distinguish between righteousness and unrighteousness, between truth and falsehood. It taught order over chaos, life over death, and separation from all that would defile their unique covenant relationship with God. Every meal was a sermon, every menu a moral choice, and every hungry stomach an opportunity to affirm, "I am the LORD your God. Consecrate yourselves therefore, and be holy, for I am holy" (Leviticus 11:44).

5.6 The Lord's Table: The Culmination of Food Theology

Beloved, the entire biblical narrative of food—from the creational menu to the manna, from the post-diluvian concession to the Levitical code—finds its ultimate fulfillment, its transcendent meaning, and its radical transformation in the person and work of Jesus Christ. He does not merely add another chapter to the story; He is the climax to which every previous detail pointed. In Him, the theology of food is taken up, transfigured, and brought to its glorious consummation, reorienting all of human existence, including our eating and drinking, around His redemptive mission. This culminates at the Lord's Table, which becomes the new hermeneutic for understanding every other table.

We see this first in the startling ministry of **Jesus the Feasting Messiah.** In stark contrast to the ascetic John the Baptist, who came "eating no bread and drinking no wine" (Luke 7:33), Jesus entered into the full fabric of human social life, and He did so most often around a table. His first public miracle was not healing the sick but providing an abundance of fine wine for a wedding feast in Cana (John 2:1-11), sanctifying human joy and celebration. He was known derisively as "a glutton and a drunkard, a friend of tax collectors and sinners!" (Matthew 11:19). This was not a mark of dissipation but a deliberate theological strategy. By feasting with sinners—with Zacchaeus, with Matthew and his friends—Jesus was enacting the gospel of the kingdom. In the eyes of the religious leaders, sharing a meal with such people was defiling; it violated the Levitical codes of separation. But Jesus redefined purity not around external dietary codes, but around His own person and mission. He was the true Temple, the source of purity. His presence at the table sanctified the meal and the guests. He declared that it is not what goes into a person from outside that defiles them, but what comes out from the heart (Mark 7:15-23). In doing so, He shifted the entire locus of holiness from the plate to the person, from the food to the heart.

This leads directly to the epochal declaration that fundamentally altered the relationship between God's people and food: **The Declaration of All Foods Clean.** In Mark's account of the same teaching, the evangelist adds a stunning parenthetical commentary: "*Thus he declared all foods clean.*" (Mark 7:19). This was a theological earthquake. The entire complex system of *kashrut*, which had served for centuries as a boundary marker separating Israel from the nations, was now, in principle, rendered obsolete. This truth was dramatically confirmed and applied to the Apostle Peter in his vision in Acts 10. As Peter prayed, he saw a sheet lowered from heaven containing all kinds of animals, both clean and unclean according to Levitical law, and heard a voice saying, "*Rise, Peter; kill and eat.*" (Acts 10:13). When Peter objected on the grounds of his observance of the dietary laws, the voice replied, "*What God has made clean, do not call common.*" (Acts 10:15).

The immediate application was not merely dietary but missiological. The vision was about people, not just food. God was showing Peter that the gospel was breaking down the dividing wall between Jew and Gentile (Ephesians 2:14). The ceremonial separation was over. The focus of holiness was now internal. The purity laws, which had served as a "guardian" (Galatians 3:24) pointing toward the need for a clean heart, had found their fulfillment in Christ, who alone can cleanse the conscience. This does not mean that all food is now morally neutral or that gluttony is acceptable. Rather, it means that no food, in and of itself, is ceremonially unclean. The distinction is no longer between clean and unclean *foods*, but between thankful and idolatrous *hearts*. We are to receive all food with gratitude, as a good gift from God (1 Timothy 4:4-5), but we are to abstain from anything that causes a brother to stumble or is explicitly offered to idols in a way that constitutes participation in demonic worship (1 Corinthians 8, 10). The boundary has moved from the plate to the conscience, empowered by the Spirit.

This radical reorientation finds its most profound and concentrated expression in **The Eucharist as the True Food.** In the sixth chapter of John's Gospel, after the feeding of the five thousand, Jesus delivers a breathtaking discourse that forever changes the meaning of eating. He declares, "*I am the bread of life; whoever comes to me shall not hunger, and whoever believes* *in me shall never thirst.*" (John 6:35). He startles and offends His listeners by insisting, "*Truly, truly, I say to you, unless you eat the flesh of the Son of Man and drink his blood, you have no life in you.*" (John 6:53). Here, Jesus identifies Himself as the true Manna, the ultimate sustenance that the wilderness bread merely foreshadowed. He is the true sustenance that nourishes the soul to eternal life. Faith itself is portrayed as a kind of eating—a receiving, ingesting, and internalizing of Christ Himself.

This spiritual reality is then sacramentally enacted at the Last Supper. On the night He was betrayed, Jesus took bread, gave thanks, broke it, and gave it to His disciples, saying, "*Take; this is my body.*" And He took a cup, and when he had given thanks he gave it to them, and they all drank of it. And he said to them, "*This is my blood of the covenant, which is poured out for many.*" (Mark 14:22-24). In this simple yet infinitely profound meal, the entire theology of food is recapitulated and elevated. The bread and wine, common elements of daily sustenance, become the vehicles of the most extraordinary grace. They are the means by which we participate in the benefits of Christ's sacrificial death—the forgiveness of sins and the establishment of the New Covenant. The Eucharist is the true food and the true drink (1 Corinthians 10:16), the nourishment for our spiritual journey, the bond of our unity as the body of Christ, and the foretaste of the heavenly banquet.

Therefore, all eating is now re-oriented around this central, sacramental meal. Our daily bread, our family dinners, our celebratory feasts—all find their ultimate meaning in relation to the Lord's Table. Every meal becomes a potential echo of the Eucharist, a reminder to receive God's gifts with gratitude, to remember Christ's sacrifice, to foster community, and to look forward in hope. For the Lord's Supper itself points beyond itself to the final, glorious consummation: the **Marriage Supper of the Lamb** (Revelation 19:9). Our communion here is a pledge and a preview of that great eschatological feast, when the people of God from every tribe and nation will sit down at the table of the King in the New Creation, and the fellowship and joy we taste now in part will be ours in full. At that table, the story that began with the trees of Eden will find its perfect and eternal fulfillment.

5.7 Conclusion: Eating as an Act of Covenantal Gratitude

Beloved, as we draw this foundational chapter on the theology of food to its culmination, we are confronted with a truth that must forever change our relationship with every morsel we consume, every meal we share, and every hunger pang we feel. The comprehensive biblical witness, from Genesis to Revelation, performs a great work of transformation upon the act of eating. It is lifted from the realm of a mere, mundane biological function—a necessary refueling of the human machine—and is instilled with profound theological and covenantal significance. Eating is revealed to be nothing less than a **covenantal practice**, a sacred drama in which our entire relationship with God, His creation, and our neighbor is enacted, expressed, and nourished. The faithful steward, having journeyed through this divine narrative, can no longer approach the table with a mindless or purely utilitarian disposition. Instead, we come with reverence, gratitude, and discernment, for we now understand that what we eat, how we eat, and why we eat speaks volumes about our deepest understanding of God, His world, and our place within it.

At its most fundamental level, this theology transforms eating into an **act of receiving God's good gifts with gratitude.** The Apostle Paul's charge to his disciple Timothy rings with this foundational truth: "*For everything created by God is good, and nothing is to be rejected if it is received with thanksgiving, for it is made holy by the word of God and prayer.*" (1 Timothy 4:4-5). This is the Christian's basic posture at the table. Before the first bite is taken, the heart is to be oriented in thanksgiving. This gratitude is not a vague, general feeling of well-being; it is a specific, targeted acknowledgment of God as the ultimate Provider. It is the recognition that the earth is the Lord's and everything in it (Psalm 24:1). The succulent fruit, the nourishing grain, the sustaining protein—all of it is a gift from our Father's hand. This practice of gratitude is a powerful antidote to the entitlement and consumerism that characterizes our age. It sanctifies the meal, setting it apart from a transaction with the grocery store or a reward for our labor, and re-establishes it as a moment of communion with the Giver of every good and perfect gift (James 1:17). To eat without gratitude is to live as a practical atheist, enjoying the gifts while ignoring the Giver.

Furthermore, our daily meals become a **discipline of trusting His daily provision.** The lesson of the manna in the wilderness is eternally relevant. We are trained, through the rhythm of our hunger and its satisfaction, to rely not on our own stockpiles and strategic plans, but on the faithful, moment-by-moment care of our Heavenly Father. Just as Israel was commanded to gather only what they needed for the day, we are taught to pray, "Give us this day our daily bread" (Matthew 6:11). This trust militates against the twin sins of anxiety and greed. It frees us from the frantic worry about tomorrow's menu and from the hoarding impulse that seeks security in abundance rather than in God's character. Every meal becomes a quiet, tangible reaffirmation of our dependence. It is a declaration that we are not self-made or self-sustained, but are creatures, beloved and cared for by our Creator. This trust transforms our relationship with food from one of control to one of reception, from striving to resting in His faithful provision.

The table is also, by God's design, a primary **celebration of community.** From the covenant-making meals of the patriarchs to the table fellowship of Jesus with sinners, to the "breaking of bread" in the early church, food is the God-appointed catalyst for relationship. It is around the table that stories are shared, burdens are lifted, laughter rings out, and the body of Christ is knit together in love. The shared meal is a powerful enactment of *koinonia*—fellowship, partnership, and communion. It is a foretaste of the heavenly banquet, where people from every nation will sit down together. This is why the isolation of the modern meal—eating alone in the car, in front of a screen, or apart from family—is so spiritually and psychologically damaging. It severs the connection between physical nourishment and relational nourishment for which we were designed. The faithful steward, therefore, prioritizes and protects shared meals, understanding that to feed the body alone is insufficient; we must also feed the soul through the ministry of presence, conversation, and mutual care that happens when we break bread together.

Ultimately, our eating is a **participation in the redemptive narrative that finds its climax in Christ.** Every meal is a small, provisional echo of the Lord's Supper. The Eucharist stands at the center of Christian life as the meal that defines all other meals. In it, we see the ultimate purpose of food: to convey grace, to commemorate a sacrifice, to establish a covenant, and to point toward a future fulfillment. When we eat the bread and drink the cup, we are participating in the very life of Christ, receiving the benefits of His broken body and shed blood. This central sacrament reorients all of our eating. Our daily food now reminds us of the True Food that gives eternal life. Our physical hunger points us to our spiritual hunger for Christ. Our shared tables point us toward the Marriage Supper of the Lamb.

Therefore, the faithful steward approaches every table—from the fast-food counter to the Thanksgiving feast—with a theological consciousness. We eat with **discernment**, not in the Levitical sense of clean and unclean animals, but in the New Testament sense of considering what is loving, wise, and edifying (1 Corinthians 10:23-31). We ask not only "Is this food healthy?" but "Does this food honor God? Does my consumption reflect a heart of self-control and temperance? Could this food cause a brother or sister to stumble?" We eat with the awareness that our bodies are temples of the Holy Spirit, and thus our food choices are an act of stewardship over that sacred dwelling. What and how we eat reflects our understanding of God as the generous Provider, of creation as His good gift to be received with thanks and cared for with wisdom, and of community as the essential context for human flourishing. To eat is to worship. To eat is to trust. To eat is to commune. To eat is to hope. Let us then go to our tables as theologians, as priests, and as grateful children, and may every meal be a sacrament of God's enduring covenant love.

CHAPTER 06

Principles of Biblically-Informed Nutrition: Macronutrients and Micronutrients

6.1 Introduction: General Revelation in the Garden

Beloved, as we transition from the grand biblical narrative of food to the practical daily choices of what we place on our plates, we must navigate a crucial intersection of divine revelation. The Scriptures provide a profound theological framework for *why* we eat—establishing food as gift, provision, community-builder, and sacrament. Yet, when we seek specific, detailed guidance on *what* to eat for optimal temple maintenance, we do not find a divinely dictated meal plan or a list of approved superfoods in the book of Leviticus. The Bible is not a nutritional textbook; its purpose is far greater—to reveal God's redemptive plan and to shape us into the image of Christ. However, to conclude that God is therefore silent on the particulars of nutrition is to embrace a dangerous false dichotomy. The Lord speaks to us through two complementary books: the Book of Scripture (Special Revelation) and the Book of Nature (General Revelation). It is in the fruitful and prayerful integration of these two divinely authored volumes that we discover a robust, biblically-informed approach to nourishing the temple of our bodies.

The doctrine of **General Revelation** teaches us that the created order itself proclaims the glory, wisdom, and character of God. As the Psalmist declares, "*The heavens declare the glory of God, and the sky above proclaims his handiwork. Day to day pours out speech, and night to night reveals knowledge.*" (Psalm 19:1-2). This revelation is not salvific—it cannot tell us of the grace found in Jesus Christ—but it is profoundly true and instructive. The intricate design of a cell, the complex interplay of ecosystems, and the very biochemical pathways that govern our metabolism all bear the fingerprints of the Divine Artisan. The modern science of nutrition, for all its secular framing, is fundamentally the study of General Revelation as it pertains to the sustenance of physical life. It is the systematic exploration of the good and purposeful design God embedded in His creation for our flourishing.

Therefore, to ignore the findings of nutritional science under the pretext of relying solely on Scripture is not piety; it is a rejection of God's general wisdom revealed in the world He made. It is akin to refusing to study engineering while building a house because the Bible doesn't specify load-bearing formulas. We are called to be stewards, and faithful stewardship requires that we understand the nature of what we are stewarding. The science of macronutrients (proteins, carbohydrates, and fats) and micronutrients (vitamins and minerals) unveils the magnificent, God-wrought complexity of the "dust" from which we are formed and the "food" by which we are sustained. This knowledge is a gift of common grace, allowing us to understand the *how* of the Creator's sustaining power, even as Scripture reveals the *Who* and the *why*.

Our task, then, is to integrate this scientific knowledge from General Revelation with the unwavering theological truths of Special Revelation. We must build a framework for nutrition that is grounded in a **biblical theology of creation, stewardship, and wisdom.**

First, a **theology of creation** establishes the fundamental goodness and intentionality of the physical world. When God surveyed everything He had made and declared it "very good" (Genesis 1:31), He was affirming the goodness of the material structures that would later be identified as amino acids, glucose molecules, and fatty acids. The building blocks of life are not accidental; they are deliberately designed. This means that the study of nutrition is, at its heart, an exploration of God's good design. It is an act of tracing the wisdom with which He constructed reality. We can approach the science of food with a sense of wonder and reverence, knowing that we are peering into the mind of God as we learn how a vitamin catalyzes a crucial reaction or how a protein repairs tissue.

Second, a **theology of stewardship** provides the imperative for applying this knowledge. As we have firmly established, our bodies are not our own; they are temples of the Holy Spirit, bought with a price (1 Corinthians 6:19-20). Therefore, we are obligated to manage them wisely. This stewardship extends to our nutritional choices. To willfully consume a diet that we know, through the study of General Revelation, leads to inflammation, disease, and impaired function is to be a poor steward of a sacred trust. It is to ignore the clear operational manual that God has written into the fabric of His creation. Understanding macronutrients and micronutrients becomes part of our priestly duty to "work and keep" the garden of our own bodies (Genesis 2:15), using the best knowledge available to maintain the temple in a state that honors its Divine Resident.

Finally, a **theology of wisdom** guides the application of this knowledge with balance, discernment, and grace. The book of Proverbs is filled with exhortations to pursue wisdom and understanding. This biblical virtue is not merely spiritual; it is intensely practical, governing every area of life, including our health. A wise approach to nutrition avoids the twin pitfalls of legalistic obsession and negligent disregard. It recognizes that while nutritional science provides invaluable principles, it is not a source of salvific law. It understands that our physical bodies exist within a fallen world, and perfect health is not attainable this side of eternity. Wisdom therefore applies nutritional knowledge with flexibility, recognizing that there is no one-size-fits-all "God's diet," but rather, general principles of wholeness, variety, and moderation that align with the Creator's design. It prioritizes the state of the heart—gratitude, self-control, and love—over rigid adherence to any particular dietary regime.

In this chapter, we will therefore explore the major categories of nutrients—proteins, carbohydrates, fats, vitamins, and minerals—through this integrated lens. We will seek to understand the magnificent divine wisdom inherent in their design and function, and we will derive stewardship principles for how we can use this knowledge to honor God with our bodies, fuel ourselves for His service, and partake of His good gifts with gratitude and joy. Let us proceed as students of both books, seeking the mind of Christ as we learn to nourish the temples He has entrusted to our care.

6.2 A Theology of Macronutrients: Energy for Service

Beloved, as we delve into the practical outworking of a biblically-informed approach to nutrition, we begin with the foundational elements that God has designed to sustain our physical existence: the macronutrients. These are not merely biochemical categories; they are the very stuff of God's provision, the tangible expression of His sustaining grace. Carbohydrates, proteins, and fats—in their magnificent diversity and specific design—reflect the creative abundance of our God and reveal His intentionality in providing for our every need. To understand them is to appreciate the wisdom of the Creator; to steward them wisely is to honor Him with the energy and strength they provide for a life of service.

Let us first consider **Carbohydrates: The Sustaining Energy of Daily Bread.** In the biochemical economy of the body, carbohydrates are the primary and most efficient source of energy. They are broken down into glucose, the fuel that powers everything from the firing of our neurons to the contraction of our muscles. This physiological reality is imbued with deep theological significance. Carbohydrates, particularly in the form of grains, are the biblical symbol *par excellence* of God's sustaining, daily provision. When our Lord Jesus taught us to pray, "Give us this day our daily bread" (Matthew 6:11), He was anchoring our most basic physical need in a posture of dependence on our Heavenly Father. The "bread" here represents not a luxury, but the foundational sustenance for life. It is the energy for the daily labor, the fuel for the journey, the strength for the task at hand. In receiving our carbohydrates, we are receiving God's gracious provision for the faithful labor to which He has called us. They are the caloric manifestation of His covenant faithfulness, a daily reminder that He knows our needs and provides for them.

This leads us to a critical point of **Wisdom in Selection.** The Bible consistently presents a strong preference for whole, complex carbohydrates. The staple foods of the biblical world were whole grains like wheat and barley, legumes, and fruits—foods that provide a slow, steady release of energy due to their fiber and complex molecular structure. This stands in stark contrast to the refined sugars and flours that dominate the modern diet, which cause rapid spikes and crashes in blood sugar. This biblical pattern aligns perfectly with the wisdom revealed in the created order. A diet centered on whole, complex carbohydrates promotes sustained energy, stable moods, and long-term health. This mirrors a profound spiritual principle found in Proverbs: "*Have you found honey? Eat only what you need, lest you have your fill of it and vomit it.*" (Proverbs 25:16). The warning is against the pursuit of fleeting, intense pleasure that leads to sickness and disgust. Refined sugars offer a fleeting "honey-like" rush, but they lack substance and lead to metabolic dysfunction. The wisdom of God, revealed in both Scripture and nature, calls us to seek lasting, substantive nourishment—the "daily bread" that truly sustains—over the empty calories that offer a momentary thrill but ultimately fail to support a life of enduring service and vitality.

Next, we turn to **Proteins: The Building Blocks of Repair and Strength.** If carbohydrates are the fuel, proteins are the architects and construction crews of the body. They are essential for building and repairing tissues, producing enzymes and hormones, and maintaining the structural integrity of our entire physical frame. This function resonates powerfully with themes woven throughout the biblical narrative. The image of rebuilding, restoration, and strength is central to God's redemptive work. We see it in Nehemiah's determination to rebuild the broken walls of Jerusalem, a project that required immense physical and communal strength. We hear it in the promise of Isaiah: "*but they who wait for the LORD shall renew their strength; they shall mount up with wings like eagles; they shall run and not be weary; they shall walk and not faint.*" (Isaiah 40:31). This renewal is not merely spiritual; it encompasses the whole person, including the physical body that God designed for action and endurance.

Furthermore, the Apostle Paul uses this very imagery to describe the church: "*In him you also are being built together into a dwelling place for God by the Spirit.*" (Ephesians 2:22). As the body of Christ, we are a living temple, constantly being repaired, strengthened, and built up. The protein we consume is the physical substrate for this ongoing work of maintenance and repair in our individual bodies, which are the constituent parts of this larger spiritual temple. A body deficient in protein is like a building with crumbling mortar; it cannot withstand stress or fulfill its purpose.

This understanding leads to a principle of **Diverse Sources and Stewardship** in our protein intake. The biblical witness presents a remarkable variety of protein sources, from the lentil stew for which Esau traded his birthright (Genesis 25:34) to the fish eaten by the disciples (Luke 24:42-43) and the meat of the fatted calf prepared for the prodigal son (Luke 15:23). This diversity itself is a gift, reflecting God's creative abundance. A biblically-informed approach, therefore, encourages variety and moderation. It invites us to be mindful stewards, considering not only our personal health but the ethical and environmental costs associated with our choices. The intensive industrial farming of animals, for instance, often involves practices that conflict with the creational mandate of compassionate dominion and environmental care. Wisdom, then, may lead us to embrace a diversity of protein sources—including plant-based options like lentils and beans—practicing moderation in our consumption of animal products and seeking out sources that align with a theology of creation care and humane treatment. Our protein choices become a practical outworking of a stewardship that considers the whole creation, not just our own plate.

Finally, we come to **Fats: The Concentrated Blessing and Anointing.** In our macronutrient trio, fats are the most energy-dense, providing more than twice the calories per gram than carbohydrates or protein. They are vital for hormone production, brain health, nerve function, and the storage of energy for future use. In Scripture, fat is consistently associated with the best portion, abundance, and joy. Joseph promised his family the "fat of the land" in Egypt (Genesis 45:18). In the sacrificial system, the fat of the offering was reserved exclusively for God, signifying the richest and best part (Leviticus 3:16). Fat was a symbol of blessing, celebration, and divine favor. This symbolism aligns with its biological role: healthy fats are a concentrated source of blessing for the body, essential for cognitive function, hormonal balance, and long-term energy storage. They are not to be feared, but received with gratitude as part of God's good provision.

However, this reception must be tempered with **Discernment Between Fats.** The biblical dietary laws, while primarily ceremonial, often displayed a pre-scientific wisdom that separated healthier options from those associated with disease. The distinction between clean and unclean animals frequently separated lean, ruminant animals (like cattle and sheep) from scavengers (like pigs) that often have higher levels of saturated fats and are more prone to carrying disease. This principle encourages a preference for the kinds of fats God's creation provides most abundantly in their healthiest forms: primarily unsaturated fats. Consider olive oil, a staple of the biblical world. It is a source of healthy monounsaturated fats, and throughout Scripture, oil is a powerful symbol of the Holy Spirit's anointing, healing, and blessing (James 5:14, Psalm 23:5). Choosing such fats over the industrially-produced trans fats and excessive saturated fats that can contribute to arterial plaque is an act of wisdom. This plaque, which hardens and narrows the arteries, is a powerful physical picture of the spiritual condition warned against in Psalm 95: "*do not harden your hearts*" (Psalm 95:8). A diet that leads to hardened arteries is a physical manifestation of a failure to steward the temple well, while a diet rich in the "anointing" of healthy fats supports the fluidity, health, and vitality of the very system that carries life throughout the body.

6.3 A Theology of Micronutrients: The Subtle Wisdom of Wholeness

Beloved, if macronutrients are the bold, structural pillars and energetic fuel of the temple, then micronutrients are the sacred, often unseen, liturgy that makes the entire sanctuary function. Vitamins and minerals, though required by the body in minuscule amounts compared to their macro counterparts, are utterly essential for the intricate symphony of physiological processes that constitute life itself. Their existence testifies to God's breathtaking attention to detail—that the Creator who hung the stars in place also ordained that a few milligrams of a specific organic compound would be the difference between vitality and systemic collapse. In this, we see a profound spiritual principle: that small, consistent, and faithful practices are the building blocks of true wholeness. The neglect of these seemingly minor elements can lead to catastrophic failure, both in the body and in the soul.

Let us first contemplate **Vitamins: Organic Catalysts for Life Processes.** Vitamins are complex organic molecules that act primarily as coenzymes—substances that enable enzymes to perform their work. They are not used for energy or structure themselves, but they make the processes of energy production, repair, and growth possible. They are the indispensable facilitators, the unseen hands that guide the machinery of life.

This function provides a powerful metaphor for **The "Unseen" Work of the Spirit.** In the spiritual life, the Holy Spirit operates in a similarly catalytic and often imperceptible manner. The Apostle Paul describes the fruit of the Spirit as "love, joy, peace, patience, kindness, goodness, faithfulness, gentleness, self-control" (Galatians 5:22-23). We do not see the Spirit directly; we see the results of His inner working. He catalyzes the transformation of our character, enabling us to produce virtues that are impossible to manufacture through mere willpower. Just as a vitamin enables a specific chemical reaction, the Spirit enables us to love the unlovable, to have peace in turmoil, and to exercise self-control in the face of temptation. The work is His; the beautiful, functional outcome is manifested in our lives.

Furthermore, the consequence of vitamin deficiency offers a sobering physical parable. Consider **Scurvy**, a disease historically devastating to sailors, caused by a lack of Vitamin C. This single, small-molecule deficiency leads to a systemic failure: bleeding gums, loose teeth, wounds that fail to heal, anemia, and eventually death. The body is receiving ample calories from macronutrients, but the absence of this one, tiny catalyst unravels the entire system. This illustrates with devastating clarity how "small" spiritual disciplines are vital for our overall spiritual health. The consistent, daily intake of Scripture (Psalm 1:2), the practice of prayer (1 Thessalonians 5:17), and the habit of gratitude (1 Thessalonians 5:18) may seem like minor, private activities. Yet, a deficiency in these spiritual micronutrients can lead to a systemic failure of faith—a soul that cannot heal from wounds, that lacks the strength to stand against temptation, and that slowly succumbs to the spiritual anemia of despair. The health of the whole person depends on these seemingly small, faithful practices.

Beyond their catalytic role, many vitamins, particularly Antioxidants like Vitamins C and E, play a critical role in combating oxidative stress. "Free radicals" are unstable molecules that damage cells, contributing to aging and disease. Antioxidants neutralize these radicals, donating electrons to stabilize them and prevent cellular havoc. This is a powerful physical metaphor for **Spiritual Warfare.** Our souls are constantly bombarded by corrosive influences—the "fiery darts of the evil one" (Ephesians 6:16). These include lies that distort our identity in Christ, temptations that erode our character, and accusations that poison our relationship with God. We need spiritual antioxidants to combat this onslaught. The Word of God is this antioxidant. When we hide Scripture in our hearts, it actively counteracts the lies of the enemy, stabilizing our soul. Prayer is an antioxidant, creating a space of grace that neutralizes the toxins of anxiety and fear. The indwelling Holy Spirit is the ultimate antioxidant, protecting the very core of our being from the corrupting power of sin. A life deficient in these spiritual antioxidants will show the signs of corrosion: cynicism, bitterness, fear, and a hardened heart.

Turning from organic compounds to inorganic elements, we encounter **Minerals: The Foundational Structure and Regulation.** Minerals provide the literal and structural backbone of the body and regulate a vast array of physiological processes, from nerve transmission to fluid balance.

Consider first the minerals that provide **The Foundation of Bones: Calcium and Phosphorus.** These minerals form hydroxyapatite crystals, the rigid matrix that gives our skeleton its strength and resilience. Our bones are the internal framework upon which the entire body is built. This physical reality finds a direct parallel in the spiritual life. In His seminal Sermon on the Mount, Jesus concludes with the parable of the two builders. The wise man, He says, "*built his house on the rock. And the rain fell, and the floods came, and the winds blew and beat on that house, but it did not fall, because it had been founded on the rock.*" (Matthew 7:24-25). Jesus identifies this rock as His own words—His teachings and commands. A life built on the foundation of Christ's teachings possesses a structural integrity that can withstand the storms of life—suffering, loss, temptation, and doubt. The teachings of Christ are the spiritual calcium and phosphorus; they provide the non-negotiable, solid framework for a resilient and upright life. Without this foundation, the soul is like a house built on sand, vulnerable to complete collapse when the rains descend.

Then there is the profound symbolism of **The Blood and Atonement: Iron.** Iron is the central atom in the heme molecule of hemoglobin, the protein in red blood cells that binds to oxygen in the lungs and carries this life-giving element to every cell in the body. Without iron, there is no oxygen transport; without oxygen, there is no cellular respiration; without respiration, there is no life. This is a stunning biochemical echo of the foundational Levitical principle: "*For the life of the flesh is in the blood...*" (Leviticus 17:11). The physical life of the body is indeed in the blood, and iron is the crucial element that makes this life-sustaining function possible. This entire system points, with prophetic clarity, to the ultimate source of spiritual life. The blood of bulls and goats could never take away sin (Hebrews 10:4), but it was a God-ordained symbol pointing to the one, final, sufficient sacrifice. The blood of Jesus Christ, shed on the cross, is the true source of spiritual life and oxygen for the soul. Just as iron-based hemoglobin carries physical life to the body, the blood of Christ carries eternal life, forgiveness, and reconciliation to all who believe. Our physical need for iron-rich blood is a daily, embodied reminder of our ultimate need for the life that is found only in the atoning blood of the Lamb.

Finally, we must consider **Electrolytes and Spiritual Balance: Sodium and Potassium.** These minerals exist in a delicate balance across cell membranes, creating an electrical potential that is essential for nerve impulse transmission, muscle contraction, and fluid balance. An imbalance—too much sodium or too little potassium—disrupts this delicate system, leading to problems ranging from muscle cramps and brain fog to cardiac arrhythmia and death. The body requires a precise, dynamic equilibrium to function.

This physiological reality powerfully **mirrors the need for balance in the spiritual life.** A healthy Christian walk is not characterized by extremism but by a Spirit-wrought equilibrium. We see this in the need for **balanced doctrine**, holding God's sovereignty and human responsibility in tension, embracing both His justice and His mercy. We see it in the balance of **grace and truth**, which were perfectly embodied in Christ (John 1:14). An excess of grace without truth leads to license and moral compromise; an excess of truth without grace leads to legalism and harsh judgment. We see it in the rhythm of **work and rest**, modeled by God Himself in creation. An imbalance toward relentless work leads to burnout and idolatry of productivity; an imbalance toward rest without purposeful work leads to sloth and futility. The electrolytes of the spiritual life are the guiding wisdom and discernment of the Holy Spirit, who helps us maintain this godly balance in all things, ensuring that our spiritual "nerve impulses"—our decisions, our emotions, our actions—are transmitted faithfully and effectively for the glory of God.

6.4 The Principle of Variety and Seasonality

Beloved, as we continue to trace the fingerprints of the Divine Artisan upon the intricate design of nutrition, we encounter a principle so fundamental to God's character and so woven into the fabric of His creation that to miss it is to risk a profound impoverishment of both body and soul. This is the twin principle of **Variety and Seasonality**. It is not merely a suggestion for culinary interest or environmentalism; it is a theological statement embedded in the very soil from which our food springs. It reflects the boundless creativity of our God, His fatherly provision for our well-being, and His pedagogical method for teaching us trust and contentment.

Consider first the breathtaking **Diversity of Micronutrients**. Step into a well-stocked farmer's market and behold the visual symphony: the deep ruby of a beet, the vibrant orange of a carrot, the sunny yellow of a bell pepper, the rich purple of an eggplant, the verdant green of spinach. This explosion of color is not arbitrary; it is a direct manifestation of a vast array of phytonutrients—antioxidants, flavonoids, carotenoids—each with a unique and vital role in protecting the plant and, when we consume it, in protecting and nourishing our bodies. The sheer, extravagant variety of these compounds, found across thousands of different edible plants, reflects God's **creative delight and generosity.** He did not create one "super-plant" that contained every nutrient we need. Instead, He scattered His wisdom and goodness across a dazzling array of creations. The God who invented the thousands of unique species of beetles, the countless varieties of orchids, and the infinite palette of a sunset, is the same God who designed the nutritional ecosystem. This diversity is a reflection of His infinite, abundant nature. It is an invitation to explore, to savor, and to give thanks for a creativity that far surpasses mere utility.

This deliberate diversity serves a profound purpose for our stewardship. A diet limited to a few staple foods, no matter how nutritious, will inevitably lead to micronutrient gaps. We require the symphony, not a solo. To consume a wide variety of colorful fruits and vegetables is to participate in God's full provision. It is to acknowledge that our need for wholeness is met by His multifaceted wisdom. The modern, monotonous diet of highly processed foods, often based on a narrow band of ingredients like corn, wheat, and soy, is a rebellion against this creational principle. It represents a human attempt to simplify, control, and homogenize God's abundant diversity. It is a nutritional reductionism that says, "We know better than the Creator's design." In contrast, a varied, whole-foods diet is an act of humble reception. It is to confess that we need the full spectrum of His creative genius to be truly nourished. Every brightly colored berry and dark leafy green is a testament to God's specific, loving forethought for our intricate physiological needs.

This principle of variety is inextricably linked to the God-ordained rhythm of **Seasonality.** The created order does not offer all things at all times. The Psalmist declares, "*You have fixed all the boundaries of the earth; you have made summer and winter.*" (Psalm 74:17). This divine fixing of boundaries extends to the harvest. There is a time for the first tender asparagus of spring, a time for the sun-ripened tomatoes of high summer, a time for the hearty squash and apples of autumn, and a time for the stored root vegetables and preserved foods of winter. This cyclical provision is not a limitation but a pedagogy. It **teaches dependence on God's cycles and rhythms.**

In a globalized food economy, we can eat strawberries in December and squash in July. While this is a testament to human ingenuity, it can also foster a spirit of autonomy and entitlement, subtly eroding our sense of dependence on God's timing and provision. The seasonal diet, by contrast, forces us into a rhythm of anticipation, reception, and gratitude. We learn to look forward to the short, precious season of peaches, to receive them with joy when they arrive, and to release them without grasping when their time has passed. This is a spiritual discipline that trains the soul in contentment. It echoes the wisdom of Ecclesiastes that there is a season for everything (Ecclesiastes 3:1). It teaches us to receive what God gives, when He gives it, and to trust that what He withholds in one season, He will provide in another. This rhythm of waiting and receiving is a master class in faith, combating the instant-gratification mindset that characterizes both our modern food culture and our spiritual lives.

Furthermore, a seasonal diet naturally encourages a diet that is **local and fresh.** Food that is grown locally and consumed in its season is typically more nutrient-dense, having been allowed to ripen fully and consumed shortly after harvest. This stands in stark contrast to the highly processed diet, which is often reliant on foods that have been transported across continents, bred for durability rather than flavor or nutrition, and processed to extend shelf life at the cost of microbial life and nutrient integrity. The processed food paradigm is fundamentally at odds with the creational model. It seeks to transcend the limits of locality and season, creating a sterile, uniform, and perpetual now. But this rejection of creational limits comes at a cost—a cost to our health, to the environment, and to our taste of God's specific, timely goodness.

Therefore, the principle of variety and seasonality is far more than a nutritional strategy. It is a spiritual practice. It is a way of aligning our lives with the grain of the universe as God designed it. It cultivates gratitude for diversity, patience in waiting, contentment in receiving, and a humble recognition that we are creatures bound by time and place, dependent on a Creator whose provision is both perfectly timed and lavishly varied. To eat with the seasons is to join creation in its groaning and its glory; to embrace variety is to partake in the joyful, abundant generosity of the God who could have made the world gray and uniform, but instead chose to make it a feast for all the senses.

Beloved, we have now arrived at the critical juncture where our lofty theological framework must descend into the daily, tangible, and often messy reality of our kitchens, our grocery stores, and our dining tables. We have spoken of temples and stewardship, of *Shalom* and the Fall, of the sacredness of the physical. But what does it all *mean* when we stand before an open refrigerator, when we peruse the endless aisles of a supermarket, when we feel the pang of hunger and the temptation of convenience? It is here, in the seemingly mundane act of choosing what to eat, that our theology is proven genuine or revealed as a mere abstraction. And it is here that we must grasp a profound truth: the choice for nourishment is not, at its deepest level, a matter of biochemistry or caloric calculation. It is, and has always been, an act of wisdom.

We are not called to a new Pharisaism, a fresh set of dietary laws to be codified and policed, a return to the Levitical purity codes that Christ Himself fulfilled and transcended. To do so would be to miss the entire point of the gospel's liberating power. No, the apostolic declaration stands firm: "Everything is indeed clean" (Romans 14:20). The issue, therefore, is not one of ceremonial cleanness or uncleaness. The issue is one of *wisdom*. The question shifts from "Is this food permitted?" to the far more demanding and nuanced question: "Is this food *wise*?" Does this particular food, consumed in this particular quantity, at this particular time, contribute to the overall health, wholeness, and functional purpose of my entire being—body, soul, and spirit—as a vessel for God's glory? This is the question of the wise steward, the question that Paul himself implicitly asks when he declares, "'All things are lawful for me,' but not all things are helpful. 'All things are lawful for me,' but I will not be dominated by anything" (1 Corinthians 6:12).

So, what is wisdom? In the biblical consciousness, wisdom is not merely intellectual knowledge or street-smart cunning. It is the skill for living in right relationship with God, with others, with creation, and with oneself. It is the ability to see the world as God sees it and to order one's life in accordance with His created design and redemptive purposes. The book of Proverbs, that magnificent treasury of divine practicalities, personifies Wisdom as the master craftsman present with God at creation, rejoicing in His inhabited world and delighting in the children of man

(Proverbs 8:30-31). To live wisely, therefore, is to live in sync with the grain of the universe. It is to align our choices with the fundamental architecture of reality as established by the Divine Architect.

When we apply this to nutrition, we are called to a *theologically-informed wisdom*. This means we read the "book of nature"—the science of nutrition, the study of human physiology—in the light of the "book of Scripture." We operate from the foundational presupposition that all truth is God's truth. The discoveries of nutritional science about the benefits of phytonutrients in colorful vegetables, the importance of omega-3 fatty acids for neurological function, the detrimental effects of chronic inflammation driven by processed sugars and industrial seed oils—these are not secular threats to a spiritual worldview. They are glimpses into the intricate, God-woven wisdom embedded within His creation. They reveal the profound ways in which the physical systems of our bodies are designed to interact with the physical systems of the world He declared "very good." To ignore this general revelation is not piety; it is folly. It is like refusing to read the instruction manual for a complex and precious piece of equipment, in this case, the human body, the temple of the Holy Spirit.

This wisdom recognizes the profound **symbolism and practical logic God has embedded in His creation.** Consider the creational menu laid out in Genesis 1:29: "And God said, 'Behold, I have given you every plant yielding seed that is on the face of all the earth, and every tree with seed in its fruit. You shall have them for food.'" The original dietary design was plant-based, a fact rich with theological significance. It paints a picture of a peaceful, non-violent sustenance, where life is nourished without the taking of other conscious, *nephesh* life. It is a system of abundance and generosity, where food comes from the fruitful, seed-bearing multiplication of plants, a reflection of God's own creative and life-giving power. The very structure of a seed—containing within itself the potential for an entire plant, a whole cycle of life—is a miniature testament to God's design for self-perpetuating abundance. To eat from this system is to participate in a rhythm of life that is fundamentally generous and sustainable.

Even after the Fall and the post-diluvian concession of meat-eating (Genesis 9:3), the wisdom principle remains. The Levitical dietary laws, while serving a primary purpose of setting Israel apart as a holy nation, also contained a layer of creational wisdom. The animals deemed "clean" were often those that functioned as natural "filters" within the ecosystem—ruminants that ate plants, fish with scales that lived in clean water. The "unclean" animals were often scavengers and predators, creatures that consumed death and disease. The law was, in a sense, steering Israel towards a diet that was, by the standards of the ancient world, safer and more aligned with the original creational order. It was a tangible way of teaching a people to choose life over death, purity over corruption, in their most basic daily act. While we are not bound by these ceremonial laws, the underlying wisdom principle—the call to choose foods that promote life and wholeness over those that promote decay and disease—is an enduring creational norm.

A wise approach to nourishment, therefore, calls for a **balanced, varied, and predominantly whole-foods diet.** Let us unpack this with the reverence it deserves.

Balance is the rejection of every form of extremism and idolatry. It is the recognition that the body is a complex system requiring a symphony of nutrients, not a monotonous fanfare of a single macronutrient. The modern dietary landscape is a carnival of fads: the ultra-low-fat zealot, the keto evangelist, the carnivore purist. Each presents itself as the one true path to salvation, complete with its own set of dogmas and heresies. But wisdom stands in the center and says, "Beware of any teaching that reduces the glorious diversity of God's provision to a single, salvific principle." Balance understands that there is a time for carbohydrates, the body's primary fuel, especially from complex sources like whole grains and tubers that provide sustained energy. There is a time for proteins, the building blocks for repair and the synthesis of essential enzymes and neurotransmitters. There is a time for fats, crucial for hormonal production, brain health, and the absorption of fat-soluble vitamins. Wisdom does not demonize any of God's good gifts in their proper context and proportion. It is the application of the principle of *moderation* that the Greek philosophers glimpsed and that Scripture sanctifies (Philippians 4:5), recognizing that our freedom in Christ is not license for excess but the power to choose the good in its right measure.

Variety is the celebration of God's creative extravagance. Why did God create not one, but thousands of edible plant species, each with a unique flavor, texture, and nutritional profile? Why the staggering diversity of colors in fruits and vegetables—the deep purple of an eggplant, the vibrant orange of a carrot, the rich green of kale, the fiery red of a pepper? This is not divine redundancy. It is a deliberate, artistic declaration of abundance and a profound biochemical strategy. Different colored plants contain different families of phytonutrients—antioxidants, flavonoids, carotenoids—that serve specific protective roles within the body. To eat a monotonous diet, even of "healthy" foods, is to ignore this creational symphony. It is to willfully blind ourselves to the rainbow of God's provision. Variety is a hedge against nutritional deficiencies and a way of ensuring a broad spectrum of these protective compounds. It is an act of humility, acknowledging that no single food created by God contains all the wisdom we need; we need the entire chorus of creation to sing the song of health into our cells. Every time we choose a new vegetable, an unfamiliar whole grain, or a different legume, we are participating in the exploration of God's generous creativity. We are, in a small way, fulfilling the cultural mandate to "subdue" the earth by discovering and gratefully receiving its hidden treasures.

Predominantly Whole Foods is the choice for integrity over disintegration. A whole food is one that is as close to its natural, God-created state as possible. It is a potato from the ground, not a potato chip from a factory. It is an apple from a tree, not an apple-flavored fruit roll-up. It is a piece of wild-caught salmon, not a fish stick composed of minced remnants and fillers. The wisdom here is profound. In its whole state, a food exists as a complex nutritional matrix, a package where fiber slows the absorption of sugars, where vitamins and minerals work in synergy, where thousands of micronutrients interact in ways that modern science is only beginning to comprehend. When we process a food—when we strip away the bran and germ from a wheat berry to make white flour, when we press olives to extract the oil and discard the pulp, when we concentrate the sugar from a cane stalk and discard the molasses—we are engaging in a form of nutritional hubris. We are presuming that we understand the food better than its Creator. We are taking a divinely designed complex system and reducing it to a few isolated components, arrogantly believing we have captured its "essence." The result is almost always a degraded, imbalanced, and inflammatory substance that the body struggles to recognize and process wisely. The epidemic of metabolic disease in the modern world is, in large part, a testament to our foolish departure from the wisdom of whole foods. To choose the whole food is to choose God's original, integrated design. It is a vote for creational integrity, a decision to consume things as they were intended to be consumed, in the form that reflects the holistic wisdom of the Maker.

This entire framework of wise nourishment is fundamentally an act of **honoring God as the source of all good gifts.** When we pause before a meal, whether in a formal prayer of gratitude or a moment of conscious reflection, we are performing a critical theological act. We are reorienting ourselves. We are breaking the spell of the modern illusion that food originates in a supermarket, that it is a product of human industry alone. We are acknowledging the ultimate source: the soil, the sun, the rain, the intricate biological processes—all sustained by the faithful, providential hand of the Creator. We are recognizing that every good gift and every perfect gift is from above, coming down from the Father of lights (James 1:17). This gratitude is the spiritual engine that drives wise stewardship. It transforms eating from a selfish act of consumption into a reciprocal act of worship. We receive the gift with thanks, and we honor the Giver by using the gift in the manner for which it was intended. To do otherwise—to mindlessly consume God's good gifts in ways that lead to gluttony, sloth, and disease—is a form of ingratitude. It is like receiving a beautifully crafted, hand-made tool from a master artisan and using it to dig a ditch until it breaks, with no regard for its design or the generosity of its giver.

Finally, and most practically, this wise nourishment is about **maintaining the temple for effective service and witness.** We must never forget the *telos*, the ultimate purpose, of this stewardship. It is not for our own self-aggrandizement, for the sculpting of a body that is an end in itself. That is the idolatry of the therapeutic-utilitarian impulse. No, the purpose is missional. A body that is well-nourished with a balanced, varied, and whole-foods diet is a body that has stable energy, a clear mind, a resilient immune system, and a balanced mood. It is a body that is prepared. Prepared for what? Prepared for the long, demanding work of love. Prepared to have the emotional and physical stamina to listen to a friend in crisis. Prepared to have the mental clarity to study the Word of God and to discern His will. Prepared to have the vitality to serve in the nursery, to volunteer in the community, to go on a mission trip. Prepared to endure suffering with greater fortitude. A body fueled by the slow-burning, nutrient-dense energy of whole foods is like a well-built furnace, providing steady heat for the long haul. A body jerked around by the sugar spikes and crashes of a processed-food diet is like a sputtering engine, unreliable and prone to breakdown just when it is needed most.

When we choose wisdom on our plates, we are making a declarative statement about what we believe this body is for. We are saying, "This body is not my own; it was bought with a price. Therefore, I will glorify God in my body" (1 Corinthians 6:19-20). I will glorify Him by ensuring it is a well-maintained, fully functioning, resilient instrument for the work of His kingdom. I will not allow it to be dulled by sloth, clouded by poor fuel, or weakened by self-indulgence. My eating is an act of preparation for the good works God has prepared for me to walk in. It is a daily, tangible way of loving the Lord my God with all my strength, and of positioning myself to love my neighbor as myself. In a world that is sick, tired, and anxious, a Christian whose life is marked by the peaceful, disciplined, and joyful wisdom of good nourishment is a walking apologetic. They testify, without saying a word, that the gospel is powerful enough to save the soul *and* to sanctify the daily habit of eating, and that the Lordship of Christ extends even to the choice between a whole apple and a processed apple pastry. This is the high and holy calling of nutritional stewardship: to eat, drink, and do all to the glory of God.

CHAPTER 07

Dietary Laws, Purity, and Contemporary Application: From Leviticus to Modern Health

7.1 Introduction: From Ceremonial Code to Wisdom Principle

Beloved, we now approach one of the most complex and often misunderstood intersections of our faith and our physical existence: the Levitical dietary laws. For the modern Christian, standing as we do on this side of Calvary and the empty tomb, the pages of Leviticus 11 and Deuteronomy 14 can feel like a foreign country, with customs and regulations that seem not only strange but utterly irrelevant to our daily lives. We read of clean and unclean animals, of creatures that chew the cud and part the hoof, of fish with fins and scales, and we are tempted to turn the page quickly, dismissing it as an archaic relic of a bygone era, a system of purity that was nailed to the cross of Christ. And in one very real sense, we would be correct to do so.

The New Testament is unequivocal: the ceremonial law, as a binding legal code that defines one's standing before God and membership in the covenant community of Israel, has been fulfilled, transcended, and rendered obsolete in the person and work of Jesus the Messiah.

Yet, I must pose a question to you, a question that probes deeper than a simple binary of "obey" or "ignore." What if God, in His infinite wisdom, was doing more than one thing at once? What if the dietary laws, while serving a primary and historically-contingent *ceremonial* function, were also encoding within their symbolic architecture a deeper, creational wisdom—a wisdom that speaks to the very nature of holiness, to the fundamental structure of a world He called "very good," and to the principles of discernment that are as vital today as they were at the foot of Mount Sinai? To dismiss these laws as *only* ceremonial is to risk throwing away a master key to understanding God's heart for how His holy people are to navigate a fallen world in their most fundamental, daily acts.

The central thesis we must grapple with in this chapter is this: **The Levitical dietary laws, in their original context, served a primary function of establishing Israel as a distinct, holy nation, set apart for Yahweh. This ceremonial and national boundary has been definitively dismantled in Christ. However, the underlying principles embedded within these laws—principles of separation from death and decay, of intentional discernment in consumption, and of a reverence for the sacredness of life—these are not abrogated. They are, rather, transfigured. They are lifted from the plane of national-ethnic identity and planted deep within the soil of the individual believer's heart, providing a**

vital, enduring framework for a contemporary theology of nutritional ethics.

To understand this, we must first immerse ourselves in the world of ancient Israel and grasp the primary, non-negotiable purpose of these laws. God's declaration to His people is thundering in its clarity: "You shall be holy, for I the LORD your God am holy" (Leviticus 19:2). This call to holiness (*qadosh*) means, fundamentally, to be set apart, distinct, consecrated for a specific purpose. The dietary laws were a primary, tangible, daily mechanism for enacting this holiness. In a world teeming with surrounding nations—Canaanites, Egyptians, Hittites—each with their own gods and their own culinary practices, what you ate was a powerful marker of identity. To refuse the pig, the shellfish, the vulture, was to make a statement with every single meal: "We are not like them. We belong to Yahweh." It was a constant, physical reminder that they were a "kingdom of priests and a holy nation" (Exodus 19:6). The boundary of the plate became the boundary of the covenant community.

This system of clean and unclean was part of a larger symbolic world, a comprehensive "symbolic universe" designed to teach Israel the fundamental categories of life and death, order and chaos, purity and defilement. The creatures deemed "clean" often embodied integrity and conformity to their created order. The land animal that both chews the cud *and* has a parted hoof is a picture of consistency, of a creature that fully embodies its creational category as a ruminant. It is a symbol of an integrated life. The clean fish, with its fins and scales, is one that can navigate the chaotic, unseen depths of the waters with purpose and direction, its scales forming a protective boundary between it and the murky environment. These animals were permitted to be brought into the sphere of the holy—into the body of the Israelite, and even onto the altar of God.

Conversely, the "unclean" animals often represented a blurring of boundaries or an association with death. The pig, for instance, has a parted hoof but does not chew the cud. It possesses the external sign of cleanness but lacks the internal reality. It is a creature of dissonance. The shellfish—lobsters, shrimp, crabs—are scavengers of the sea floor, bottom-feeders that thrive on detritus and decay. The birds of prey and the carrion-eaters—the vulture, the eagle, the raven—are creatures whose very existence is predicated on death. They consume that which is already dead and decaying. To ingest these animals was, symbolically, to ingest death itself. It was to introduce the chaos and defilement of the fallen world directly into the sanctuary of the body, which was meant to be a microcosm of the holy camp of Israel.

Therefore, the primary function of these laws was pedagogical and boundary-forming. They were a divine object lesson, teaching a fundamentally spiritual reality—the need for separation from the spiritual death and moral chaos of the pagan world—through the most visceral and daily of physical acts: eating. They were a form of "training wheels" for holiness, a tangible curriculum for a people learning what it meant to be distinct unto the Lord.

But then came the Christ-event. And with it, a seismic shift that redefined the very meaning of purity, holiness, and the people of God. The pivotal moment is recorded for us in Acts 10, in the vision given to the Apostle Peter. He sees a great sheet lowered from heaven, filled with all manner of animals, reptiles, and birds—a veritable catalogue of the unclean from Leviticus 11.

And a voice commands him, "Rise, Peter; kill and eat." Peter, the good Jew, recoils: "By no means, Lord; for I have never eaten anything that is common or unclean." And the voice responds with a declaration that shatters the old paradigm: "What God has made clean, do not call common" (Acts 10:13-15).

This was not merely a lesson about dietary liberalism. This was a theological earthquake. The vision was immediately interpreted as pertaining to people—to the Gentiles, who were previously considered "unclean" and outside the covenant community. The death and resurrection of Jesus had broken down the dividing wall of hostility (Ephesians 2:14). The Holy Spirit was poured out on all flesh. The criteria for membership in the people of God was no longer ethnic descent and adherence to the ceremonial law, but faith in the Messiah and regeneration by the Spirit. The external, national boundary was dissolved. This truth is sealed by the apostolic decree in Jerusalem (Acts 15) and expounded theologically by Paul, who states unequivocally, "I know and am persuaded in the Lord Jesus that nothing is unclean in itself" (Romans 14:14), and "Everything created by God is good, and nothing is to be rejected if it is received with thanksgiving, for it is made holy by the word of God and prayer" (1 Timothy 4:4-5). So, is that the end of the story? Do we simply close Leviticus 11 and move on, free to eat anything and everything without a second thought? To do so would be to ignore the profound wisdom principle that undergirds the ceremonial code. While the *specific regulations* are fulfilled and set aside, the *creational logic and theological principles* they embody are not. They are, I contend, transfigured. They are lifted from the external, national plane and internalized, spiritualized, and universalized for the New Covenant believer, who is indwelt by the Holy Spirit and called to work out their salvation with fear and trembling.

The principle of **separation from death and decay** remains. For the Old Testament saint, this meant not eating the scavenger that fed on carcasses. For the New Testament saint, this principle is elevated. We are called to separate ourselves not from certain animals, but from spiritual death and moral decay in all its forms. "Therefore go out from their midst," says the Lord, "and be separate from them... and touch no unclean thing" (2 Corinthians 6:17). This "unclean thing" is now clearly defined as idolatry, sexual immorality, greed, slander, and malice (Ephesians 4:25-32; 1 Corinthians 6:9-11). But does this principle have no physical application? If our bodies are temples of the Holy Spirit, is there not a wisdom in choosing foods that are life-giving, that promote vitality and health, over those that are known to promote disease, inflammation, and cellular decay—the very physical analogues of death? To choose, by wisdom, to nourish our bodies with foods that are "clean" in the sense of being pure, wholesome, and health-promoting, is a modern application of this ancient principle. It is a way of physically enacting our separation from the corruption of the Fall, of defying the entropy that sin introduced into creation.

The principle of **intentional discernment** remains. The Israelite had to stop and think, to examine the animal: Does it chew the cud? Does it have a parted hoof? This forced a pause, a moment of discernment before consumption. It was a divinely mandated interruption to mindless appetite. For the New Covenant believer, the call to discernment is even more profound. We are to "test everything; hold fast what is good" (1 Thessalonians 5:21). We are to have our powers of discernment "trained by constant practice to distinguish good from evil" (Hebrews 5:14). This applies directly to our consumption. In a world of industrialized food systems, of hyper-palatable processed creations designed to hijack our brain's reward centers, the call to intentional discernment is critical. We are to pause and ask not, "Is this ceremonially unclean?" but the more demanding, wisdom-oriented questions: "What is the source of this food? How was it produced? What is its effect on the temple of my body? Does its consumption align with the principles of love for neighbor and care for creation?" This is the Levitical pause, baptized into Christ and applied to the globalized food economy of the 21st century.

The principle of **reverence for life** remains. The original creational ideal was a plant-based diet (Genesis 1:29). The permission to eat meat came after the Fall and the Flood (Genesis 9:3), a concession in a world now marred by violence and death. The Levitical laws, with their intricate rules for slaughter and the prohibition against consuming blood ("for the life of the flesh is in the blood," Leviticus 17:11), instilled a profound reverence for the life that was being taken. It was a graphic reminder that sustenance came at a cost, that life was sacred. For the Christian, this principle is not abolished. While we are permitted to eat all meats, we are not permitted to be cavalier about the life that was given for our nourishment. This principle can lead us to ethical considerations about animal welfare, about the horrors of industrial factory farming, which stands in stark contrast to the reverence for life modeled in the Levitical code. It calls us to receive our meat with gratitude and a sober recognition of the cost, a recognition that finds its ultimate fulfillment in the One who said, "This is my body, broken for you," and "This is my blood of the covenant, poured out for many." Our eating of any food, but especially of meat, can become a sacrament of remembrance, pointing us to the ultimate sacrifice that truly gives life.

Therefore, the journey from the ceremonial code of Leviticus to a contemporary Christian nutritional ethic is not a journey of abolition but of transfiguration. We move from a holiness defined by external, national boundaries to a holiness defined by the internal, transformative work of the Spirit, which then expresses itself in all of life, including our physical consumption. We move from a law that said, "Do not eat the unclean creature," to a wisdom that asks, "How can my eating, in this complex modern world, best reflect the holy, life-affirming, discerning character of the God I serve?" The dietary laws are not our rulebook, but they are a profound repository of divine wisdom, teaching us that even something as mundane as our diet is a theatre for working out our salvation, a daily opportunity to choose life, to practice discernment, and to honor the God of life with our whole being, body and spirit.

7.2 The Original Purpose of the Kashrut Laws

Beloved, to truly grasp the significance of the Levitical dietary code, we must journey back in our imaginations to the base of Mount Sinai, to a people freshly liberated from the polytheistic, animistic stew of Egyptian culture. We must see the *Kashrut* laws not as an arbitrary list of divine prohibitions, but as a multifaceted and brilliant pastoral strategy, a divine curriculum designed to shape a slave people into a holy nation. The purpose of these laws was not monolithic but rather threefold, weaving together threads of ceremonial identity, practical health, and profound moral and spiritual formation into a single, cohesive tapestry of holiness. To isolate one thread from the others is to unravel the entire garment. We must, therefore, examine each strand with care, understanding how they worked in concert to accomplish Yahweh's ultimate goal: a people set apart for Himself.

First, and most fundamentally, we confront the **Ceremonial Purpose: The Sanctification of the Common Life.** The thundering declaration of Exodus 19:5-6 forms the indispensable foundation: "Now therefore, if you will indeed obey my voice and keep my covenant, you shall be my treasured possession among all peoples, for all the earth is mine; and you shall be to me a kingdom of priests and a holy nation." This identity as a *goy qadosh*—a holy nation—was not a vague spiritual ideal; it was to be embodied in the concrete, daily reality of their corporate life. Holiness (*qedushah*) in the Hebrew mind was not primarily a moral quality but a state of being—a state of being set apart, consecrated, designated for a specific purpose. The entire Levitical system was an elaborate mechanism for creating and maintaining this state of separation, and the dietary laws were its most intimate and frequent application.

Imagine the life of an Israelite family. Several times a day, at every single meal, they were faced with a choice. The pig was a common feature in the diets of their Canaanite neighbors. The shellfish were abundant in the coastal regions. To refuse these foods was to make a tangible, costly, and continuous declaration of allegiance. It was to say, with every bite, "We are not Egyptians. We are not Canaanites. We are not like the other nations. We belong to Yahweh." The dinner table became a miniature sanctuary, the plate an altar, where their distinct identity was rehearsed and reinforced. This was not about earning salvation through dietary rigor; it was about living out the salvation already granted by Yahweh's gracious deliverance from Egypt. It was an act of covenantal fidelity.

This ceremonial function created a tangible boundary that protected the community from assimilation. Intermarriage and shared meals were the primary social mechanisms by which ancient cultures syncretized and lost their distinct identity. By making shared table fellowship with pagans impossible on the basis of their divinely mandated diet, God erected a protective fence around the spiritual and genetic integrity of the messianic line. The *Kashrut* laws were, in effect, a divinely instituted immigration and customs policy for the soul of the nation. They were a constant, physical reminder that they were guests in Yahweh's land, living under Yahweh's rule, and that their most basic appetites were to be submitted to His sovereign will. The holiness of God was not to be confined to the Tabernacle; it was to permeate the camp, and indeed, the very bodies of the people. Their physical digestion was to be a mirror of their spiritual discernment—taking in that which was clean, holy, and life-giving, and rejecting that which was unclean, common, and associated with death.

Secondly, we must consider the **Health and Hygienic Purpose: The Divine Wisdom of Preventive Care.** While it is a reductionist error to claim that the dietary laws were *merely* about health, it is an act of theological negligence to ignore the profound layer of creational wisdom and protective care embedded within them. We worship the God who created the human body with intricate, functional systems, and who understands its vulnerabilities in a fallen world. The *Kashrut* laws can be seen, in part, as a divinely provided public health code, a form of preventive medicine that protected Israel from many of the health scourges that afflicted their contemporaries.

Let us take the most famous example: the prohibition of the pig (Leviticus 11:7-8). In the ancient Near East, the pig was a creature of the filth, a scavenger that would consume anything, including its own waste and carrion. It is a hot-blooded mammal, but unlike ruminants, it does not sweat through its skin, leading to a concentration of toxins in its fat and tissues. The pig is a primary host for a plethora of parasites and pathogens, most notably the trichinella spiralis parasite, which causes trichinosis—a debilitating and potentially fatal disease. The life cycle of this parasite is broken precisely by the act of cooking, a technology that was not universally reliable or practiced in the ancient world. By simply prohibiting the consumption of pork altogether, God provided a foolproof safeguard against this and other porcine-borne illnesses.

Similarly, consider the laws regarding shellfish (Leviticus 11:9-12). Shellfish such as shrimp, lobster, crabs, and clams are bottom-feeders and filter-feeders. They function as the ocean's sanitation system, consuming decaying organic matter, bacteria, and toxins from the water. In doing so, they bio-accumulate these harmful substances, including viruses like hepatitis, and pathogens like vibrio vulnificus, which can cause severe gastrointestinal distress and even fatal sepsis. In an era without refrigeration or modern understanding of foodborne illness, the simple prohibition of all creatures without fins and scales was a breathtakingly effective public health measure. It protected the community from "red tide" poisoning and a host of other maritime health hazards.

The prohibition of consuming blood (Leviticus 17:10-14) is another prime example. The blood is the medium of life, but in a fallen world, it is also the medium for a host of blood-borne diseases. Furthermore, the intricate rules of slaughter (*shechita*), which involved a rapid, deep incision across the throat to ensure rapid and complete drainage of blood, produced meat that was not only ritually clean but also far less likely to harbor bacteria

that thrive in pooled blood. This method, though its primary purpose was theological ("for the life of the flesh is in the blood"), resulted in a safer, more sanitary meat product.
We must be careful not to interpret this through a purely modern, scientific lens. The Israelites were not given a microbiology textbook. They were given divine commands. Yet, in His gracious providence, the God who designed the human body also prescribed a way of eating that would protect and preserve it. This reveals a God who cares not only for the state of our souls but also for the well-being of our physical frames. The health benefits were a secondary, yet very real, manifestation of God's creational wisdom and His fatherly care for His people. It was a form of common grace, a protective hedge that allowed the nation to flourish in a world teeming with unseen physical dangers, just as the ceremonial law protected them from unseen spiritual dangers.

Finally, and perhaps most profoundly for our ongoing spiritual formation, we encounter the **Symbolic and Moral Purpose: The Pedagogy of Discernment.** The *Kashrut* laws were a divine training program for the conscience, a daily drill in the fundamental spiritual discipline of distinguishing between the holy and the common, the clean and the unclean. God was not merely creating a people with a peculiar diet; He was forging a people with a peculiar way of *seeing* the world. He was inculcating a habit of mind, a default setting of discernment that would equip them to make righteous judgments in every area of life.

The system itself was a masterpiece of symbolic theology. The criteria for land animals—that they must both part the hoof *and* chew the cud—is rich with meaning. An animal that only does one but not the other is incomplete, a symbol of hypocrisy or a lack of integration. The pig, with its parted hoof but its failure to chew the cud, became the archetype of the unclean—a creature that presents an external sign of order but lacks the internal reality of reflection and rumination. It is the symbol of the person who has the outward form of godliness but denies its power (2 Timothy 3:5). To reject the pig was to reject a life of dissonance between appearance and reality.

The clean animals, the ruminants, by contrast, embody a principle of reflection. They consume the raw material of the field, then they retreat, they rest, and they patiently, methodically chew the cud, breaking it down, extracting its nourishment, and integrating it into their very being. This is a powerful picture of the spiritual life. We are to consume the Word of God, but we are not to swallow it whole and move on. We are to meditate upon it day and night (Psalm 1:2), to "chew the cud," to ruminate on its truths until they are fully digested and become the source of our spiritual strength and vitality. The dietary law, therefore, was a constant, physical parable about the proper way to feed one's soul.

Furthermore, the fundamental categories of "clean" and "unclean" were teaching Israel to associate with life and shun death. The clean animals were typically herbivores, pasture-fed, and associated with life and vitality. The unclean animals were very often scavengers, predators, and carrion-eaters—creatures whose existence was intimately tied to death, decay, and the consumption of that which was already dead. To eat a vulture or a crab was to ingest the principle of death itself. It was to symbolically unite oneself with the realm of chaos and corruption that stands opposed to the God of life and order. This symbolic association was meant to train their moral and spiritual instincts. If they were to be so careful about what they allowed into their physical bodies, how much more careful should they be about what they allowed into their minds, their hearts, and their community? The habit of discernment practiced at the dinner table was meant to translate into discernment in relationships, in business, in worship, and in ethics. It was a school for the soul, teaching them that not everything that is permissible is beneficial, and that holiness requires the constant, conscious exercise of choice, rejecting the toxic and embracing the pure. This symbolic pedagogy was, in essence, preparing the heart of Israel for the ethical teachings of the prophets and the ultimate call of the gospel to be living sacrifices, holy and acceptable to God.

7.3 The New Testament Fulfillment and Abrogation

Beloved, we now arrive at the great theological pivot point, the moment in the divine drama where the shadows cast by the Levitical law are flooded with the brilliant, clarifying light of the Gospel of Jesus Christ. To remain within the confines of the old covenant's dietary boundaries is to stand in the courtyard after the veil of the temple has been torn in two from top to bottom. It is to cling to the scaffolding after the magnificent edifice of God's redemptive purpose has been completed and unveiled. The New Testament does not merely suggest a relaxation of the *Kashrut* laws; it proclaims, with apostolic authority and Christological finality, their decisive fulfillment and abrogation as a binding ceremonial code. This was not a minor adjustment to the law, but a cosmic shift in the very definition of purity, holiness, and the people of God. To understand this is to be liberated from a yoke that neither we nor our fathers were able to bear, and to be launched into the vast, Spirit-led freedom of the new creation.

The first and foundational crack in the edifice of the old dietary code appears not from Paul or Peter, but from the lips of the Lord Jesus Himself. The confrontation is recorded in Mark 7, a pivotal moment where the theological legalism of the Pharisees collides with the revolutionary authority of the Incarnate Word. The Pharisees, ever vigilant in their externalism, notice that some of Jesus' disciples are eating with hands that are "defiled," that is, unwashed according to the tradition of the elders. This was not about hygiene, but about ritual purity, a complex web of man-made regulations that had encrusted the simpler Torah commands. Jesus seizes this moment to deliver a thunderous blow to the entire system of external purity that had come to define Second Temple Judaism. He declares, "Hear me, all of you, and understand: There is nothing outside a person that by going into him can defile him, but the things that come out of a person are what defile him" (Mark 7:14-15).

The disciples, still thinking within the old paradigm, are perplexed. So, privately, Jesus explains the parable, and in doing so, He annuls the Levitical food laws with a stunning, parenthetical declaration from the Gospel writer himself. "Do you not see that whatever goes into a person from outside cannot defile him, since it enters not his heart but his stomach, and is expelled?" And then comes the earth-shattering clause, a theological bombshell placed in the text by the inspired evangelist: "(*Thus he declared all foods clean*)" (Mark 7:18-19). The Greek here is breathtaking in its finality: *katharizōn panta ta brōmata*. It is a present active participle, indicating a declarative act with ongoing, permanent effect. "Making all foods clean." In this one divine pronouncement, the entire complex system of clean and unclean animals, the very foundation of Israel's daily dietary holiness, is rendered null and void. The source of defilement, Jesus insists, is not external, entering the body from without. Defilement is internal, moral, and spiritual, bubbling up from the fallen human heart—from evil thoughts, sexual immorality, theft, murder, adultery, coveting, wickedness, deceit, sensuality, envy, slander, pride, foolishness (Mark 7:21-22). The locus of the battle for holiness has shifted decisively from the plate to the heart. The temple to be purified is no longer primarily the physical body of Israel as a nation, but the inner person of every individual believer, Jew and Gentile alike, who would be indwelt by the Holy Spirit.

This theological foundation laid by Christ finds its dramatic, historical outworking in the event that forever changed the complexion of the church: the conversion of the Gentile Cornelius, as orchestrated through the Apostle Peter. The account in Acts 10 is one of the most carefully narrated in the entire New Testament, a sign of its supreme importance. Peter, the devout Jew, goes up on the housetop to pray and falls into a trance. He sees heaven opened and something like a great sheet descending, lowered by its four corners to the earth. Inside are all kinds of animals and reptiles and birds—a veritable catalogue of the unclean from Leviticus 11. And a voice commands him, "Rise, Peter; kill and eat."

Peter's response is instinctive, conditioned by a lifetime of Levitical observance and a deep, pious desire to remain undefiled: "By no means, Lord; for I have never eaten anything that is common or unclean" (Acts 10:14). The voice responds a second time with a declaration that shatters Peter's theological world: "What God has made clean, do not call common" (Acts 10:15). This happens not once, but three times, a divine emphasis that echoes Peter's own triple denial and later restoration, underscoring the completeness of this new revelation.

We must not miss the profound Christological symbolism here. The vision occurs while Peter is praying, and he is hungry. His physical hunger mirrors the spiritual hunger of the nations, represented by the Gentile Cornelius who is simultaneously seeking God. The sheet is lowered from *heaven*, signifying that this new reality is a divine initiative, not a human innovation. The contents of the sheet—the amalgamation of clean and unclean beasts—represent the entire human race, Jew and Gentile, now to be united in one new people. The command to "kill and eat" is a command to annul the old separations, to embrace what God has now declared acceptable. Peter's initial refusal represents the stubborn resistance of the early Jewish church to this radical inclusion. The triple repetition signifies the thoroughness with which God intends to dismantle this barrier. The vision is not, in its primary intent, about dietary law; it is about people. It is about the gospel breaking out of its ethnic prison. But the mechanism for this breakthrough is the abolition of the food laws that had served as the primary social barrier between Jew and Gentile. You cannot have table fellowship with a Gentile if you believe his food, and by extension his very household, is unclean. By declaring all foods clean, God was tearing down the middle wall of partition, creating in Himself one new humanity in place of the two (Ephesians 2:14-15). The abrogation of the dietary code was the necessary precondition for the Gentile mission and the catholicity of the Church.

This newfound freedom, however, was not without its pastoral challenges and potential for misuse, which brings us to the profound and nuanced treatment of the issue by the Apostle Paul, particularly in his letter to the Romans. The church in Rome was a mixed community of Jewish and Gentile believers, each with different backgrounds, consciences, and levels of understanding regarding their freedom in Christ. Some, the "strong" in faith (often Gentiles), fully embraced the truth that all foods were clean and felt free to eat anything, including meat that had been sacrificed to idols and then sold in the marketplace. Others, the "weak" in faith (often Jewish believers or Gentile God-fearers steeped in synagogue culture), were scandalized by this. Their consciences, trained for years under the Levitical system or in a context that abhorred idolatry, were defiled by the mere thought of eating such food.

Into this tense situation, Paul brings a masterful pastoral theology that upholds the objective truth of freedom while prioritizing the higher law of love. In Romans 14, he makes the objective, theological reality perfectly clear: "I know and am persuaded in the Lord Jesus that nothing is unclean in itself" (Romans 14:14). This is a direct, apostolic reaffirmation of the declarations of Jesus and the vision given to Peter. The ceremonial law is abrogated. The kingdom of God, Paul insists, is not a matter of food and drink—it is not about external observances and dietary regulations. The essence of the Kingdom is "righteousness and peace and joy in the Holy Spirit" (Romans 14:17).

But then Paul introduces the crucial, governing principle for the exercise of this freedom: love for one's brother. "But if your brother is grieved by what you eat, you are no longer walking in love. By what you eat, do not destroy the one for whom Christ died" (Romans 14:15). Here, the focus shifts entirely from the objective status of the *food* to the subjective state of the *brother's conscience* and the ultimate imperative of *love*. For Paul, to flaunt one's freedom in a way that causes a weaker brother to stumble—to act against his own conscience—is to sin against Christ Himself. This is the great transfiguration of the principle of holiness. Under the old covenant, holiness was maintained by separating from unclean *things*. Under the new covenant, holiness is expressed by lovingly limiting one's freedom for the sake of unclean *consciences*, for the building up of the body of Christ. The call to discernment, once focused on the hoof and the cud, is now focused on the needs and vulnerabilities of one's neighbor. The goal is no longer personal, ceremonial purity, but corporate, relational *Shalom*. Therefore, while the dietary law as a binding code is abrogated, its underlying spirit—the spirit of discernment, of setting oneself apart for the good of God's people and His purposes—is taken up, internalized, and elevated to a new and more demanding plane. The Christian is free to eat all things, but they are bound by the law of love to sometimes *choose* not to, for the sake of the gospel and the unity of the church. This is the true fulfillment of the law: not its letter, but its heart, which is love for God and love for neighbor, now empowered by the indwelling Spirit of Christ.

7.4 Translating Principles for a Modern Context: A Hermeneutic of Wisdom

Beloved, having established the decisive New Testament abrogation of the Levitical dietary code as a binding ceremonial law, we now face the most pressing pastoral and practical question: what do we *do* with Leviticus now? Do we simply close the book, consigning its intricate statutes to the archives of a bygone dispensation? Such an approach, while theologically correct in one sense, would be an act of profound spiritual poverty. It would be like discovering that the detailed architectural plans for the Tabernacle are no longer the blueprint for our church buildings, and therefore concluding that the principles of sacred space, of intentionality in worship, and of God's glorious presence dwelling among His people are also irrelevant. No, the ceremonial specifics have been fulfilled in Christ, but the eternal wisdom principles embedded within them have not been annulled; they have been unleashed, universalized, and transfigured. They await a new application, a contemporary incarnation, guided not by the letter of the law but by the Spirit of wisdom. We are called to exercise a *hermeneutic of wisdom*, a Spirit-led discernment that extracts the enduring creational and theological logic from its ancient, culturally-bound shell and translates it into a faithful witness in the complex global food system of the twenty-first century.

The first and most vital principle to be translated is **The Principle of Discernment: From External Ordinance to Internal Wisdom.** The entire Levitical system was a divine pedagogy in discernment. It forced the Israelite, multiple times a day, to pause and ask a fundamental question: "Is this clean? Is this acceptable? Does this conform to the Lord's standard?" This was a spiritual discipline of the highest order, training the people of God to see the world through a theological lens, to make choices based on divine revelation rather than mere appetite or cultural convention. The specific object of that discernment—the cloven hoof, the ruminant stomach—has passed away. But the *habit of mind*, the *discipline of holy discernment*, is an eternal principle. It is the very essence of what it means to have a renewed mind, to prove what is the good and acceptable and perfect will of God (Romans 12:2).

So, what is the modern landscape upon which this Spirit-trained discernment must now operate? It is no longer a simple binary of pig versus lamb. It is a dizzyingly complex, globalized, and industrialized food system. The Christian is therefore called to exercise discernment not about *kinds* of animals in the old sense, but about *qualities* and *systems* of food production. We must learn to ask a new set of wisdom-oriented questions, questions that apply the ancient principle of "testing everything" (1 Thessalonians 5:21) to our modern plates.

We are called to discern between the **processed and the whole**. Where the Levitical law separated the clean from the unclean based on the animal's nature and habits, we are now called to separate foods based on their degree of creational integrity. A whole food—a vegetable from the garden, a piece of fruit from a tree, a grain in its kernel—is a direct gift from God's creation, bearing the imprint of His creative wisdom. A highly processed food—a sugar-laced cereal, a chemically-preserved snack, a lab-created meat analogue—is a product of human ingenuity that has often been stripped of its God-given nutritional matrix and laden with substances that the human body, the temple, was not designed to process in quantity. Discernment here asks: Does this food resemble something that God made, or is it primarily a product of a factory? Does it promote vitality and health, or does it contribute to inflammation and disease? This is not a new legalism of "thou shalt not eat processed food," but a call to wise stewardship that prioritizes the foods that best nourish the temple.

We are called to discern between the **nutrient-dense and the calorie-dense**. The Levitical laws guided Israel toward foods that were, in their context, generally safer and more healthful. Our discernment must now operate in an environment of caloric abundance but nutritional poverty. Many modern foods are "empty calories"—providing energy but few of the essential vitamins, minerals, and phytonutrients required for the body's intricate systems to function optimally. To choose nutrient-dense foods—leafy greens, colorful vegetables, lean proteins, healthy fats—is to honor the temple's need for high-quality building materials. It is a practical outworking of the understanding that our bodies are not our own, and that we are called to offer them as living sacrifices, which requires that they be in the best possible state of repair for service.

Furthermore, we are called to discern the **source and system of our food**. This is perhaps the most sophisticated application of the principle. The ancient Israelite knew the shepherd; we are often separated from our food by a vast, opaque industrial complex. Discernment now asks: What is the environmental impact of this food's production? Does it come from a system that exploits workers or treats God's creation with contempt? Was this animal raised in a manner that respects its God-given nature, or was it subjected to the cruel confinements of a factory farm? By choosing locally-sourced, sustainably-grown, and ethically-produced foods when possible and prudent, we are enacting a modern form of holiness. We are separating ourselves not from unclean *things*, but from unclean *systems*—systems of exploitation, environmental degradation, and cruelty that stand in opposition to the creational *Shalom* God intends. Our grocery choices become a tangible, albeit small, vote for a world that more closely reflects the justice, mercy, and goodness of the Kingdom of God.

The second principle demanding translation is **The Principle of Separation: From National Identity to Counter-Cultural Witness.** The *Kashrut* laws were the primary mechanism for making Israel's holiness visible. They were a nation set apart by what they refused to eat. For the New Covenant believer, the call to be "a chosen race, a royal priesthood, a holy nation, a people for his own possession" (1 Peter 2:9) remains. But our separation is no longer ethnic or national; it is moral, spiritual, and cultural. We are to be in the world but not of it. And in a culture characterized by a deeply disordered relationship with food, our "separation" must manifest as a radical departure from the prevailing norms.

The modern food culture is, in many ways, a culture of death disguised as a culture of consumption. It is a culture of **gluttony**, which is not merely about quantity but about a heart-attitude that seeks comfort, fulfillment, and identity in food rather than in God. It is a culture of **addiction**, engineered by food scientists to create products that override our God-given satiety signals, keeping us coming back for more of that which does not satisfy. It is a culture of **haste and distraction**, where meals are consumed alone, in front of screens, rather than in community as a sacred time of fellowship and gratitude. It is a culture that promotes **health-destroying patterns**, contributing to an epidemic of obesity, diabetes, and heart disease that cripples the Church's capacity for mission and service.

Therefore, the modern application of the principle of separation is a conscious, deliberate disengagement from this spirit of the age. It is a commitment to **temperance and self-control** (a fruit of the Spirit, Galatians 5:22-23) in the face of relentless temptation. It is a separation from the mindless consumption that surrounds us. It can manifest as the discipline of fasting, not as a public display of piety, but as a tangible declaration that "man shall not live by bread alone, but by every word that comes from the mouth of God" (Matthew 4:4). It manifests as the intentional choice to eat in a way that promotes health and vitality, thereby separating oneself from the chronic fatigue and disease that plague our society. It manifests as the commitment to shared, leisurely meals with family and community, creating a small pocket of *Shalom* that stands in stark contrast to the fragmented, hurried nature of modern life. In this way, our eating habits become a silent but powerful sermon. They proclaim that our appetites are under the lordship of Christ, that our bodies are destined for resurrection, and that our true sustenance comes not from the bread that perishes, but from the Bread of Life.

Finally, we come to the profound and challenging principle of **Reverence for Life: From Ritual Prohibition to Ethical Stewardship.** The Levitical prohibition against consuming blood was rooted in the foundational theological declaration: "For the life of the flesh is in the blood, and I have given it for you on the altar to make atonement for your souls, for it is the blood that makes atonement by the life" (Leviticus 17:11). This law instilled a sacred reverence for the life that was being taken to provide sustenance. It was a graphic, daily reminder that their nourishment came at a cost, that a life had been given so that they might live.

In Christ, the ultimate atonement has been made by His own blood. The ritual prohibition is thus fulfilled. However, the underlying principle—the sacredness of the life that God has created—is not only upheld but intensified. We live in a creational order that, though groaning, still bears the marks of its Maker. The dominion granted to humanity in Genesis 1:28 was not a license for tyrannical exploitation, but a call to a priestly stewardship, to "work and keep" the garden (Genesis 2:15). The Proverbs remind us that "the righteous care for the needs of their animals, but the kindest acts of the wicked are cruel" (Proverbs 12:10).

A modern application of this reverence for life, therefore, leads us into a thoughtful **ethical consideration of animal welfare**. This is not a call for universal vegetarianism, but a call to reject a posture of indifference toward the suffering of creatures under our dominion. The horrors of the industrial concentrated animal feeding operation (CAFO), where intelligent, feeling creatures are subjected to lives of intense confinement, mutilation, and stress, stand in direct opposition to the principle of reverent stewardship. To choose, when possible, to source meat, eggs, and dairy from farms that allow animals to express their God-given behaviors—to root, to peck, to graze, to socialize—is a modern act of "reverence for life." It is a tangible way of acknowledging that these creatures are part of God's good creation, and that our dominion over them is accountable dominion, to be exercised with wisdom and compassion, not with brutalizing efficiency.

This principle also cultivates a general **posture of gratitude rather than entitlement**. The Israelite, forbidden from eating the blood, was constantly reminded to be grateful for the life given. We, in our abundance, are prone to a spirit of entitlement, thoughtlessly consuming without a moment of reflection on the sun, soil, rain, and life that was expended for our meal. To pause and give thanks before eating is not a empty formality; it is a radical act of reorientation. It is to acknowledge the Giver in the gift. It is to recognize the chain of life that sustains our own, and to receive our food as a sacred trust. This posture of gratitude naturally extends to a care for the entire created order—the soil, the water, the air—that God has entrusted to our care. Our eating, when guided by this transfigured principle, becomes an act of worship that encompasses all of creation, a small but significant participation in the redemption of all things, groaning as they wait for the revealing of the sons of God.

7.5 Case Studies in Contemporary Application

Beloved, having established the hermeneutic of wisdom by which we translate the enduring principles of the Levitical code into our modern context, we must now descend from the heights of theory into the practical, often muddy, terrain of daily decision-making. It is one thing to affirm the principles of discernment, separation, and reverence for life in the abstract; it is quite another to apply them to the specific, concrete choices that confront us in the grocery aisle, at the restaurant, and in our own kitchens. To that end, let us engage in a series of case studies, examining particular foods and dietary trends through the lens of our transfigured theological framework. In doing so, we will see that the ancient wisdom of the *Kashrut* does not provide us with a simple list of "eat this, not that," but rather equips us with a discerning mind and a sanctified conscience to navigate the complexities of our time with gospel-informed wisdom.

Let us begin with what is perhaps the most iconic of the biblically prohibited foods: **The Pork Question.** For the first-century Jewish believer, the declaration that all foods were clean was most shockingly demonstrated by the inclusion of pork. The pig was the quintessential unclean animal, the very symbol of everything from which a devout Jew separated themselves. For us today, the theological question is settled: pork is ceremonially clean. There is no sin in eating a properly cooked pork chop, a slice of bacon, or a ham sandwich. The blood of Christ and the voice from heaven to Peter have secured our freedom.

However, to move immediately from "it is permitted" to "therefore I will consume it without reflection" is to abandon the hermeneutic of wisdom for a libertine folly. The principle of discernment calls us to ask a deeper set of questions. We are to pursue not only what is permissible, but what is *beneficial* (1 Corinthians 6:12), and indeed, what is "most excellent" (1 Corinthians 12:31) in our stewardship of the temple. When we apply this lens to modern pork, a more nuanced picture emerges.

First, we must consider **modern production methods.** The pig of the ancient world was a forager, a creature of the forest and the field. The pig of the modern industrial system is often a creature of the CAFO—the Concentrated Animal Feeding Operation. Confined in crowded, stressful conditions, these animals are routinely administered antibiotics to prevent the diseases that flourish in such environments, and they are fed a diet of genetically modified corn and soy, which alters the fatty acid profile of their meat. The result is a product that is different from its pre-modern counterpart, often higher in pro-inflammatory omega-6 fatty acids and potentially containing traces of pharmaceuticals. Discernment here does not declare the food "unclean," but it may lead one to ask: Does this production system align with the principle of reverence for life and care for creation? If one has access to pork from a farm that raises pigs on pasture, allowing them to express their God-given rooting behaviors, the wisdom calculation may shift.

Second, we must consider its **nutritional profile.** Pork, particularly in its processed forms like bacon, sausage, and ham, is often high in saturated fat and sodium. In a context of caloric abundance and sedentary lifestyles, the consistent, high consumption of such foods has been linked through general revelation (i.e., nutritional science) to an increased risk of cardiovascular disease and other health complications. Therefore, the wisdom principle does not say, "You must not eat pork." It says, "As a wise steward of the temple, how does this food, in this quantity and frequency, fit into a pattern of eating that promotes vitality and longevity for the service of the Kingdom?" For some, the answer may be to enjoy it on occasion as part of a balanced diet. For others, particularly those with specific health concerns, the most excellent way of stewardship may be to abstain. The key is that the decision is made not out of a slavish fear of an old law, but out of a loving, intelligent desire to glorify God in one's body. The pork is clean, but my consumption of it must be governed by the higher law of love for the Lord and for the temple He has entrusted to me.

Our second case study takes us from the land to the sea, to consider **Seafood and Environmental Toxins.** The Levitical law prohibited all aquatic creatures that lacked both fins and scales, a category that includes shellfish like shrimp, lobster, crab, and clams, as well as bottom-feeders like catfish. The ancient wisdom, as we have seen, likely provided a health safeguard against pathogens and toxins that these filter-feeders and scavengers could accumulate. Today, we have the tools of modern science to detect dangers that the ancient Israelite could not see, and the principle of discernment demands that we pay attention.

The Levitical prohibition finds a striking modern parallel in public health advisories regarding **mercury in certain fish.** Large, predatory fish such as shark, swordfish, king mackerel, and tilefish sit at the top of the aquatic food chain. Over their long lifespans, they bio-accumulate mercury, a potent neurotoxin, from the polluted waters of a fallen creation. For a pregnant woman, a nursing mother, or a young child, the consumption of these fish poses a significant risk to neurological development. Here, the creational wisdom principle screams through the data of modern science. The discerning Christian, seeking to steward the temple—especially the vulnerable temples of the young—will exercise caution. They will choose lower-mercury options like salmon, sardines, or cod. This is not because a swordfish is ceremonially unclean, but because the principle of discernment, now illuminated by general revelation, leads us to make choices that protect life and health.

Similarly, the concern about **toxins in shellfish** from polluted waters is a direct modern analogue to the ancient risk. Shellfish are still nature's filtration systems, and in waters contaminated with industrial runoff, sewage, or "red tide" algae blooms, they can concentrate dangerous bacteria, viruses, and biotoxins. A government warning to avoid harvesting shellfish from a certain bay is not a revival of the Mosaic code; it is a contemporary application of the same creational wisdom that underpinned it. The discerning believer will heed such warnings, not out of legalism, but out of a wise desire to avoid introducing known toxins into the temple of the Holy Spirit. In this case, the object of discernment has shifted from the *kind* of creature to the *environment* from which it comes, but the underlying principle of separating oneself from potential harm remains powerfully relevant.

Finally, let us consider the phenomenon of modern dietary patterns, specifically the **"Paleo" and "Whole30" Diets.** These are secular, popular dietary frameworks that have gained widespread followings. They are not Christian programs, and they often come with their own ideological baggage, sometimes promoting a quasi-worship of a romanticized "natural" state. However, from our perspective of theological wisdom, we can evaluate them not as new laws to be slavishly followed, but as potential, albeit imperfect, *applications* of the wisdom principles we have been discussing.

At their core, these diets advocate for the elimination of highly processed foods, refined sugars, industrial seed oils, and often, certain grains and legumes. They encourage the consumption of whole, nutrient-dense foods: meats, fish, eggs, vegetables, fruits, and healthy fats. When we look at this through our hermeneutic of wisdom, we see a striking resonance. The call to eliminate processed foods is a modern enactment of the principle of **discernment**, choosing the whole over the fragmented, the creational over the industrial. It is a deliberate separation from the very food systems that contribute to inflammation and disease. This aligns with our call to be "set apart" from the health-destroying patterns of the prevailing food culture.

Furthermore, the emphasis on high-quality animal proteins, when coupled with an concern for sourcing from pasture-raised and grass-fed operations, can be seen as an application of the principle of **reverence for life**. It is a move away from supporting the cruel and degrading systems of the CAFO and toward a model of animal husbandry that more closely respects the creature's God-given nature. It is a dietary pattern that, perhaps unintentionally, points toward a more holistic and creational vision of *Shalom*.

However, the Christian must engage with these diets with continued discernment. We must reject any underlying narrative that suggests we can achieve salvation or perfect health through our dietary choices—a form of works-righteousness. We must be wary of a spirit of elitism or judgmentalism toward those who do not eat this way. And we must remember that "the earth is the Lord's and the fullness thereof" (1 Corinthians 10:26), and that all foods are to be received with thanksgiving. These diets can be excellent *tools* for a season of resetting one's health and cultivating better habits, but they must not become a new source of identity or a new law that binds the conscience. They are a potential application of wisdom, not a replacement for the gospel of grace. In them, we see the world groping, often unknowingly, for the very principles of creational order and holistic well-being that God revealed to His people millennia ago, and which find their true fulfillment and motive power in the redemption and lordship of Jesus Christ.

7.6 The Danger of a New Legalism

Beloved, as we have journeyed together through the profound wisdom of the Levitical dietary code and its transfigured application for the New Covenant believer, we now stand at the most treacherous precipice in our entire exploration. It is the point where a holy and noble pursuit—the wise stewardship of our bodies as temples—can, with a subtle and almost imperceptible shift in the heart, curdle into one of the most insidious and soul-crippling perversions of the gospel: the creation of a new Christian dietary legalism. The enemy of our souls is a master alchemist, and his favorite trick is to take the pure gold of God's truth and transform it into the leaden weight of human self-righteousness. He will gladly have us eating kale and quinoa if, in the process, we begin to look down upon our brother who, in faith and gratitude, enjoys a cheeseburger. This is a danger we must name, confront, and vigilantly guard against, for it strikes at the very heart of the freedom for which Christ has set us free.

The apostolic warning thunders across the centuries, as urgent today as it was in the first-century church of Corinth and Rome. The Apostle Paul, navigating the minefield of food sacrificed to idols, lays down a foundational principle of Christian liberty that must govern all our nutritional discernment: "Eat whatever is sold in the meat market without raising any question on the ground of conscience. For 'the earth is the Lord's, and the fullness thereof.' If one of the unbelievers invites you to dinner and you are disposed to go, eat whatever is set before you without raising any question on the ground of conscience" (1 Corinthians 10:25-27). Do you hear the glorious, liberating scope of this command? The believer is to move through the world with a fundamental posture of freedom and gratitude. The food itself is neutralized as a source of spiritual defilement. The world is God's, and everything in it is a potential gift from His hand to be received with thanksgiving. To approach the marketplace or a dinner table with a spirit of anxious scrutiny, with a checklist of approved and forbidden items born of our own new tradition, is to functionally deny the all-encompassing lordship of Christ and the comprehensive cleansing He has achieved. It is to rebuild the very walls of separation that He died to tear down.

This new legalism can manifest in a multitude of subtle and deadly forms. The most obvious is the sin of **pride and spiritual elitism.** This occurs when our successful adherence to a particular dietary pattern—be it Paleo, Vegan, Keto, or a self-styled "Biblical" diet—becomes a source of identity and a metric of our spiritual maturity. We begin to look at our plate and then at our brother's plate, and in that glance, a Pharisee is born. We thank God that we are not like other men—gluttonous, undiscerning, defiling their temples with processed junk. This is the very essence of the prayer of the Pharisee in Luke 18:11-12. It is a soul-destroying poison that replaces dependence on grace with confidence in the flesh. It mistakes physical discipline for spiritual sanctification. The fruit of the Spirit is not a gluten-free diet; it is love, joy, peace, patience, kindness, goodness, faithfulness, gentleness, and self-control (Galatians 5:22-23). A person can have a perfectly "clean" diet and be filled with bitterness, judgment, and pride, thereby defiling the temple far more grievously than any non-organic strawberry ever could. Closely linked to pride is the sin of **judgment.** Paul's exhortation in Romans 14 is the definitive pastoral treatment of this peril. "Do not, for the sake of food, destroy the work of God. Everything is indeed clean, but it is wrong for anyone to make another stumble by what he eats. It is good not to eat meat or drink wine or do anything that causes your brother to stumble" (Romans 14:20-21). The "weak" brother here is not weak in willpower, but weak in faith. His conscience, perhaps newly converted from a background of paganism or still informed by a Jewish upbringing, is troubled by certain foods. If you, the "strong" believer, flaunt your freedom in front of him, you are not demonstrating your superior spirituality; you are committing an act of violence against his conscience. You are tempting him to act against his own faith, which is sin for him (Romans 14:23). To cause a brother for whom Christ died to stumble over something as secondary as dietary preference is a catastrophic failure of love. It elevates personal freedom to an idol and sacrifices the unity of the body of Christ on its altar. The truly strong believer is not the one who eats everything with a defiant air, but the one who lovingly, joyfully, and voluntarily restricts their freedom for the sake of the weaker conscience next to them. The goal is not to see how much we can get away with, but how much love we can demonstrate.

This new legalism also creates a **stumbling block for the gospel itself** to a watching world. When the world looks at the church and sees not a community of joyful, free, and grateful people, but a collection of anxious, rule-bound, and judgmental dietary sects, the gospel is obscured. The message becomes, "Come to Jesus and learn the 17 rules for righteous eating," rather than, "Come to Jesus and find rest for your souls." We must never forget that the Kingdom of God is not a matter of eating and drinking, but of righteousness, peace, and joy in the Holy Spirit (Romans 14:17). If our primary witness to our neighbors is about our superior food choices rather than the surpassing worth of Christ, we have become salt that has lost its savor, fit only to be thrown out and trampled underfoot.

Furthermore, this legalistic spirit fundamentally **misunderstands the nature of the temple and its defilement.** Under the Old Covenant, defilement was primarily external and symbolic. A person could be rendered ceremonially unclean by touching a dead body, by a bodily discharge, or by eating the wrong food. This system was a pedagogical tool pointing to the true, internal defilement of sin. In Christ, the locus of defilement has been decisively relocated. As Jesus Himself declared, "It is not what goes into the mouth that defiles a person, but what comes out of the mouth; this defiles a person... For out of the heart come evil thoughts, murder, adultery, sexual immorality, theft, false witness, slander. These are what defile a person" (Matthew 15:11, 19-20). To re-erect a system of external dietary purity is to reverse the work of the gospel. It is to suggest that the temple can be defiled by a non-organic apple or a piece of conventional bread, thereby shifting the focus from the idolatry, malice, and pride in our hearts to the contents of our refrigerator. This is a demonic distraction, a theological regression that pulls us back into the elementary principles of the world from which we have been freed.

So how do we navigate this tension? How do we passionately pursue wise, holistic stewardship of our bodies without falling into the snare of a new law? The answer lies in constantly

recentering ourselves on the **motivating virtues of the Christian life: faith, love, and gratitude.**
Our eating must be an act of **faith.** It is faith that receives all food as a gift from the Father's hand. It is faith that trusts the Holy Spirit to guide us into wise choices without giving us a specific, universal list. It is faith that believes our acceptance before God is based solely on the righteousness of Christ, not on the purity of our diet. We make our choices from a position of secure sonship, not anxious striving.

Our eating must be governed by **love.** Love for God, which desires to honor Him with our whole being, including our bodies. Love for our neighbor, which refuses to let our food become a source of offense or a barrier to fellowship. Love for the body of Christ, which prioritizes unity and the building up of one another over our personal dietary preferences. The most excellent way of 1 Corinthians 13 must be the sauce that seasons every meal.

And finally, our eating must be saturated with **gratitude.** The act of giving thanks before a meal is a theological act of the highest importance. It is the moment we reorient our hearts, acknowledging the ultimate source of our provision and sanctifying the meal by the word of God and prayer (1 Timothy 4:4-5). A grateful heart is the surest antidote to a judgmental and prideful spirit. It is impossible to simultaneously look down on another's plate and be truly thankful for your own.

The goal, therefore, is not a new code, but the cultivation of a wise, temperate, and loving character. It is to be a person who can, with the same heart of faith and gratitude, enjoy a celebratory feast at a wedding and also practice the discipline of fasting. It is to be a person whose freedom is so secure in Christ that they are utterly liberated to limit that freedom for the sake of others. It is to understand that while the temple is sacred, the final and definitive sacrifice for its cleansing has already been made, and no dietary regimen can add one cubit to our standing before a holy God. We are to steward the temple with wisdom, but we are to worship the God of the temple with a spirit of glorious, unshackled freedom.

7.7 Conclusion: Freedom Informed by Wisdom

Beloved, as we draw our extensive exploration of the Levitical dietary code to its culmination, we find ourselves standing not before a list of regulations to be reinstated, but before a profound and enduring vision of what it means to live as God's holy people in a created, yet fallen, world. The journey through Leviticus has not been an archaeological dig to unearth obsolete artifacts, but a mining operation to extract the timeless veins of divine wisdom that run through its very bedrock. The specific statutes concerning the cloven hoof and the ruminant stomach, the fins and the scales, have passed away, their ceremonial and national purpose gloriously fulfilled in the cross of Christ and the birth of the universal Church. But the spiritual and creational logic that animated them—the principles of holiness, discernment, and reverence for life—these have not been abrogated. They have been transfigured, liberated from their national-ethnic confines, and unleashed upon the whole people of God, to be applied by the Spirit-led conscience in the bewildering complexity of the modern world. The Levitical law thus guides the contemporary Christian not as a binding statute, but as a masterclass in divine wisdom, a sacred curriculum teaching us to approach the most fundamental act of eating with the mind of Christ.

This wisdom begins with a fundamental reorientation of our entire perspective on consumption. The Levitical code forced intentionality. It mandated a pause, a moment of examination and discernment before the act of eating. In a culture of drive-thrus, mindless snacking, and food consumed as entertainment, this call to intentionality is a prophetic word. It summons us out of our passivity and calls us to be active, conscious stewards of the appetites God has given us. We are to eat with our eyes open, not merely with our taste buds activated. This intentionality is the practical outworking of Paul's command to "present your bodies as a living sacrifice" (Romans 12:1). A sacrifice is an intentional act. It involves the conscious selection of the offering and its deliberate presentation to God. So too, our eating is to be a daily, living sacrifice. Each meal is an opportunity to consciously offer our bodies back to God, not as a grim duty, but as a grateful response to His grace. This intentionality transforms the dinner table from a mere refueling station into a sanctuary of stewardship, where we acknowledge that even our most basic physical needs are a realm in which we can glorify God.

At the heart of this intentionality lies the principle of **discernment**, which was the very soul of the *Kashrut* system. The ancient Israelite was trained to ask, "Is this clean? Does this conform to God's standard?" For us, the question has been transfigured. It is no longer about the biological classification of an animal, but about the theological and creational implications of our food choices. We are now called to exercise a more demanding, Spirit-led discernment that asks a more complex set of questions: Does this food contribute to the health and vitality of the temple of the Holy Spirit? Does its production system reflect the justice, mercy, and creational care of the Kingdom of

God? Does my consumption of it support practices that honor life or that perpetuate cruelty and exploitation? This is the "renewal of the mind" (Romans 12:2) applied to our pantries. It is the freedom in Christ to choose not merely what is permissible, but what is "excellent" (Philippians 1:10), what is "beneficial" (1 Corinthians 6:12), and what is "fitting" for a citizen of heaven. This discernment is not a cold, clinical calculation, but a spiritual discipline, a way of loving the Lord our God with all our mind, even in the grocery aisle. It requires us to be students of both Scripture and creation, to listen to the voice of the Spirit and the data of general revelation, weaving them together into a tapestry of wise living.

Furthermore, the Levitical code, with its profound prohibition against consuming blood, instilled a deep-seated **reverence for the life** that God creates and sustains. Every meal involving meat was a solemn reminder that sustenance comes at a cost, that a life was given so that their life might continue. This principle, too, finds its ultimate fulfillment in Christ, the true Lamb whose blood was shed for the life of the world. Yet, it also finds a continued application in our posture toward all of creation. Our freedom in Christ is not a license for a cavalier, entitled disregard for the lives—plant and animal—that sustain our own. A wisdom-informed freedom cultivates a spirit of profound gratitude and humility. It leads us to consider the ethical dimensions of our food, to prefer systems of production that treat animals with the dignity due to creatures under our dominion, and to be mindful of the environmental impact of our dietary choices. It calls us to receive our food with thanksgiving, not as a right, but as a gift, recognizing the intricate web of life—the soil, the sun, the rain, the farmer—that God employs to provide our daily bread. This reverence sanctifies the act of eating, turning it into a Eucharistic practice, a continual remembrance of the God who is the source of all life and the ultimate sustainer of our own.

Therefore, the glorious freedom we possess in Christ, the freedom that declares all foods clean, is a particular kind of freedom. It is not, as the world would have it, the freedom to indulge every appetite without restraint. That is not freedom; it is slavery to desire, the very bondage from which Christ came to liberate us. The freedom of the gospel is the *freedom to choose wisely.* It is the liberation from the enslaving power of sin and the oppressive weight of the law, which then empowers us to willingly, joyfully, and intelligently choose the good, the true, and the beautiful. It is the freedom to say "no" to the gluttonous, addictive patterns of our culture, not because we are forced to, but because we are free to pursue a higher good. It is the freedom to choose a whole food over a processed one, not out of legalistic obligation, but out of a loving desire to maintain the temple in good repair. It is the freedom to occasionally enjoy a celebratory feast without guilt, and the freedom to fast without self-righteousness. This is a freedom that requires more of us, not less. It demands spiritual maturity, self-control, and a conscience trained by the Word and the Spirit.

This entire endeavor—this intentional, discerning, and reverent approach to eating—has one ultimate, unifying end: **the glory of God and the good of His temple.** The telos of our nutritional stewardship is doxological. We care for our bodies, we exercise discernment in our consumption, we cultivate a spirit of gratitude, not as an end in itself, but so that this physical vessel, this earthenware jar, might be a fit dwelling for the transcendent power of the Holy Spirit (2 Corinthians 4:7). We do it so that we might have the energy, clarity, and vitality to love God with all our strength and to love our neighbor as ourselves.

A body wracked by the consequences of foolish consumption is a body with diminished capacity for service. A mind fogged by inflammatory foods is a mind with diminished capacity for prayer and discernment. Our stewardship is for mission. It is about positioning ourselves to be more effective instruments of righteousness, more enduring runners in the race set before us, more ready servants in the Kingdom of our Lord. When we understand this, our eating is no longer a merely personal or private matter. It is integrated into the great drama of redemption. It becomes part of our participation in the ongoing work of the Spirit, who is renewing all things, beginning with us. We steward these temporary, earthly bodies in hopeful anticipation of the day when they will be redeemed and transformed into glorious, imperishable bodies, fully and finally suited for an eternity in the presence of God. Until that day, we walk in the glorious, wisdom-informed freedom of the children of God, offering every bite, every meal, as an act of worship to the One who is both the Creator of our food and the Redeemer of our souls.

CHAPTER 08

Ethical Consumption and Fasting: Spiritual Disciplines for Physical and Spiritual Health

Beloved, we now embark upon a profound expansion of our vision, moving from the inner sanctum of the individual temple to the vast, interconnected web of relationships in which that temple exists. Our exploration of Embodied Stewardship has thus far focused primarily on the personal, physical, and spiritual implications of what we choose to consume. We have established that the body is a temple, that our eating is a theological act, and that wisdom must guide our choices. But a temple does not exist in a vacuum. It is situated within a city, within a creation, and its maintenance requires resources drawn from a wider world. To stop at the boundary of our own skin is to embrace a truncated, ultimately Gnostic gospel that fails to account for the cosmic scope of Christ's redemption. True holistic discipleship recognizes that our most personal acts—our eating and our drinking—ripple outward with ethical and spiritual consequences. Therefore, we must now turn our attention to the twin disciplines that frame our relationship with food in its fullest context: the discipline of **ethical consumption**, which considers the impact of our appetites on God's world and our global neighbors, and the discipline of **fasting**, the sacred art of restraining our appetites for the sake of spiritual clarity and dependence upon God. These are not separate concerns but two sides of the same coin, both essential for a faith that seeks to love God with all our strength and our neighbor as ourselves.

8.1 Introduction: The Ethics of the Appetite

We begin by confronting a foundational, yet often unexamined, truth: **our appetite is never a purely private matter.** In the modern, industrialized West, we are conditioned to think of our food choices as expressions of personal preference, budget, or health goals. We operate as sovereign consumers in a marketplace of endless options. But this is an illusion, a fiction of affluence. From a biblical perspective, every act of consumption is an act of participation in a complex system of creation, labor, and distribution. It is a moral and theological act with a chain of consequences that extends from the soil to the soul, from the feedlot to the family table, from the migrant worker to the global climate.

The creational mandate given to humanity in Genesis 1:28—to "subdue" the earth and have "dominion" over its creatures—was not a license for exploitation, but a call to a priestly stewardship. The Hebrew words *kabash* (to subdue) and *radah* (to have dominion) in their ideal sense imply a bringing of order and a exercising of righteous rule, much as a wise king cares for his realm. This dominion was to be exercised within the context of the garden that God had planted, a context of abundance and harmony. The Fall catastrophically corrupted this dominion, twisting it into a relationship of toil, frustration, and exploitation (Genesis 3:17-19). The ground is cursed because of us, and our relationship with the creation becomes one of struggle.

The gospel of Jesus Christ, however, announces the redemption of all things (Colossians 1:20). This includes the redemption of our relationship with creation and our mode of dominion. We are no longer to operate according to the pattern of the fallen "subdue and exploit," but according to the pattern of the Second Adam, who came not to be served but to serve (Mark 10:45). Our consumption, therefore, must be re-imagined as an aspect of our redeemed dominion. It is an exercise of power, and like all power, it must be wielded with justice, mercy, and humility.

This is where the concept of **ethical consumption** emerges as a non-negotiable dimension of Embodied Stewardship. It is the conscious and prayerful effort to align our eating habits with the values of the Kingdom of God. It asks not only, "Is this good *for me*?" but also, "Is this good *for the world God loves*?" This involves a multi-faceted discernment:

First, it considers **the treatment of animals.** The Proverbs tell us that "the righteous care for the needs of their animals, but the kindest acts of the wicked are cruel" (Proverbs 12:10). While we are permitted to eat meat, we are not permitted to be indifferent to the suffering of creatures under our dominion. The industrialized factory farming system, with its intense confinement, mutilation, and systemic cruelty, stands in stark contrast to the vision of a shepherd-king like David, who risked his life for his sheep. Ethical consumption leads us to ask: Does the meat, dairy, and eggs I consume come from systems that honor the life of the creature, or from systems that treat it as a mere unit of production? This is an application of the Levitical principle of reverence for life, transposed into a modern industrial context.

Second, ethical consumption considers **the treatment of people.** The food on our plate is the product of human labor—farmers, pickers, processors, truckers, and grocery workers. Are the people in this supply chain treated with dignity and paid a just wage? Or does our demand for cheap food depend on the exploitation of vulnerable labor, often hidden from our view? The prophets thunder against those who "trample the head of the poor into the dust of the earth" (Amos 2:7). When we consume without consideration for the hands that harvested our food, we risk participating in this trampling. Ethical consumption seeks to support systems of fair trade and just labor practices, recognizing the image of God in every person involved in bringing sustenance to our table.

Third, it considers **the health of the creation itself.** Our agricultural practices have a profound impact on the soil, the water, and the climate—all part of the "very good" world God entrusted to our care. Does the production of this food degrade the soil through erosion and chemical dependency? Does it pollute waterways with pesticide runoff? Does it contribute disproportionately to the greenhouse gases that are destabilizing the global climate upon which the poor are most dependent? To care for the creation is an act of worship to the Creator, and a practical outworking of the command to love our global neighbor.

Simultaneously, we must recover the ancient, foundational discipline of **fasting.** If ethical consumption is about *how* we eat in a redeemed way, fasting is about the God-given power to *not eat* for a higher purpose. In a culture of instant gratification and constant stimulation, the voluntary restraint of our most basic appetite is a radical, counter-cultural act of defiance. It is a tangible declaration that "man shall not live by bread alone, but by every word that comes from the mouth of God" (Matthew 4:4).

Fasting is the spiritual discipline of abstaining from food (and sometimes drink) for a set period of time to heighten our spiritual focus and express our dependence on God. It is not a spiritualized diet plan. Its primary goal is not physical detoxification, though that may be a side benefit. Its goal is to create a space of heightened spiritual awareness. When the pangs of hunger strike, they become a trigger for prayer. They are a physical reminder of our spiritual poverty and our ultimate dependence not on physical sustenance, but on God Himself. In fasting, we consciously disrupt the automatic rhythm of consumption to ask the deeper questions: What am I truly hungry for? In whom do I truly trust?

Fasting is a weapon against the idolatry of the appetite. It exposes the ways we use food not merely for nourishment, but for comfort, for escape, for boredom, and for control. By saying "no" to a legitimate good (food), we strengthen our spiritual muscles to say "no" to illegitimate desires. It is a form of "training in godliness" (1 Timothy 4:7-8), teaching us that we are not slaves to our stomachs, but are, in Christ, masters of our appetites.

Together, ethical consumption and fasting form the complete arc of a Christian theology of food. One directs our engagement with the world, ensuring that our participation in the systems of consumption is just, merciful, and humble. The other directs our engagement with God, ensuring that our hearts are not captive to those very systems, but are rooted in the One who is the true Bread of Life. One is an expression of love for neighbor and creation; the other is an expression of love for God. To pursue one without the other is to fall into either a secular activism devoid of spiritual power or a pietistic withdrawal devoid of tangible love. Holistic discipleship requires both: a fork that is guided by justice and a heart that is disciplined by prayerful abstinence. This is the sacred, integrated practice of the ethics of the appetite.

8.2 Ethical Consumption: Loving Our Neighbor Through Our Plate

Beloved, we now press into one of the most demanding and far-reaching implications of our doctrine of Embodied Stewardship. The great commandment, to "love your neighbor as yourself" (Mark 12:31), is not a sentiment to be confined to our personal relationships or charitable donations. It is a comprehensive ethical principle that must govern every sphere of our existence, including the most mundane and daily of our activities: our eating. To sever our dietary choices from their ethical consequences is to practice a form of spiritual schizophrenia, where our faith is compartmentalized from the tangible impact of our lives in the world. The food on our plate is the end product of a vast, global network of ecological and economic relationships. Every time we eat, we are casting a vote for the kind of world we want to live in—a world that reflects the justice, mercy, and *Shalom* of God's kingdom, or a world characterized by exploitation, degradation, and indifference. Therefore, loving our neighbor through our plate requires a conscious, prayerful, and often costly realignment of our consumption with the creational and redemptive purposes of God.

First, we must consider our **Stewardship of Creation.** The Genesis mandate to "work and keep" the garden (Genesis 2:15) establishes humanity's original vocation as priestly stewards of God's good earth. The words *avad* (to work/serve) and *shamar* (to keep/guard) imply a relationship of nurturing care and protective custody. The Fall corrupted this vocation, turning it into painful toil and introducing a tendency toward exploitation (Genesis 3:17-19). Much of modern industrial agriculture is a manifestation of this fallen dominion. It is a system often characterized by massive monocultures that deplete soil health and biodiversity; by the prolific use of pesticides and herbicides that poison waterways and harm pollinators; and by the confinement of animals in conditions that deny them the possibility of expressing their God-given *nephesh*, or creaturehood.

A biblically-informed approach to consumption, therefore, must ask a piercing question of every food choice: **Does this contribute to the flourishing of God's creation, or to its exploitation?** Does my demand for this product support agricultural practices that "keep" the garden, or that strip-mine it? When we choose to support local, sustainable, and regenerative farming practices, we are engaging in a tangible act of creational stewardship. We are aligning our economic power with systems that build topsoil, protect water quality, and enhance biodiversity. We are participating in a form of environmental *Shalom*. When we seek out meat, eggs, and dairy from farms that practice humane animal husbandry—where chickens can peck, pigs can root, and cattle can graze—we are honoring the principle of Proverbs 12:10, which declares that "the righteous care for the needs of their animals." We are acknowledging that these creatures are not merely production units, but living beings under our dominion, for whose well-being we will give an account. This is not a romanticized return to a non-existent agrarian past; it is a prophetic, practical commitment to a mode of consumption that reflects our God-given role as image-bearers tasked with cultivating a creation that groans for its redemption (Romans 8:22). To willfully ignore the ecological and ethical cost of our food is to fail in our creational priesthood.

Second, our plate becomes a matter of **Global Justice and the Poor.** The prophetic literature of the Old Testament reserves its most scathing condemnations for economic systems that grind the faces of the poor. The prophet Amos delivers a word from the Lord that cuts to the heart of our modern globalized food economy: "Hear this, you who trample the needy and bring the poor of the land to an end, saying, 'When will the new moon be over, that we may sell grain? And the Sabbath, that we may offer wheat for sale, that we may make the ephah small and the shekel great, and deal deceitfully with false balances, that we may buy the poor for silver and the needy for a pair of sandals and sell the chaff of the wheat?'" (Amos 8:4-6). The sin here is a relentless drive for profit that exploits the most vulnerable, using dishonest measures to maximize gain from those who can least afford it.

This ancient indictment finds a chilling resonance in our world today. Our insatiable Western demand for cheap food—for out-of-season produce, for inexpensive coffee, for bargain-bin chocolate—often depends on a supply chain built on the back of profound human suffering. It can depend on the campesino in a foreign land paid a pittance for his harvest, on the child laborer forced to work on a cocoa plantation, on the factory farm worker subjected to dangerous conditions and poverty wages. When we purchase these products without a thought for their origin, we become complicit in a system that "tramples the needy." We are, in effect, seeking to "buy the poor for silver."

Therefore, loving our global neighbor requires a new kind of economic discernment. It may lead us to actively seek out and support **fair-trade certified products.** The fair-trade model is not a perfect solution, but it is a tangible attempt to rectify the imbalances of global trade by ensuring that farmers and workers receive a living wage, work in safe conditions, and have access to community development funds. To choose fair-trade coffee or chocolate is a small but significant act of economic justice. It is a way of saying that the person who grew my food is my neighbor, and I will not allow my appetite to contribute to their oppression.

Furthermore, a commitment to global justice must confront the scandal of **food waste.** In a world where millions face hunger, the fact that nearly a third of all food produced is wasted is a moral obscenity. In the wisdom of Scripture, waste is a sign of folly and a failure of stewardship (John 6:12). To consciously reduce our food waste—through careful meal planning, proper storage, and using leftovers—is a practical, daily act of solidarity with the hungry. It is a declaration that the resources God has provided are sacred and are to be used with reverence and responsibility, not squandered in a culture of abundance. Every scrap of food saved is a small rebellion against the systemic injustice that allows some to feast while others starve.

Finally, and most intimately, ethical consumption must shape **The Body of Christ and Community Health.** The Apostle Paul provides a devastating case study in the failure of ethical consumption within the church itself. In 1 Corinthians 11:17-22, he confronts the Corinthian believers over their behavior during the Lord's Supper, which was then a full, communal meal. He writes, "When you come together, it is not the Lord's supper that you eat. For in eating, each one goes ahead with his own meal. One goes hungry, another gets drunk. What! Do you not have houses to eat and drink in? Or do you despise the church of God and humiliate those who have nothing?" (1 Corinthians 11:20-22).

The sin here is not merely bad manners; it is a profound theological failure. The wealthy members of the congregation were arriving early, consuming their lavish provisions, and even becoming drunk, while the poorer members—likely slaves who could not get away from work—arrived later to find nothing left. Their gluttony and cliquishness were desecrating the very symbol of Christian unity and equality at the foot of the cross. They were using the table of the Lord to reinforce social divisions and to "shame those who have nothing." Their consumption was a direct violation of the law of love.

This passage stands as a permanent warning to the church. Ethical consumption within the body of Christ means that our shared meals—whether the Eucharist, a potluck, or a coffee hour—must be laboratories of the Kingdom. They must be characterized by **radical hospitality, generosity, and a preferential option for the poor.** It means ensuring that no one in our fellowship goes hungry while others have plenty. It means that our church budgets and our potluck sign-ups should reflect a conscious care for the economic diversity of our members. It means that our celebrations are not occasions for showcasing our wealth, but for sharing our blessings. When we gather around food, we are to do so in a way that visibly demonstrates the reconciling power of the gospel, where there is no Jew or Greek, slave or free, rich or poor, but all are one in Christ Jesus (Galatians 3:28). Our table fellowship must be a foretaste of the Messianic banquet, where the last are first and where every need is met in the abundance of God's grace. To fail in this is to preach a hollow gospel, one that has power to save the soul but not to transform the social and economic relationships of the body.

8.3 The Biblical Theology of Fasting

Beloved, we now turn from the outward-facing discipline of ethical consumption to the inward-facing, deeply personal, and profoundly powerful discipline of fasting. If ethical consumption is about sanctifying our *engagement* with the world through our appetites, fasting is about sanctifying our *detachment* from the world for the sake of a deeper engagement with God. In an age of instant gratification and sensory overload, the voluntary, temporary abstinence from food for spiritual purposes stands as a radical, counter-cultural act. It is a tangible declaration of war against the tyranny of the flesh and a profound affirmation that our ultimate sustenance is not physical, but spiritual. Fasting is not, as it is often misconstrued in our modern context, a spiritualized diet plan or a technique for physical detoxification. While it may have secondary physical benefits, its primary purpose is always and unequivocally spiritual. It is a spiritual weapon, a response to grievous sacred moments, a pathway to humility, and a means of intensifying our prayer and focus on God. To understand its true power, we must immerse ourselves in the rich tapestry of its biblical theology, observing how God's people have used this discipline across the sweep of salvation history.

We begin at the very foundation of the covenant, with **Moses on Sinai (Exodus 34:28)**. The context is one of supreme theological significance. Moses has just witnessed the catastrophic sin of the golden calf, he has shattered the tablets of the Law in righteous anger, and he has interceded for the people, pleading with God for their forgiveness. Now, he is called back up the mountain to receive the Law a second time. The text tells us, "He was there with the LORD forty days and forty nights. He neither ate bread nor drank water. And he wrote on the tablets the words of the covenant, the Ten Commandments." This fast was not an act of penance imposed by God, but a response—a necessary, human response—to the overwhelming gravity of the moment. In the presence of the holy, speaking God, the ordinary needs of the body faded into insignificance. This fast signifies a state of **total dependence and singular focus on God's word.** Moses was being sustained not by bread, but by the very glory and voice of Yahweh. His physical hunger became a symbol of his spiritual receptivity. He was emptying himself of physical sustenance to be completely filled with divine instruction. This teaches us that fasting is a fitting preparation for receiving revelation from God. When we need to hear God's voice with clarity, when we are seeking His will on a matter of great importance, fasting creates a space of spiritual attentiveness, quieting the clamor of our physical needs to amplify the still, small voice of the Spirit.

From the mountain of covenant law, we descend into the depths of a penitent heart with **David's Penitential Fast (Psalm 35:13)**. Here, fasting takes on a different hue. It is not about receiving revelation, but about expressing the most profound grief and contrition. David, speaking of his enemies, says, "But I, when they were sick—I wore sackcloth; I afflicted myself with fasting; I prayed with head bowed on my chest." The Hebrew word for "afflicted myself" is *'innah*, which carries the meaning of humbling, oppressing, or mishandling the soul. David's fasting was an external manifestation of an internal state of brokenness. He was not trying to manipulate God; he was giving physical expression to the agony of his spirit. This is fasting as a language of lament, a somatic prayer when words are inadequate. It is the body joining the soul in its grief, its repentance, or its intercession. When we are confronted with the gravity of our own sin, or when we are burdened by the suffering of others, a plate of food can seem trivial, even offensive. To eat would be to deny the reality of the spiritual crisis at hand. Fasting, in this context, is a way of "putting on" the reality of our spiritual poverty, of agreeing with God about the seriousness of a situation. It is the physical embodiment of James's command: "Be wretched and mourn and weep. Let your laughter be turned to mourning and your joy to gloom. Humble yourselves before the Lord, and he will exalt you" (James 4:9-10).

A different dimension of fasting is revealed in the exile, through the prophet **Daniel's Partial Fast (Daniel 10:2-3)**. "In those days I, Daniel, was mourning for three weeks. I ate no delicacies, no meat or wine entered my mouth, nor did I anoint myself at all, for the full three weeks." This was not a complete abstinence from all food, but a selective fasting from "choice food," from the rich and pleasant things. Daniel was not in a state of abject penitence, but of intense spiritual seeking. He was mourning over the state of his people in exile and seeking understanding from God regarding a vision he had received. His fast was one of **solemn seeking and heightened spiritual sensitivity.** By denying himself the pleasures of the king's table, he was creating a context of heightened spiritual alertness. He was declaring that his desire for God's answer, for God's presence, was greater than his desire for the comforts and luxuries of Babylon. This teaches us that fasting can be a form of spiritual warfare against the seductive power of a comfortable, assimilated life. It is a way of setting ourselves apart, of saying "no" to the world's delights so that we can say a more wholehearted "yes" to the God who reveals mysteries. Daniel's fast shows us that the discipline is adaptable; it is not an all-or-nothing proposition, but can be tailored to the specific spiritual objective and the leading of the Holy Spirit.

The theology of fasting finds its ultimate paradigm and validation in the life of our Lord, **Jesus in the Wilderness (Matthew 4:1-2)**. "Then Jesus was led up by the Spirit into the wilderness to be tempted by the devil. And after fasting forty days and forty nights, he was hungry." This passage is of monumental importance. First, note that Jesus' fast was Spirit-led. It was not a self-generated act of asceticism, but a deliberate obedience to the Father's will for a specific season of His life. Second, the fast was preparatory for spiritual warfare. Immediately following this period of consecration and dependence, Jesus faced the direct, frontal assault of the tempter. The enemy's first temptation was precisely targeted at Jesus' physical hunger: "If you are the Son of God, command these stones to become loaves of bread" (Matthew 4:3). Jesus' response, "Man shall not live by bread alone, but by every word that comes from the mouth of God," is the definitive theological statement on the meaning of His fast, and of all Christian fasting. The fast was a physical enactment of this very truth. By enduring hunger, Jesus was reaffirming His absolute dependence on the Father and the primacy of spiritual sustenance over physical need. He was demonstrating that His identity and power were not derived from meeting His own physical needs, but from His obedient relationship with the Father. In this, Christ sanctified fasting, transforming it from a mere religious ritual into a Christological pattern of dependence and obedience. Our fasting, then, is to be done in union with Christ, following His example, and for the purpose of strengthening our spirit to resist temptation and to walk in greater obedience.

Finally, we see the discipline carried forward into the life of the newborn church in **The Early Church (Acts 13:2-3)**. "While they were worshiping the Lord and fasting, the Holy Spirit said, 'Set apart for me Barnabas and Saul for the work to which I have called them.' Then after fasting and praying they laid their hands on them and sent them off." Here, fasting is integrated into the very fabric of corporate worship and mission. It is a community discipline, not just a private one. The church at Antioch was engaged in worship and fasting, creating a collective posture of humility, attentiveness, and surrender. In this context, the Holy Spirit spoke clearly, directing the first great missionary endeavor. The fast was both a preparation for hearing God's voice and a consecration of the ones being sent. This teaches us that fasting is a vital component of the church's discernment process. When we face major decisions as a body—calling a pastor, launching a new ministry, seeking revival—corporate fasting is a powerful means of silencing our own agendas and attuning our collective heart to the mind of the Spirit. It is a way of saying, "This decision is too important to be made on full stomachs and with clear-headed human logic alone. We need to hear from God, and we are willing to set aside our physical comfort to seek His face together." In the early church, fasting was not a relic of the Old Covenant; it was a vital, ongoing practice of a Spirit-filled community, essential for guidance and for setting apart workers for the harvest.

8.4 The Purposes and Benefits of Fasting

Beloved, having traced the biblical-theological landscape of fasting, we must now descend from the panoramic view to the intimate, personal terrain of its purpose and effect in the life of the believer. Why do we fast? What is God's intended design for this ancient discipline? It is not a meritorious work to earn God's favor, nor is it a manipulative tool to force God's hand. Rather, it is a God-ordained means of grace, a spiritual instrument designed to recalibrate our entire being—spirit, soul, and body—toward its true north: communion with the living God. The purposes and benefits of fasting are multifaceted, operating on spiritual, psychological, and even physical levels, all converging to produce a more integrated, disciplined, and God-dependent disciple. Let us explore these profound dimensions, understanding that in this sacred practice, the grace of God meets the intention of the human will to produce transformative results.

First and foremost, fasting is a powerful catalyst for **Intensifying Prayer.** There are moments in the life of faith when ordinary prayer feels insufficient to carry the weight of our burden, our need, or our desperation. In such times, fasting becomes the physical amplifier of our spiritual cry. We see this powerfully demonstrated in the life of Ezra. As he prepared to lead a vulnerable caravan of returning exiles from Babylon to Jerusalem, carrying vast treasures for the temple, he proclaimed, "Then we proclaimed a fast there, at the river Ahava, that we might humble ourselves before our God, to seek from him a safe journey for ourselves, our children, and all our goods. For I was ashamed to ask the king for a band of soldiers and horsemen to protect us against the enemy on our way, since we had told the king, 'The hand of our God is for good on all who seek him, and the power of his wrath is against all who forsake him.' So we fasted and implored our God for this, and he listened to our entreaty" (Ezra 8:21-23). Ezra's fast was an expression of radical dependence. It was a way of putting "skin in the game," of demonstrating with their bodies the absolute seriousness of their petition. The physical hunger pangs became a constant, bodily reminder to pray, a trigger that turned every stomach rumble into a silent intercession. Fasting, in this sense, adds an exclamation point to our prayers. It says to God and to our own souls, "This matter is of utmost importance. We are not just casually mentioning this to You; we are staking our physical comfort on Your answer." It creates a sacred synergy where the body's deprivation fuels the spirit's intensity, focusing our entire being like a laser beam on the throne of grace.

This leads directly to the second purpose: **Humbling the Soul.** Fasting is the God-appointed means of physically embodying our spiritual poverty. The Psalmist cries out, "I humbled my soul with fasting" (Psalm 35:13, KJV). The Hebrew word here, *'anah*, means to afflict, to humble, to bow down. When we fast, we voluntarily take upon ourselves a state of physical affliction. We choose weakness. We choose hunger. We choose the growling stomach and the lightheadedness. Why would we do such a thing? Because it is a tangible, undeniable reminder of our creatureliness. In a culture that prizes self-sufficiency, control, and satiety, fasting is a radical act of deconstruction. It forcibly reminds us that we are not self-sustaining. We are fragile, dependent beings who cannot go for more than a few weeks without food. This physical humbling has a profound spiritual corollary. It exposes the illusion of our autonomy and drives us to our knees in dependence. It starves the arrogant, self-reliant flesh and feeds the spirit that cries, "Abba, Father." When we are sated and comfortable, it is easy to forget our need for God. But when we are hungry, the reality of our dependence is inescapable. Fasting, therefore, is a divinely prescribed medicine for the soul-sickness of pride. It is a way of "putting on" humility, of allowing the body to tutor the soul in the fundamental truth that "apart from [Christ] you can do nothing" (John 15:5).

Thirdly, fasting is an indispensable discipline for **Seeking God's Guidance.** Our minds are often clouded by a cacophony of voices—the clamor of our own desires, the opinions of others, the relentless noise of media, and the distracting demands of our appetites. When we face a critical crossroads, a major decision, or a season of confusion, we need clarity. We need to hear the still, small voice of God above the din. Fasting is a way of turning down the volume on the world and turning up the receiver of our spirit. By temporarily setting aside the pursuit of physical satisfaction, we create a cognitive and spiritual space for heightened receptivity. The energy typically devoted to digesting food, planning meals, and experiencing the pleasure of eating is redirected toward prayer and listening. The early church understood this. In Acts 13, it was while they were "worshiping the Lord and fasting" that the Holy Spirit spoke clearly about setting apart Paul and Barnabas for mission. Their collective fast created a corporate environment of such spiritual sensitivity that the voice of God was unmistakable. Fasting clears the static from the line. It is like defragmenting a hard drive, allowing the core data—the will of God—to be accessed with greater speed and clarity. It is a way of telling God, "Your direction is more important to me than my next meal."

Fourth, fasting is a master class in **Exercising Self-Discipline.** The Christian life is a race, a fight, a long obedience. To persevere, we must train. The Apostle Paul, using the metaphor of an athlete, declares, "But I discipline my body and keep it under control, lest after preaching to others I myself should be disqualified" (1 Corinthians 9:27). The word he uses for "discipline" is *hupōpiazō*, a brutal word from the boxing ring that means to strike under the eye, to give a black eye, to subdue. Paul is describing a vigorous, intentional warfare against the rebellious desires of the flesh. Fasting is one of the primary ways we practice this spiritual pugilism. It is the gym where we strengthen the muscle of self-control. Every time we feel a hunger pang and choose not to break the fast, we are landing a blow against the tyranny of our appetites. We are training the body to obey the spirit, rather than the spirit being dragged along by the body's every whim. This discipline cultivated in the realm of food then spills over into every other area of life. The same will that is strengthened to say "no" to a sandwich is the will that can more effectively say "no" to lust, to greed, to anger, and to laziness. Fasting weakens the power of fleshly desires by repeatedly denying them their automatic satisfaction, thereby reinforcing the sovereignty of the spirit, which is submitted to Christ.

Finally, we must acknowledge what modern science has revealed about the **Physiological Resetting** that occurs during a fast. While this must never be our primary motive, it is a fascinating example of God's creational wisdom, where a spiritual discipline is woven into the very fabric of our biological design. When we abstain from food for a period, the body undergoes a remarkable metabolic shift. Insulin sensitivity improves dramatically, allowing for better blood sugar control. The body begins to switch its primary fuel source from glucose to ketones, derived from stored fat, which can lead to enhanced mental clarity and sustained energy. Most remarkably, the process of *autophagy* is significantly upregulated. Autophagy, from the Greek for "self-eating," is the body's innate cellular housecleaning process. During a fast, cells break down and recycle old, damaged proteins and cellular components, clearing out the metabolic debris that can lead to inflammation, dysfunction, and disease. This is a physical "reset," a deep, systemic cleansing at the cellular level. We can see this as a creational gift, a built-in benefit of a spiritual discipline. It is as if God, in His wisdom, designed our bodies to experience a form of physical renewal and purification when we engage in the spiritual work of fasting. The physical "reset" becomes a powerful metaphor and even a parallel experience to the spiritual renewal we seek—the putting off of the old, corrupted self and the putting on of the new, vibrant life in the Spirit. Thus, in fasting, the spiritual and the physical, grace and nature, divine command and creational design, beautifully and mysteriously converge for the holistic good of the whole person, body and soul.

8.5 The Practice of Fasting: Wisdom and Caution

Beloved, having been captivated by the profound theology and transformative potential of fasting, we must now pivot to the critically important, practical application of this discipline. To rush headlong into a fast without prayerful preparation and godly wisdom is to risk turning a means of grace into an occasion of folly, or worse, physical harm. The same Apostle Paul who so vigorously disciplined his body also exhibited immense pastoral caution, recognizing the God-given limits of our physical frames and the paramount importance of love and sound judgment. Fasting is a spiritual weapon of great power, but like any powerful tool, it must be handled with care, humility, and a deep reliance on the Holy Spirit's guidance. It is not a spiritual competition, nor a badge of holiness to be displayed. It is a deeply personal, intimate journey of the soul into deeper dependence upon God, and as such, it must be approached with both faith and wisdom, with passion and prudence.

First and foremost, we must address the issue of **Medical Consultation and Health Conditions.** The body is the temple of the Holy Spirit, and our stewardship of it requires that we honor its God-given design and its vulnerabilities. Fasting places a unique physiological stress upon the body. For most healthy individuals, this stress is beneficial, triggering the adaptive responses we have discussed. However, for those with specific medical conditions, this stress can be dangerous. It is an act of profound spiritual and physical wisdom, not a lack of faith, to seek counsel from a physician before undertaking a significant fast.

This is especially crucial for individuals with conditions such as **diabetes,** particularly those who are insulin-dependent. The dramatic shift in blood glucose levels during a fast can lead to dangerous hypoglycemic episodes, with potential for confusion, seizures, or loss of consciousness. The management of insulin and other medications requires careful, professional supervision that cannot be set aside by spiritual zeal. Similarly, those with a history of **eating disorders** such as anorexia or bulimia must exercise extreme caution. For them, the line between a spiritually-motivated fast and a psychologically-driven relapse into disordered patterns can be perilously thin. The discipline of fasting is meant to liberate us from the tyranny of the flesh, not to provide a religiously-sanctioned framework for a pathology of self-punishment or body-image distortion. In such cases, the more excellent spiritual discipline may be the difficult work of learning to eat regularly and healthily as an act of worship and self-care, thereby "fasting" from the destructive patterns of the disorder.

Other conditions, such as pregnancy, breastfeeding, advanced age, or chronic illnesses affecting the kidneys, liver, or heart, also demand careful medical evaluation. The principle here is one of stewardship. We are called to offer our bodies as *living* sacrifices (Romans 12:1). A fast that willfully endangers the life or health of the temple is a contradiction in terms. It is to treat the body with the same contempt the Gnostics did, by ignoring its legitimate needs. Therefore, if you have any underlying health concerns, the first step of your fast should be a conversation with a healthcare professional who understands and respects your spiritual commitments. This is not a compromise with the world's wisdom, but a submission to the God who created the intricate systems of the body and who calls us to love Him with all our strength—a strength that must be responsibly preserved.

Assuming one is medically cleared, the next principle is that of a **Gradual and Incremental Approach.** The spiritual life is a marathon, not a sprint. We do not begin weight training by attempting to lift 500 pounds, nor should we begin the discipline of fasting by attempting a 40-day absolute fast. Such an approach is a recipe for failure, discouragement, and potential harm. The path of wisdom is to start small and build spiritual and physical endurance over time.

A wise beginning is to start with **short, single-meal fasts.** Perhaps you feel led to skip lunch one day a week. Use that time that would have been spent preparing and eating food for focused prayer and Scripture reading. This allows your body and your mind to become accustomed to the sensation of hunger without being overwhelmed by it. You learn to recognize the physical signals and to redirect the mental energy toward God. After several weeks of this, you may feel led to progress to a **24-hour fast,** perhaps from sunset to sunset, or from breakfast to breakfast. This longer period allows the body to more fully enter into the metabolic state of ketosis and deepens the spiritual intensity of the experience. Only after one has become comfortable with these shorter fasts and has a clear sense of God's leading should one consider a **multi-day fast.** Even then, it is wise to have a plan for breaking the fast gently with broths and easily digestible foods to avoid shocking the system. This gradual approach honors the body as a creation of God, recognizing that spiritual disciplines are meant to train and sanctify our physicality, not to brutalize or destroy it. It is the practical outworking of Paul's instruction to Timothy: "For while bodily training is of some value, godliness is of value in every way" (1 Timothy 4:8). The training has value, but it is the godliness that is the ultimate goal.

A critical component of safe fasting, especially for fasts beyond 24 hours, is the principle of **Adequate Hydration.** The human body can survive for weeks without food, but only for a few days without water. Dehydration is a serious and rapid-onset danger. Therefore, for most people undertaking an extended fast, a **water fast** is the most prudent and sustainable model. This involves abstaining from all solid food and caloric beverages while drinking plenty of pure water throughout the day. Some may also choose to include non-caloric electrolytes to maintain mineral balance. This is distinct from an **absolute fast,** or a "dry fast," which involves abstaining from both food and water. Absolute fasts are exceedingly rare in Scripture (Moses and

Elijah on Mount Sinai being notable exceptions) and are typically of very short duration, as they pose significant health risks. Unless one receives a very specific, undeniable, and miraculous leading from the Holy Spirit to undertake such a fast, the path of wisdom is to maintain hydration. To willfully dehydrate the temple of the Holy Spirit is an act of poor stewardship, not great faith. The water fast preserves the physical vessel while still accomplishing the primary spiritual purpose of denying the body its solid sustenance and focusing the mind on God.

Finally, and most importantly, we must guard our **Motivation and Heart Posture.** The Lord Jesus Christ Himself delivered the definitive teaching on this matter in the Sermon on the Mount: "And when you fast, do not look gloomy like the hypocrites, for they disfigure their faces that their fasting may be seen by others. Truly, I say to you, they have received their reward. But when you fast, anoint your head and wash your face, that your fasting may not be seen by others but by your Father who is in secret. And your Father who sees in secret will reward you" (Matthew 6:16-18). Here, Jesus exposes the deepest peril of the discipline: the temptation to use it for self-glorification. The "hypocrites" of His day had turned fasting into a public performance, a means of cultivating a reputation for extreme piety. They "disfigured their faces"—making a show of their discomfort and sacrifice so that others would be impressed by their spiritual dedication.

Jesus's instruction is radical: "Anoint your head and wash your face." In other words, make a conscious effort to appear normal. Do not draw attention to your fast. Do not complain about your hunger to elicit sympathy or admiration. Do not post about it on social media. Fasting is a private transaction between the soul and God. It is a secret discipline. The moment it becomes a source of pride, a point of comparison, or a means of gaining spiritual status, it ceases to be a fast unto the Lord and becomes a work of the flesh. The reward of the hypocrite is the fleeting admiration of people; the reward of the secret faster is the intimate approval and blessing of the Father who sees in secret. This requires rigorous self-examination. We must constantly ask ourselves: *Why am I doing this?* Is it to draw closer to God, to humble myself before Him, to seek His face in a matter of urgency? Or is there a hidden desire to feel spiritually superior, to prove my dedication to myself or others, to manipulate God into answering my prayer? True fasting springs from a heart of love for God and a desperate desire for more of Him, not from a heart that seeks to accumulate spiritual merit. It is an act of love, not leverage. It is a response to grace, not an effort to earn it. By keeping our fast a secret matter between us and our Father, we protect our hearts from this most subtle and deadly form of pride and ensure that our reward is the one that truly matters: a deeper, more authentic communion with God Himself

8.6 The Synergy of Ethical Consumption and Fasting

Beloved, as we stand at the confluence of these two mighty rivers of spiritual discipline—ethical consumption and fasting—we must behold the powerful, dynamic synergy that is created where they meet. To consider them in isolation is to grasp only half of the gospel's transformative power over our appetites. One directs our engagement with the world; the other, our detachment from it for the sake of God. One sanctifies our *participation* in the systems of creation; the other sanctifies our *abstention* for the sake of communion. Together, they form a pincer movement, a spiritual strategy that attacks the idolatry of the appetite from two flanks, reorienting our entire relationship with food away from the black hole of self-centered consumption and toward the luminous, others-focused reality of God-centered stewardship and worship. They are the practical, daily outworking of the Great Commandment: we love the Lord our God with fasting, and we love our neighbor through our plate.

Consider this: ethical consumption, at its core, is an outward-facing discipline of **love for neighbor and creation.** It is the conscious, often costly, decision to allow the law of love to govern our economic and dietary choices. When we choose to buy fair-trade coffee, we are loving the unseen farmer in a distant land, ensuring they receive a just wage. When we select meat from a local farm that practices humane animal husbandry, we are loving the creature under our dominion and honoring the Creator who made it. When we reduce our food waste, we are loving the global poor and acting as faithful stewards of the abundance God has provided. This discipline forces us to look beyond the confines of our own plate and our own palate to see the vast, interconnected web of relationships—human, animal, and ecological—that are affected by our consumption. It is the tangible application of Paul's command: "So, whether you eat or drink, or whatever you do, do all to the glory of God" (1 Corinthians 10:31). It is eating and drinking as an act of justice, mercy, and humble walking with our God (Micah 6:8).

Fasting, by beautiful and necessary contrast, is an inward and upward-facing discipline of **love for God.** It is the voluntary, temporary renunciation of the good gift of food to declare, with our bodies, that the Giver is more precious than the gift. It is the physical enactment of the truth that "man shall not live by bread alone, but by every word that comes from the mouth of God"

(Matthew 4:4). When we fast, we are not saying that food is bad; we are saying that God is better. We are creating a sacred space of emptiness, a vacuum in the center of our physical being, which can only be filled by the presence and sustenance of the Holy Spirit. Fasting is the ultimate expression of "as the deer pants for flowing streams, so my soul pants for you, O God" (Psalm 42:1). It turns the natural hunger of the stomach into a spiritual catalyst, a constant reminder to pant after God. It is the discipline that starves the flesh of its automatic gratification and feeds the spirit on the bread of heaven.

The synergy between these two is profound and essential. If we practice ethical consumption *without* fasting, we run a grave risk. We risk developing a new form of works-righteousness, a secularized activism fueled by self-will and a subtle pride in our own moral purity. We can become crusaders for a cause, but lose the intimate, dependent connection with the God for whom the cause exists. Our consumption may become ethically pristine, but our hearts may become far from God, trusting in our own righteous choices rather than in His grace. We may love the creation but forget the Creator.

Conversely, if we practice fasting *without* ethical consumption, we risk falling into a detached, Gnostic spirituality. We can become so focused on our private, vertical relationship with God that we neglect the horizontal implications of that relationship. We might seek profound spiritual experiences in our closet while remaining willfully ignorant of the suffering embedded in the supply chain of the food we consume when we are not fasting. We can love God in the abstract while failing to love the neighbor we can actually see and impact through our economic choices. This was the sin of the Pharisees, who tithed mint and dill but neglected the weightier matters of justice and mercy (Matthew 23:23).

But when these two disciplines are held together in dynamic tension, they form a complete and robust Christian spirituality. **Ethical consumption provides the "what" and "how" of our loving engagement with the world, while fasting provides the "why" and the power.** Fasting constantly re-centers our ethical choices in a posture of dependence upon God. It reminds us that our ability to make just and merciful choices is itself a gift of grace, and it purifies our motives, ensuring that our activism flows from a heart of love for God, not a desire for self-justification. It is the spiritual engine that drives the car of ethical consumption.

Simultaneously, **ethical consumption provides the tangible, practical outworking of the humility and love cultivated in fasting.** The self-denial practiced in the secret place must manifest in a life of justice and mercy in the public square. The love for God that is intensified through fasting must inevitably express itself in love for the neighbor whom He has placed in our path, even if that neighbor is a nameless farmer thousands of miles away. Fasting that does not lead to a more compassionate and just mode of life is a fasting that has missed its target.

Together, these disciplines perform a powerful work of liberation. They **break the tyrannical power of food to function as a master.** In a culture of consumerism, food is often more than fuel; it is comfort, entertainment, identity, and addiction. It can master us, dictating our moods, our schedules, and our spending. Ethical consumption dethrones food as a mere object of personal pleasure by forcing us to consider its true cost. Fasting dethrones food by demonstrating that we can, by the Spirit's power, live without it for a season. It proves that we are not slaves to our stomachs. In this liberated space, we are free to enjoy food as the good gift it is meant to be, without being enslaved by it.

Ultimately, this synergistic work re-establishes God as the sole source of our satisfaction. The Psalmist declares, "For he satisfies the longing soul, and the hungry soul he fills with good things" (Psalm 107:9). Ethical consumption and fasting are the twin disciplines that train our souls to find their ultimate satisfaction in God alone. One does so by directing our satisfied hunger toward the good of others, and the other by embracing holy hunger to be satisfied by God Himself. They re-orient our entire existence from a self-referential orbit around our own appetites to a theocentric orbit around the glory and goodness of God. In this sacred rhythm—of receiving with gratitude and ethical care, and of abstaining with faith and spiritual focus—we truly learn to glorify God in our bodies, whether we eat or drink, or whatever we do. We become living sacrifices, our very appetites transformed into instruments of worship.

8.7 Conclusion: Mastering the Appetite for the Master's Use

Beloved, we have journeyed to the very heart of what it means to live an embodied faith, a faith that does not seek to escape the physical realities of hunger and consumption but seeks to redeem them, to harness them, to direct every pang and every pleasure toward a single, glorious end: the glory of God and the advancement of His Kingdom. The disciplined stewardship of our consumption—a stewardship that finds its full expression in the twin pillars of ethical extension and holy restraint—is not a peripheral spiritual hobby for the especially devout. It is, rather, a profound and non-negotiable mark of genuine spiritual maturity. It is the tangible evidence that the gospel has penetrated beyond the realm of our abstract beliefs and has taken captive our most basic, primal drives. It is the lived-out declaration, screamed not from a pulpit but from a dinner table and an empty stomach, that "man shall not live by bread alone, but by every word that comes from the mouth of God" (Matthew 4:4). This is the final and ultimate synthesis of our theology of Embodied Stewardship: the mastery of the appetite for the Master's use.

Consider the profound theological statement we make when we bring our eating under the lordship of Christ through these disciplines. We are asserting, against the screaming testimony of our own biology and the relentless pressure of our consumer culture, that our deepest identity is not that of *consumer*, but of *image-bearer* and *temple-dweller*. The world tells us that our appetites define us—that we are what we eat, that our desires are the ultimate compass for our lives. The gospel tells us a more glorious and liberating truth: we are who God says we are—redeemed, adopted, and indwelt. Our appetites, therefore, are not our masters; they are resources to be managed, instruments to be tuned, channels to be directed. When we choose ethical consumption, we are using our God-given appetite as a force for *Shalom* in the world. When we choose to fast, we are using the temporary suspension of that appetite as a force for intimacy with God. In both cases, the appetite is dethroned. It is no longer an autonomous tyrant, but a servant to the spirit, which is itself submitted to the Holy Spirit.

This mastery is an active, lifelong participation in the process of sanctification. The redemption we have in Christ is not merely a forensic declaration; it is an invasive, transformative power that seeks to reclaim every square inch of our fallen humanity. Our disordered appetites, curved in upon themselves since the Fall, are a primary battlefield in this war of redemption. The practice of ethical consumption is a strategic campaign on this battlefield. It is the conscious retraining of our consumption habits away from the pattern of "what is cheapest and most pleasurable for me" and toward the pattern of "what is most just, merciful, and creational for God's world." It is the hard, daily work of bending our economic power back toward its original, God-honoring design. It is the practical outworking of being "transformed by the renewal of your mind" (Romans 12:2) in the realm of the marketplace.

Simultaneously, the practice of fasting is the direct assault on the fortress of self-gratification. It is the voluntary embrace of weakness to prove the surpassing power of Christ. It is in the crucible of hunger that we discover the flimsiness of our self-sufficiency and the rock-solid reliability of God's sustaining grace. Each successfully resisted temptation to break a fast prematurely is a victory in this war of redemption. It is a small but significant reclaiming of territory from the flesh and a planting of the flag of the Spirit. In this sacred rhythm—of engaging the world with ethical intentionality and then withdrawing from it in focused dependence—we are quite literally working out our salvation with fear and trembling, knowing that it is God who works in us, both to will and to work for his good pleasure (Philippians 2:12-13).

Therefore, the body and its needs are never an end in themselves. They are a means to a far greater end. The food we eat is not ultimately for our own pleasure or even for our own sustenance; it is fuel for the mission of God. The hunger we feel is not merely a problem to be solved; it is a tutor pointing us to our true source of life. When we grasp this, the entire paradigm shifts. A meal becomes more than a meal; it is an act of preparation. It is the taking on of supplies for the journey of discipleship. We eat to have the strength to serve, to love, to pray, to endure. We eat so that the temple might be maintained in good repair for the work of the Priest who dwells within it. Conversely, the fast becomes more than a fast; it is a strategic withdrawal for intelligence and orders from the Commander. It is a clearing of the deck for action, a silencing of the lower frequencies so that the higher frequency of the Spirit's voice can be heard with clarity.

In this divine economy, nothing is wasted—not a single calorie, not a single hunger pang. Everything is taken up into the grand narrative of God's redemptive purpose. The choice for a fair-trade product becomes a small but real participation in God's justice. The decision to abstain from meat for a day becomes a tangible act of dependence on God's word. This is holistic discipleship in its most potent form. It is a faith that connects the grocery cart to the Great Commission, the hunger in our stomach to the hunger for righteousness in our spirit. It is the demonstration that the lordship of Christ is not a compartmentalized truth, but a totalizing reality that demands and enables the mastery of every appetite, for the Master's own glorious use. This is our high calling: to so master our appetites through the power of the indwelling Spirit that every meal and every missed meal becomes a doxology, a testament to the all-sufficiency of the God who satisfies our deepest longings and who uses our most basic needs as a canvas upon which to display the beauty of His redeeming grace.

PART III

MENTAL AND EMOTIONAL WELL-BEING: THE RENEWED MIND

CHAPTER 09

The Psychology of Scripture: Mental Health in the Lives of Biblical Figures

Beloved, we now turn our theological gaze to one of the most pastorally urgent and often misunderstood dimensions of our embodied existence: the landscape of the human mind and its afflictions. In our modern, hyper-clinical age, we have constructed a rigid and artificial dichotomy between the "spiritual" and the "psychological." We have compartmentalized the soul, assigning despair to therapists and sin to pastors, creating a schism in the human person that the biblical witness simply does not recognize. This fragmentation is a legacy of a Cartesian and post-Enlightenment worldview, not a Hebrew one. Scripture presents us with a holistic anthropology, where the *nephesh*—the living being—is an inextricable unity of inner and outer, of emotion, body, and spirit. To impose our modern categories upon the sacred text is to do violence to its profound and integrated realism. The Bible does not shy away from the raw, unvarnished reality of mental and emotional anguish. Its heroes are not stained-glass saints with perpetually serene expressions; they are flesh-and-blood individuals whose walks with God are often punctuated by seasons of debilitating depression, paralyzing anxiety, and soul-crushing despair. Their stories are not presented as tales of failed faith, but as sacred testimonies that the path of covenant faithfulness often leads directly through the valley of the shadow of death.

9.1 Introduction: Affliction in the Cloud of Witnesses

We must begin by demolishing the idol of a faith that is immune to psychological distress. This pervasive and pernicious idea—that strong belief should inoculate one against depression, anxiety, or trauma—finds no support in the great cloud of witnesses that surrounds us (Hebrews 12:1). On the contrary, this cloud is filled with the groans, the laments, and the desperate prayers of men and women who loved God deeply yet found themselves in the grip of profound mental and emotional suffering. Their affliction was not a sign of God's absence, but often the very context in which His presence was most profoundly sought, questioned, and sometimes, mysteriously, felt.

The biblical narrative is shockingly honest about the psychological toll of a life lived in a fallen world, often in direct service to a holy God. We see leaders buckling under the weight of their responsibility, prophets grappling with burnout and suicidal ideation, and poets giving voice to the deepest caverns of human despair. This is not a record of failure; it is a divine revelation of the true nature of the *via dolorosa*, the way of the cross, which every disciple is called to walk. To ignore this dimension of Scripture is to create a church that is ill-equipped to deal with the silent epidemic of mental anguish in its own pews. It produces a community that, when faced with internal suffering, can only offer shallow platitudes, calls to "pray more," or worse, accusations of hidden sin—responses that only deepen the isolation and shame of the sufferer.

A pastoral and theological analysis of these accounts is therefore not an academic exercise. It is a critical ministry of normalization and compassion. It is to look into the canon of Scripture and say to the struggling believer, "You are not alone. Your dark night of the soul is not a foreign country in the economy of God. Look, here is Elijah, a mighty prophet, wishing for death under a broom tree. Here is David, a man after God's own heart, crying out that his bones are troubled. Here is Job, righteous and blameless, cursing the day of his birth. Here is Jeremiah, the weeping prophet, feeling deceived and overwhelmed. You are in venerable company."

This analysis allows us to develop a robust theology of suffering that can hold the tension between the "already" of God's redeeming grace and the "not yet" of our ongoing sanctification and the world's brokenness. It affirms that mental affliction can be, and often is, a complex interplay of physiological, psychological, spiritual, and circumstantial factors. It can be the result of sheer physical exhaustion, as with Elijah. It can be the neurochemical aftermath of trauma, as perhaps with many of the Psalmists. It can be the righteous response to an overwhelming and evil world, as with Jeremiah. It can be a mysterious, sovereignly permitted trial, as with Job. And yes, it can sometimes be exacerbated by personal sin or a crisis of faith. But to reduce it to a single cause is to ignore the complex, psychosomatic unity of the human person as God created us.

Therefore, this chapter will serve as a guided tour through the shadowed valleys of the biblical landscape. We will sit with Moses in his overwhelm, Elijah in his despair, David in his penitential agony and his existential terror, Job in the abyss of his grief and physical torment, and Jeremiah in the torrent of his lament. We will listen to their cries not as problems to be solved, but as sacred texts to be reverenced. We will seek to understand how their faith was not a shield that protected them from psychological pain, but the very rope they clung to in the midst of it. Our goal is to cultivate a church that is a true sanctuary—a place where the weary and heavy-laden can bring their whole, fractured selves, including their anxious minds and depressed spirits, and find not judgment, but the compassionate, understanding gaze of the Christ who Himself was "a man of sorrows, and acquainted with grief" (Isaiah 53:3). For it is in acknowledging the fullness of the affliction present in our cloud of witnesses that we can begin to extend the same grace to ourselves and to one another, and truly learn what it means to bear one another's burdens, and so fulfill the law of Christ.

9.2 The Anatomy of Despair: Elijah under the Broom Tree (1 Kings 19)

Beloved, we now come to one of the most starkly realistic and pastorally profound case studies in all of Scripture: the prophet Elijah, collapsed in a heap of utter desolation beneath a solitary broom tree in the wilderness. This narrative, recorded in 1 Kings 19, provides a masterclass in the anatomy of despair, a meticulous dissection of how a human soul—even a great and faithful soul—can unravel under the cumulative weight of exhaustion, fear, and isolation. It is a passage that shatters any romantic illusion of prophetic ministry or unwavering faith, revealing instead the fragile psychosomatic unity of the prophet himself. Here, we do not find a stained-glass saint, but a man whose spiritual and emotional reserves have been completely depleted, leading him to the very brink of self-annihilation. His story is not one of failure, but a sacred revelation of God's compassionate response to the brokenness of His servants.

To understand the depth of Elijah's collapse, we must first consider **The Precipitating Factors.** This was not a sudden, inexplicable descent into melancholy. It was the predictable, almost inevitable, result of a perfect storm of physiological, emotional, and spiritual exertion. Immediately prior, in 1 Kings 18, Elijah had experienced the supreme triumph of his ministry. He had confronted the 450 prophets of Baal on Mount Carmel, called down fire from heaven, and executed the false prophets. This victory was followed by a fervent prayer that ended a three-and-a-half-year drought, and then he outran King Ahab's chariot in a supernatural sprint from Carmel to Jezreel. Consider the immense toll of these events: the psychological intensity of a public spiritual showdown, the adrenal fatigue following a life-or-death contest, the physical exhaustion of a marathon run. His entire being—nervous system, endocrine system, muscular system—would have been pushed to its absolute limit.

Into this state of profound depletion comes the death threat from Queen Jezebel: "So may the gods do to me and more also, if I do not make your life as the life of one of them by this time tomorrow" (1 Kings 19:2). This threat was not an abstract danger; it was a direct, credible promise of brutal retaliation from the most powerful and vengeful person in the kingdom. The combination is critical: **catastrophic collapse often occurs not in the midst of the battle, but in its immediate aftermath, when the adrenaline subsides and the body and soul must reckon with the cost of the fight.** Elijah's spirit, which had been supernaturally upheld during the contest, now crashes. The towering prophet of fire becomes a fugitive of fear. This teaches us a vital pastoral principle: times of great spiritual victory and intense ministry output can be periods of extreme vulnerability. The soul' defenses are down, and the smallest threat can feel like an insurmountable catastrophe.

The text then lays out a devastatingly clear portrait of his **Symptomatology,** a clinical picture that aligns precisely with what we would now recognize as a severe depressive episode or a state of acute burnout.

First, we see **Fear and Flight.** "Then he was afraid, and he arose and ran for his life" (1 Kings 19:3). This is not the courageous flight of a strategist; it is the panic-driven flight of a traumatized man. The Hebrew word for "afraid" (*yare*) carries the sense of terror, of being utterly dismayed. The same man who stood unflinching before hundreds of false prophets now flees from a single woman's words. This reveals a core truth about psychological distress: it can utterly re-wire our perception of threat, making us incapable of accessing the faith and courage we possessed only days before. It is not a sin to be condemned, but a symptom to be understood.

Second, and most poignantly, we witness **Suicidal Ideation.** "But he himself went a day's journey into the wilderness and came and sat down under a broom tree. And he asked that he might die, saying, 'It is enough; now, O LORD, take away my life, for I am no better than my fathers'" (1 Kings 19:4). This is the cry of a soul that has reached its absolute limit. The phrase "It is enough" (*rav*) signifies a state of being sated, but not with food—with suffering. He is filled to the brim with anguish. His request for death is not a theological argument; it is the raw, desperate expression of a pain that has become unbearable. He sees no future, no hope, no way out. This is the very essence of clinical despair, and the Bible records it without flinching, offering no immediate rebuke, but rather, a divine response of pure grace.

Third, we observe **Social Withdrawal and Anhedonia.** The text notes that he "left his servant there" (1 Kings 19:3). In his state of profound depletion, he severs his last human connection. He journeys alone into the desert, a powerful symbol of his internal state of isolation. He withdraws from community, from responsibility, from relationship. This is a classic symptom of depression—the loss of pleasure (anhedonia) and the drive to isolate. The very things that could potentially help him—community, support, shared burden—are the very things his afflicted mind tells him to flee.

Finally, we see a profound **Cognitive Distortion.** When God finally asks him what he is doing, Elijah's response is a fixed, repetitive mantra of isolation: "I have been very jealous for the LORD, the God of hosts. For the people of Israel have forsaken your covenant, thrown down your altars, and killed your prophets with the sword, and I, even I only, am left, and they seek my life, to take it away" (1 Kings 19:10, 14). His perception is absolute: "I, even I only, am left." This is a textbook cognitive distortion known as "all-or-nothing thinking" and "catastrophizing." He has generalized the failure of the nation to a total failure, and he has personalized it into his own solitary burden. His thinking is rigid, repetitive, and factually incorrect, as God will later reveal that there are 7,000 who have not bowed the knee to Baal (v.18). But in the depths of his despair, he cannot see this. His cognitive lens is darkened.

The heart of this passage, and its enduring gift to the church, is **The Divine Intervention – A Model of Care.** God's response to Elijah's breakdown is a masterful, compassionate protocol for healing that begins not with the spirit, but with the body.

First, **Somatic Care First.** An angel of the Lord does not appear with a sermon or a rebuke. The angel touches him and says, "Arise and eat" (1 Kings 19:5). Elijah finds a cake baked on hot stones and a jar of water. He eats, drinks, and lies down again. The angel returns a second time and commands him to eat again, "for the journey is too great for you" (1 Kings 19:7). This is a breathtaking theological moment. God, through His messenger, validates the physical basis of Elijah's despair. The journey *was* too great for him. His exhaustion was real. God's first prescription is not prayer, but sleep; not a spiritual exhortation, but nourishing food. This provides a foundational principle for pastoral care: we must honor the profound connection between the physical body and the state of the mind. Chronic sleep deprivation, poor nutrition, and physical exhaustion can create a physiological substrate upon which anxiety and depression readily flourish. To address the spiritual while ignoring the somatic is to build a house on sand.

Second, **Gentle Inquiry.** Only after this period of physical restoration—a forty-day journey's worth of strength from that food—does God speak to him. And His question is not an accusation: "What are you doing here, Elijah?" (1 Kings 19:9, 13). It is an invitation. It is a therapeutic question, allowing the prophet to articulate his narrative of distress, to give voice to the broken record playing in his mind. God listens to the same distorted complaint twice without immediate interruption or correction. He creates a space for Elijah to be heard, which is the first step toward healing a fractured sense of self.

Third, **A New Revelation.** God then reveals Himself, but not in the dramatic modes of wind, earthquake, and fire that characterized the Carmel victory. These were the modalities of Elijah's former, powerful ministry. Now, in his depleted state, God comes in a "low whisper" (1 Kings 19:12), a "still, small voice." God meets Elijah not in the mode of power he has lost, but in the mode of gentle presence that his broken soul can actually bear. This tells us that God adapts His communication to our capacity to receive it. In our exhaustion, He does not shout; He whispers. He communicates in the quiet language of presence, meeting us in our vulnerability, not our strength.

Finally, **Re-orientation to Purpose.** God does not leave Elijah in the cave of his introspection. He gives him three concrete, manageable tasks: anoint Hazael king over Syria, anoint Jehu king over Israel, and anoint Elisha as his own successor (1 Kings 19:15-16). This is a profound therapeutic move. God re-engages Elijah with the world, giving him a sense of purpose that extends beyond his own suffering. He is reconnected to a timeline and a community. He is given a successor, Elisha, breaking his terrible sense of isolation. God's healing involves moving us from the paralyzing introspection of despair back into the stream of purposeful action and relational connection. In this, we see the complete picture of God's care for the despairing soul: He restores the body, listens to the pain, reveals Himself in gentle presence, and re-engages the will with purposeful mission.

9.3 The Lamenting Soul: The Diagnostic Precision of the Psalms

Beloved, if the narrative of Elijah provides us with a clinical case study of depressive collapse, then the Psalter provides us with nothing less than the divinely inspired, canonical language for the entire spectrum of human emotional and psychological experience. It is God's gift to a suffering humanity—a sacred textbook of the soul's anatomy in distress. Within its pages, we find no sanitized spirituality, no forced piety that denies the reality of anguish. Instead, we are given permission—more than permission, a divine mandate—to bring our whole, fractured, and fearful selves into dialogue with God. The Psalms are the therapeutic vocabulary for the soul in crisis, offering a diagnostic precision for mental and emotional states that rivals any modern psychological manual, all while grounding that experience in the unwavering context of covenant relationship with Yahweh.

Let us first immerse ourselves in the profound depths of **Psalm 42-43: The Cry of the Depressed Soul.** These two psalms, likely originally a single composition, form one of the most exquisite and detailed maps of a soul navigating the treacherous terrain of depression. The psalmist begins with a powerful somatic and spiritual image: "As a deer pants for flowing streams, so pants my soul for you, O God" (Psalm 42:1). This is not the gentle longing of a contemplative; this is the desperate, physiological gasping of a creature in a state of dehydration and existential crisis. The soul itself is portrayed as having a primal, life-or-death need for God, a need that is going unmet. This is the core ache of depression—a profound spiritual and emotional thirst in a perceived desert of divine absence.

The psalmist then articulates the external and internal symptoms of his condition. Externally, his lived experience is one of relentless sorrow: "My tears have been my food day and night" (Psalm 42:3). This is a powerful metaphor for the way grief and despair can consume one's entire existence, replacing sustenance with sorrow, turning the very act of living into a cycle of feeding on pain. He is taunted by adversaries, whose question, "Where is your God?" (Psalm 42:3, 10), echoes his own deepest, most terrifying internal doubt. This external pressure exacerbates the internal wound, a dynamic familiar to anyone who has felt the sting of well-meaning or malicious questions about their faith in the midst of suffering.

Internally, the psalmist performs a remarkable act of self-diagnosis and soul-care. He names his condition with stunning clarity: "Why are you cast down, O my soul, and why are you in turmoil within me?" (Psalm 42:5, 11; 43:5). The Hebrew word for "cast down" (*shachach*) means to be bowed down, prostrated, sunk into the depths. "Turmoil" (*hamah*) signifies a roaring, a loud agitation, like the crashing of waves. This is the internal noise of anxiety and despair—a chaotic, roaring storm within the psyche. But notice what the psalmist does. He does not merely succumb to this state. He engages in a deliberate, internal dialogue. He talks to his own soul. This is a profound cognitive and spiritual technique. He is externalizing his pain, objectifying it, and then speaking truth to it. The refrain is the turning point: "Hope in God; for I shall again praise him, my salvation and my God."

This is not a glib denial of his feelings. It is a defiant act of memory and will. He is commanding his soul to hope based not on his present emotional state, but on the unchanging character of God as his *salvation*. He actively recalls a different reality:

"These things I remember, as I pour out my soul: how I would go with the throng and lead them in procession to the house of God with glad shouts and songs of praise" (Psalm 42:4). He is fighting the cognitive distortion of depression—which tells him the past was worthless and the future is hopeless—by forcibly recalling a time of genuine joy and connection. He is, in essence, practicing cognitive behavioral therapy under the inspiration of the Holy Spirit, challenging the automatic negative thoughts of his despair with the objective truth of God's past faithfulness and future hope. The psalms teach us that faith in the midst of depression is not the absence of dark feelings, but the persistent, often grueling, work of speaking truth to our own souls until our emotions eventually realign with reality.

If Psalms 42-43 represent a struggle with a glimmer of hope, then **Psalm 88: The Psalm of Unrelieved Darkness** stands as the most daring and pastorally crucial prayer in the entire canon. This psalm is unique, a stark monument in the landscape of Scripture, for it is the only psalm that begins in lament and ends in unmitigated darkness. There is no redemptive turn, no "but I will trust," no final verse of praise. It is a cry that descends into the abyss and remains there.

The psalmist, Heman the Ezrahite, holds nothing back. He describes his life as drawing near to Sheol, the realm of the dead (v.3). He feels "like a man without strength," a corpse among the dead (v.4-5). He attributes his suffering directly to God's actions: "You have put me in the depths of the pit, in the regions dark and deep. Your wrath lies heavy upon me, and you overwhelm me with all your waves" (v.6-7). This is the experience of what St. John of the Cross would later call the "dark night of the soul," where God's presence is felt only as an absence, His favor only as wrath.

The relational devastation is complete: "You have caused my beloved and my friend to shun me; my companions have become darkness" (v.18). This is the ultimate isolation. Not only has God seemingly withdrawn, but human comfort has also evaporated. His closest companions have become "darkness" itself—they are not just absent, but their absence is a active, oppressive force. The psalm ends here, with this devastating final line. There is no resolution.

And this is its profound, divine gift. By including Psalm 88 in the inspired text, God is validating the experience of those for whom despair feels absolute and unending. He is sanctifying the cry of those who cannot find a way to hope, who feel utterly abandoned by God and man. This psalm gives permission to pray from the absolute bottom of the well, where no light penetrates. It teaches us that raw, honest, even accusatory lament is a legitimate form of prayer. It is faith that continues to address God even when it can only say, "Why have you rejected me?" (v.14). To the person trapped in the unrelenting darkness of clinical depression, chronic pain, or profound grief, Psalm 88 says, "Your voice belongs here. Your pain has a place in the prayer book of God's people. You do not need to fake a resolution you do not feel. You can bring your unedited despair to the foot of the throne and know that you are heard." This psalm is a brutal refutation of any theology that demands premature praise or forced cheerfulness. It stands as a permanent witness that God is big enough to handle our anger, our confusion, and our most hopeless cries. The very act of praying this psalm, of screaming its words into the seeming void, is an act of faith—a faith that clings to God even when it cannot feel Him, trusting that the act of crying out is itself a form of holding on. In the Psalter, God has given us not only the songs of Zion's joy but also the grammar of the abyss, ensuring that no matter how deep our suffering, we are never without a language to bring it before the One who, in Christ, Himself descended into the deepest darkness of all.

9.4 The Man of Sorrows: The Mental Anguish of Christ

Beloved, we now arrive at the theological and pastoral heart of our entire exploration of mental affliction in Scripture. All the despair we have witnessed in the prophets and the psalmists finds its ultimate meaning, its profound validation, and its only true hope in the person and work of Jesus Christ. The writer of Hebrews declares that we do not have a high priest who is unable to sympathize with our weaknesses, but one who in every respect has been tempted as we are, yet without sin (Hebrews 4:15). This "every respect" must include, with stunning force, the realm of psychological and emotional suffering. The Gospels do not present a stoic, detached Savior who floats serenely above the turmoil of human emotion. They reveal to us the Man of Sorrows, *vir dolorum*, who was intimately acquainted with the deepest grief and the most profound mental anguish (Isaiah 53:3). In His passion, Christ did not merely endure physical torture; He willingly entered into the full psychological horror of the human condition in a fallen world, thereby sanctifying our own suffering and demonstrating that mental anguish is not a mark of faithlessness, but a facet of the mortal existence He came to redeem.

We begin in the quiet, shadowed olive grove of **Gethsemane's Agony (Matthew 26:36-38)**. The scene is one of almost unbearable psychological intensity. On the eve of the culmination of His cosmic mission, Jesus confesses to His closest friends, "My soul is very sorrowful, even to death" (Matthew 26:38). The Greek word for "sorrowful" here is *perilypos*, meaning encompassed by grief, deeply distressed, utterly consumed by sorrow. This is not a passing sadness. He describes its intensity as "even to death"—a sorrow so profound it feels fatal, as if the very weight of it could crush the life from His body. This is the language of a soul under maximum existential pressure, a prelude to the physical crucifixion that is itself a psychological torment of unimaginable scale.

The physical manifestation of this inner turmoil is recorded by the physician Luke: "And being in agony he prayed more earnestly; and his sweat became like great drops of blood falling down to the ground" (Luke 22:44). This description is highly suggestive of a rare but documented physiological phenomenon known as hematidrosis, or hematohidrosis. Under conditions of extreme psychological stress and terror, the capillary blood vessels that supply the sweat glands can rupture, causing a person to literally sweat blood. This is not a symbolic flourish; it is a clinical observation of a body pushed to its absolute psychological and emotional limit. The incarnate Son of God, in His full humanity, experienced a stress response so severe that it broke the boundaries between His circulatory and integumentary systems.

The theological implication of this is earth-shattering. **In Gethsemane, Christ's mental anguish was not a sin.** His dread, His sorrow, His plea for the cup to pass from Him—these were not failures of faith or a lack of resolve. They were the authentic, sinless responses of a perfect human nature facing the abyss of divine wrath and the horror of bearing the sin of the world. By experiencing this, Christ forever dismantles the heresy that anxiety, dread, or profound sorrow are inherently sinful. He sanctifies the experience of psychological distress by passing through its darkest valley Himself. He was, as the writer of Hebrews says, "made perfect through suffering" (Hebrews 2:10), and part of that perfection as our sympathetic High Priest is His firsthand, experiential knowledge of what it means for a human soul to be "sorrowful, even to death." When we feel our own souls buckling under the weight of dread or despair, we can look to Gethsemane and know that our Savior has been there before us, that He understands not from a distance, but from the intimate, bloody, anguished reality of His own experience.

This psychological descent reaches its horrifying climax on the cross, in **The Cry of Dereliction (Matthew 27:46)**. After three hours of supernatural darkness, Jesus cries out with a loud voice, "Eli, Eli, lema sabachthani?" that is, "My God, my God, why have you forsaken me?" This is the central, paradoxical mystery of the atonement. It is not merely a recitation of the first line of Psalm 22, though it is that. It is the experiential reality of the sin-bearing Lamb of God. At that moment, the One who had eternally existed in the perfect, blissful, unbroken communion of the Trinity was, for the first and only time, severed from that communion. The Father poured out the full cup of His righteous wrath against sin upon the Son, and part of the torment of that wrath was the conscious, psychological experience of abandonment.

This is the ultimate depth of human despair. All human feelings of abandonment—by family, by friends, by God—are but faint echoes of this primal, cosmic dereliction. Christ did not merely sympathize with our feeling of God-forsakenness; He was actually forsaken by the Father *for us*. He entered the absolute spiritual and psychological isolation that is the rightful due of a sinful humanity. The German theologian Dietrich Bonhoeffer, from his Nazi prison cell, wrote that God "lets himself be pushed out of the world on to the cross. He is weak and powerless in the world, and that is precisely the way, the only way, in which he is with us and helps us... Christ helps us, not by virtue of his omnipotence, but by virtue of his weakness and suffering."

In this cry, Christ fully identifies with the psalmist of Psalm 88, with Elijah under the broom tree, with every human soul that has ever screamed into the silence and felt no answer. He validates the reality of this experience not as an illusion, but as a potential dimension of a fallen existence, one that He Himself endured to its bitter end. He was not play-acting. The anguish was real. The sense of abandonment was real. The psychological torment of being cut off from the source of all life and love was the true hell He endured for our sake.

Therefore, the Man of Sorrows does not simply observe our mental suffering from a throne of serene detachment. He descends into the very pit of it. He experiences the somatic terror of Gethsemane and the existential horror of Calvary. In doing so, He accomplishes two things of inestimable value for the believer struggling with mental anguish. First, He **destroys its ultimate power.** Because He entered the deepest darkness of God-forsakenness and emerged victorious in the resurrection, He has broken the power of despair to have the final word over us. Our own dark nights, however long and deep, are now contained within the greater narrative of His passion and resurrection. Second, He **establishes an unbreakable bond of solidarity.** We can come to Him in our pain, our anxiety, our depression, and our feeling of abandonment, and know that we are not speaking to a deity who cannot understand. We are speaking to a wounded Healer, a scarred Savior, who knows the territory of our suffering intimately because He has mapped it with His own blood and tears. Our psychological pain is not a sign that He has abandoned us; it is precisely the arena in which we can most deeply experience His empathetic and victorious presence, for He is the one who was forsaken so that we might never be.

9.5 The Apostle's Thorn: Paul's Unanswered Prayer (2 Corinthians 12:7-10)

Beloved, we now turn from the foundational sufferings of Christ and the patriarchs to a deeply personal and pastoral case study that speaks directly to the experience of chronic, unrelenting affliction in the life of a believer. The Apostle Paul, that towering figure of missionary zeal and theological genius, was not exempt from the kind of persistent, debilitating struggle that can color an entire life. In his second letter to the Corinthian church, he unveils a profound personal mystery—his "thorn in the flesh" (2 Corinthians 12:7). This passage provides a critical theological framework for understanding persistent suffering, particularly the kind that does not yield to fervent prayer and seems to have no redemptive purpose in itself. It is a word for those who have prayed for healing from depression, anxiety, or other mental health conditions and have found the thorn remains, a constant, unwelcome companion.

The identity of this "thorn" (*skolops te sarki*) has been the subject of extensive scholarly debate for two millennia. The Greek word *skolops* can mean a stake or a splinter—something sharp, painful, and deeply embedded. Paul specifies it is "in the flesh" (*te sarki*), emphasizing its tangible, bodily, and likely debilitating nature. The church fathers and subsequent interpreters have proposed a myriad of possibilities: a chronic eye condition (based on Galatians 4:13-15), recurrent malarial fevers, a speech impediment, severe migraines, or even a persistent, harassing opponent. While we cannot be dogmatic, it is entirely plausible, given the holistic Hebrew anthropology Paul operated within, that this affliction had a significant psychological or neurological component. It could have been a condition that produced chronic pain, which in turn leads to depression and anxiety; or it may have been a primary affliction of his mental state itself—a "spirit of oppression" or a temperamental tendency toward despair that he experienced as a relentless, Satanic harassment. The very ambiguity of the thorn is a gift, for it allows every sufferer to see their own chronic struggle reflected in Paul's—be it physical, mental, or, as is often the case, a complex intertwining of both.

The origin of this thorn is as theologically significant as its nature. Paul is unequivocal: it was "a messenger of Satan, to harass me" (2 Corinthians 12:7). This is a crucial distinction. Paul does not say, "God gave me this thorn." He identifies its source as adversarial, as part of the evil, broken, and hostile spiritual and physical reality of a fallen world. It is a "messenger" (*angelos*) of the kingdom of darkness, sent to harass, to buffet, to strike him repeatedly (*kolaphizō*). This acknowledges the genuine reality of evil as a cause of suffering. Yet, in the very same breath, Paul places this adversarial action within the sphere of God's sovereign permission. It was given to him "*so that* (*hina*) I would not become conceited because of the surpassing greatness of the revelations." Here is the profound mystery of divine sovereignty at work. God, in His infinite wisdom, did not prevent this satanic harassment. Instead, He *permitted* it, and then *harnessed* its destructive intent for a sanctifying purpose in Paul's life: to crush spiritual pride. This provides a vital pastoral lens for viewing mental affliction. It may have its proximate cause in any number of factors—genetic predisposition, chemical imbalance, childhood trauma, or direct spiritual oppression. Yet, for the believer, this thorn does not fall outside the sovereign and loving purview of God. It is not meaningless chaos. Even the attacks of the enemy can be sovereignly woven into the fabric of God's purpose to cultivate humility and dependence in His children.

This leads us to the heart of the passage, and its most challenging and glorious truth: **The Purpose of Weakness.** Paul, in his distress, did what any faithful believer would do: he prayed. And he prayed not just once, but three times, with fervor and faith, for the Lord to remove it from him. This was not a prayer of weak faith, but of persistent, passionate pleading. The answer he received was not the one he wanted, but it was the one he needed. The Lord said to him, "My grace is sufficient for you, for my power is made perfect in weakness" (2 Corinthians 12:9).

This divine response is one of the most transformative statements in all of Scripture for a theology of suffering. God does not explain the thorn. He does not justify its existence. Instead, He offers His presence and power *within* the context of the thorn. The Greek word for "sufficient" (*arkei*) means "it is enough." It is a present-tense, ongoing reality. His grace is not a one-time pardon, but a continuous, flowing supply of divine enablement that meets the need of the moment, day after painful day. It is the strength to endure, the peace that surpasses understanding, the glimmer of hope in the darkness—all provided in real time.

And then comes the stunning, counter-intuitive logic of the Kingdom: "for my power is made perfect in weakness." The word "made perfect" (*teleitai*) means to be brought to its goal, to be completed, to be fully expressed. God is saying that the very weakness of the thorn—its persistent, debilitating, humiliating presence—is the ideal vessel, the perfect platform, for the most brilliant and authentic display of Christ's resurrection power. When we are strong, competent, and healthy, our accomplishments can easily be attributed to our own gifts and energies. But when we are weak, and yet are sustained, when we are in despair and yet do not give up, when we are anxious and yet find a moment of peace, it is undeniably the power of Christ at work. The thorn creates a permanent space of acknowledged weakness, which in turn becomes a permanent theater for the demonstration of divine grace.

This provides a profound theodicy—a defense of God's goodness—for persistent mental health struggles. For the believer wrestling with chronic depression, the question is not necessarily, "Why won't God heal me?" but can become, "How can Christ's power be perfected in this very weakness?" The affliction itself becomes the context for a unique and profound testimony. It is not that God is absent or powerless; it is that He is choosing to manifest His sustaining grace in a way that would be impossible if the struggle were simply removed. Paul's radical conclusion is therefore not a grim resignation, but a boast: "Therefore I will boast all the more gladly of my weaknesses, so that the power of Christ may rest upon me. For the sake of Christ, then, I am content with weaknesses, insults, hardships, persecutions, and calamities. For when I am weak, then I am strong" (2 Corinthians 12:9-10). This is the ultimate transfiguration of suffering. The thorn is not removed, but its meaning is utterly transformed. It is no longer merely a "messenger of Satan"; it is now a commissioned ambassador for the power of Christ. For the one with a mental health condition, this means their daily battle is not a wasted life or a failed prayer. It is a sacred, if painful, arena where the sufficiency of Christ's grace can be displayed in its most raw and authentic form, proving that His strength is indeed made perfect in our most profound and persistent weaknesses.

9.6 Conclusion: Solidarity in Suffering and the Path to Hope

Beloved, as we draw our exploration of the psychology of Scripture to a close, we are left not with a set of simplistic answers, but with a profound and enduring vision of divine solidarity and covenantal faithfulness in the very heart of human brokenness. The biblical witness, in its unflinching honesty, systematically dismantles the pervasive and destructive heresy that deep, genuine faith should—or even can—act as a spiritual vaccine against the ravages of mental and emotional distress. This toxic fiction, which has inflicted untold guilt and isolation upon suffering believers, is annihilated by the sacred testimony of the cloud of witnesses. We have walked with them through the shadowed valleys, and in their cries, we have heard an echo of our own, and in God's response to them, we have found a template for our own hope.

The overarching theme that emerges from Elijah's collapse, the Psalmist's despair, Christ's agony, and Paul's thorn is one of profound **Solidarity and Validation.** The canon of Scripture itself stands as a monumental act of validation. By including the raw, unfiltered anguish of its greatest heroes, God is declaring to every generation that the experience of psychological suffering is not a foreign country in the landscape of faith, but a well-traveled—though arduous—stretch of the narrow road.

When you feel the terror that sent Elijah fleeing into the desert, you are not a faithless coward; you are in the company of a prophet of fire. When your soul is cast down and in turmoil, and you can only manage to whisper, "Why, my soul?" you are not failing at prayer; you are praying in the inspired language of the Psalter. When you feel the dread of Gethsemane or the cry of dereliction, you are not abandoned; you are walking a path that the Son of God Himself trod. And when you plead for a thorn to be removed and find it remains, you are not experiencing a denial of your faith; you are being invited into the apostolic mystery of sufficient grace. This solidarity is the first and perhaps most crucial pastoral gift of these scriptures. It normalizes the struggle and silences the accuser who would have us believe our pain is a unique sign of God's displeasure or our own spiritual failure.

Furthermore, Scripture provides us with an indispensable **Language for Suffering.** In a world—and sadly, often in the church—that encourages the suppression of negative emotions in favor of a facade of victorious living, the Bible gives us a sacred grammar for grief. The Psalms, in particular, function as a divine permission slip to feel deeply and to express those feelings honestly to God. They teach us that lament is a legitimate, God-honoring form of worship. It is faith that holds on to God with one hand while shaking its fist at the heavens with the other. It is the stubborn refusal to let go of the covenant relationship, even when that relationship is experienced as absence, silence, or wrath. This holy language prevents our suffering from turning inward into self-destructive silence or toxic bitterness. It externalizes the pain, giving it voice and direction, channeling it toward the only One who can ultimately bear it. For the person whose own mind has become a prison of chaotic, inarticulate pain, the Psalter offers a vocabulary that can structure the chaos and frame the cry, transforming solitary despair into a communal, centuries-old dialogue between a suffering people and their covenant-keeping God.

Beyond solidarity and language, the biblical narrative models a **Holistic Approach to Care** that is desperately needed in our fragmented modern world. We see this most vividly in God's treatment of Elijah. The divine protocol for a prophet in suicidal despair was not a sermon, a rebuke, or an exorcism alone. It was, first and foremost, *somatic*: sleep and food. God honored the profound, inextricable link between the physical body and the state of the soul. This provides a crucial corrective to a spirituality that is purely "spiritual." It calls the church to a ministry that understands that a malnourished body, a sleep-deprived brain, and a dysregulated nervous system can be significant contributors to a state of mental anguish. True pastoral care must encompass a concern for the whole person, advocating for medical care, nutritional support, and rest as acts of spiritual obedience, not as a compromise with secularism. At the same time, the model is not reductionist. After caring for Elijah's body, God engaged his soul with gentle inquiry, a new revelation of divine presence, and a reorientation to purpose. The model is both/and: both somatic and spiritual, both practical and mystical, acknowledging that we are psychosomatic unities whose healing requires attention to every dimension of our being.

Ultimately, the path through the wilderness of mental suffering, as charted by Scripture, leads us to a specific and profound **Encounter with God.** The hope held out is not a guarantee of immediate healing or a quick escape from the darkness. The hope is the promise of a presence. It is the "low whisper" that meets our depletion when we can no longer bear the wind and fire. It is the "grace that is sufficient" for the unremitting thorn. It is the God who, in Christ, did not remain distant from our pain but descended into the very abyss of it, experiencing the ultimate psychological torment of God-forsakenness so that in our own felt forsakenness, we might know we are not alone. The hope is that our suffering is not a meaningless void, but can become, as it did for Paul, a platform for the power of Christ. Our weakness does not disqualify us from service; it qualifies us for a unique manifestation of divine strength. Our desperation does not prove our faith is weak; it proves that His grace is strong enough to hold us even when our own grip fails.

Therefore, the journey through the psychology of Scripture does not end with a neat, resolved conclusion where all pain is erased. It ends with a sober, realistic, yet profoundly hopeful vision. It ends with the understanding that the life of faith is not a bypass around the valley of the shadow of death, but a journey straight through it. And we are able to walk this path without fear, not because the valley is any less dark, but because we have the testimony of prophets, kings, apostles, and the Son of God Himself that we do not walk it alone. The God of the Scriptures is the God who meets us in the darkness, who hears our laments, who tends to our bodies, who whispers to our souls, and whose power is made perfect not in the absence of our weakness, but in its very midst. This is the hope that does not disappoint—a hope rooted not in the cessation of our struggle, but in the character of the God who walks with us in it.

CHAPTER 10

The Philippians 4:8 Principle: Cognitive Stewardship and the Battle for the Mind

Beloved, we now turn our attention to one of the most critical and contested arenas of our embodied stewardship: the human mind. If the body is the temple of the Holy Spirit, then the mind is its inner sanctum, the command center from which the whole of our existence—our affections, our decisions, our words, and our actions—is directed. For too long, the Church has often ceded the territory of the mind to secular psychology, treating it as a neutral space or, worse, as a purely biological machine. But Scripture unveils a far more dramatic and urgent reality: the Christian life is not a passive state of being, but an active, relentless war of worldviews, fought primarily on the battlefield of the mind. It is a cosmic conflict between the kingdom of light and the kingdom of darkness, and the primary beachhead in this war for every individual believer is the space between their own ears.

10.1 Introduction: The Mind as a Sanctified Battlefield

The Apostle Paul, a spiritual general who understood the topography of this conflict better than most, issues a foundational military command in his letter to the Romans: "Do not be conformed to this world, but be transformed by the renewal of your mind, that by testing you may discern what is the will of God, what is good and acceptable and perfect" (Romans 12:2). This verse is a theological declaration of war against passivity. The "world" (*aion*), meaning the present age with its fallen patterns, values, and systems of thought, exerts a constant, conforming pressure upon us. It seeks to squeeze us into its mold, to shape our thinking according to the principles of autonomy, materialism, sensuality, and cynicism. This conformity is not primarily about external behavior; it is about internal cognition. It is about accepting the world's narratives about identity, success, happiness, and truth.

Against this relentless pressure, Paul commands not a minor adjustment, but a radical "transformation" (*metamorphoō*), a word that denotes a change of essential form, as profound as a caterpillar's metamorphosis into a butterfly. And he locates the engine of this transformation squarely in "the renewal of your mind" (*tē anakainōsei tou noos*). The Greek word for "renewal" (*anakainōsis*) implies a continual, back-to-the-source kind of renovation. It is not a one-time event at conversion, but an ongoing process of having the mind restored, refreshed, and recalibrated according to its original, creational design in the *Imago Dei*. This renewal is the prerequisite for true discernment. A mind still patterned after the world cannot accurately discern the will of God. It will misinterpret His character, misunderstand His commands, and mistake cultural trends for divine leading.

Therefore, we must posit that **cognitive stewardship—the intentional, prayerful, and disciplined management of our thought life—is a non-negotiable spiritual discipline.** It is as essential to the health of the soul as prayer, fasting, and the study of Scripture, because it is the very mechanism through which these other disciplines take root and produce fruit. To neglect the stewardship of our thoughts is to leave the gates of the city undefended, allowing the enemy to plant his lies, his fears, and his accusations deep within our cognitive framework. It is to allow the "spirit of the age" to build strongholds—fortified patterns of thinking—that stand opposed to the knowledge of God (2 Corinthians 10:4-5).

In this great battle for the mind, the world offers its own solutions. One of the most prominent and effective in secular psychology is Cognitive Behavioral Therapy (CBT). CBT operates on the sound principle that our emotions and behaviors are largely determined by our thoughts, or "cognitions." It teaches individuals to identify their "automatic negative thoughts" and to challenge the cognitive distortions—like catastrophizing, black-and-white thinking, and overgeneralization—that lead to emotional distress. There is much to appreciate in this model, as it reflects the general revelation of how God has wired the human person.

However, the biblical approach, supremely encapsulated in Philippians 4:8, offers something far more profound and foundational than CBT. It provides a **divine protocol for cognitive renewal** that transcends the secular model in two crucial ways. First, while CBT is ultimately a self-help technique aimed at achieving personal emotional equilibrium, the Philippians 4:8 principle is an act of worship aimed at knowing and glorifying God. Its goal is not merely to feel better, but to think truly—to align our minds with the ultimate reality of God's character and His created order. Second, and most importantly, Philippians 4:8 grounds its cognitive framework not in subjective, therapeutic utility, but in objective, transcendent reality. The secular therapist asks, "Is this thought helpful?" The Apostle Paul commands, "Is this thought *true*? Is it honorable? Is it just? Is it pure? Is it lovely? Is it commendable? Does it have virtue? Is it worthy of praise?" These are not subjective categories of mental comfort; they are objective attributes rooted in the very nature of God Himself. We are to dwell on these things not because they make us less anxious (though they often do), but because they reflect the reality of the Kingdom we serve. This is cognitive stewardship baptized into Christ—a deliberate, Spirit-empowered effort to tear down every mental argument that sets itself up against the knowledge of God and to take every thought captive to obey Christ (2 Corinthians 10:5). The mind is not a neutral space; it is a sanctified battlefield, and Philippians 4:8 is our divine field manual for its liberation.

10.2 Exegetical Foundation: The Context of Peace in Philippians 4:4-9

Beloved, to wield the powerful weapon of Philippians 4:8 with precision and spiritual force, we must first understand its place in the apostle's strategic argument. The command to dwell on whatever is true, honorable, just, pure, lovely, commendable, excellent, and praiseworthy is not a free-floating piece of spiritual advice, a mere cognitive technique for positive thinking. It is, rather, the powerful, culminating application in a carefully constructed logical and theological sequence that begins in verse 4. To pluck verse 8 from this rich soil is to risk turning it into a new law, a checklist for mental purity that we strive for in our own strength. But when we see it as the Spirit-inspired conclusion to a progression of grace, it becomes a liberating and achievable pathway to a guarded and peaceful mind. Let us, therefore, walk deliberately through this sequence, for each step is a divine prerequisite for the next, building a fortress of peace around the soul.

The foundation of the entire structure is laid in verse 4 with the command, **"Rejoice in the Lord always; again I will say, rejoice."** This is the bedrock upon which all cognitive stewardship is built. Notice carefully the object and the constancy of this command. The object is not in our circumstances, which are as changeable as the wind, but "in the Lord." Our joy is anchored in the unchanging character, the finished work, and the sovereign faithfulness of Jesus Christ. This is a volitional, theological joy, not an emotional reaction. It is a conscious choice to find our delight and our identity in who God is, regardless of what is happening around us or within us. The doubling of the command, "again I will say, rejoice," underscores its non-negotiable importance and its difficulty. It is the defiant act of the will that declares, "Even here, in this prison cell, facing potential death, my joy is found in the Lord, and therefore it cannot be taken from me." This God-centered rejoicing is the fuel for the renewed mind. A mind focused on its own anxieties cannot rejoice; a mind rejoicing in the Lord cannot remain captive to those anxieties for long.

From this foundation of volitional joy flows the next characteristic: **"Let your reasonableness be known to everyone. The Lord is at hand" (v.5).** The Greek word translated "reasonableness" (*epieikes*) is profound and difficult to capture in a single English word. It signifies a gentle forbearance, a gracious fairness, a magnanimity of spirit that does not insist on its own rights for the sake of peace. It is the opposite of a rigid, harsh, or combative demeanor. How does this relate to the mind? A mind that is truly rejoicing in the sovereignty and goodness of the Lord is liberated from the need to be defensive, to control outcomes, or to prove itself right. It can afford to be gentle, because its security is not in its own intellectual prowess or its ability to win an argument, but in the nearness of the Lord. "The Lord is at hand" is the reason for this reasonableness. It is the reminder of both His imminent return and His ever-present help. This gentle, reasonable disposition is the first visible fruit of a mind that is being renewed and anchored in joyful trust.

This leads us directly to the pivotal battlefield command in verse 6: **"Do not be anxious about anything, but in everything by prayer and supplication with thanksgiving let your requests be made known to God."** Here, Paul moves from the general disposition to the specific, universal human experience of anxiety. The command "do not be anxious" (*mēden merimnate*) is not a simplistic dismissal of a complex emotion. It is a call to action. The Greek present imperative here, used with a negative, often means to stop an action already in progress. "Stop continuing to be anxious." But how? The antidote is not willpower or positive thinking. The antidote is worship. Paul provides the divine methodology: "but in everything by prayer and supplication with thanksgiving let your requests be made known to God."

This is a three-part spiritual transaction. First, **prayer and supplication**—this is the act of transfer. It is the conscious, verbal unloading of our burdens, our fears, and our "what-ifs" onto the shoulders of the One who is strong enough to bear them. It is the practical outworking of casting all our anxiety on Him, because He cares for us (1 Peter 5:7). Second, and critically, **with thanksgiving**—this is the act of recalibration. Thanksgiving is the lens of faith that looks at a troubling situation and, even before it is resolved, thanks God for His character, His past faithfulness, and His promise to work all things for good. It is the spiritual warfare that disarms anxiety by focusing on the evidence of grace. This prayerful, thankful transfer is the mechanism that actively displaces anxious thoughts.

The glorious result of this transaction is described in verse 7: **"And the peace of God, which surpasses all understanding, will guard your hearts and your minds in Christ Jesus."** This is not merely a feeling of calm; it is a divine, supernatural impartation. This peace "surpasses all understanding"—it transcends human logic and circumstance. It is a peace that can exist even in the midst of the storm. And its function is active and military: it "will guard" your hearts and minds. The Greek word *phroureō* means to garrison, to stand guard as a sentinel, to protect by a military presence. The peace of God does not just gently soothe; it actively stations itself at the gates of our heart (the seat of our affections and will) and our mind (the seat of our intellect and thoughts). It screens the incoming traffic of worries, fears, and lies, and it contains the internal turmoil, preventing it from spiraling out of control.

It is in this context—a context of volitional joy, gracious reasonableness, prayerful transfer, and a garrisoned peace—

that we finally arrive at the command of verse 8. **Philippians 4:8 is the proactive, ongoing strategy for maintaining this garrisoned peace.** It is the daily discipline that reinforces the guard. If verses 6-7 are about what to do *when* anxiety assaults the gates, verse 8 is about how to fortify the citadel *so that* it is less vulnerable to assault. It is the positive programming of the mind that crowds out the space where anxious and corrupting thoughts would otherwise take root. The command to dwell on the things that are true, honorable, just, pure, lovely, commendable, excellent, and praiseworthy is the means by which we actively, intelligently, and spiritually cooperate with the guarding peace of God. It is the mental hygiene that ensures the garrison has a clean, well-provisioned, and defensible position to hold. The sequence is therefore a complete system: Rejoice to establish your footing, be reasonable as your outward testimony, transfer anxiety through thankful prayer to receive God's garrisoning peace, and proactively guard that peace by diligently curating the content of your thoughts. This is the exegetical foundation that transforms a list of virtues from an impossible ideal into a grace-empowered pathway to a mind kept secure in Christ Jesus.

10.3 A Theological and Psychological Analysis of the Philippians 4:8 Virtues

Beloved, having established the strategic context of peace in which the command of Philippians 4:8 is given, we must now drill down into the profound theological and psychological richness of the virtues themselves. This is not a random list of positive adjectives. It is a divinely-inspired taxonomy of thought, a comprehensive curriculum for the renewed mind. Each term represents a specific category of cognition that, when deliberately cultivated, aligns the inner workings of our consciousness with the very character of God and the fundamental fabric of His Kingdom. To dwell on these things is to mentally inhabit the reality of the New Creation, even while we physically reside in the present evil age. Let us examine each virtue with the care and reverence it deserves, for in them we find the architecture of a sanctified intellect.

First and foundational is the command to dwell on **Whatever is True (*alēthē*)**. In our postmodern age, truth has been tragically reduced to subjective preference, to "my truth" versus "your truth." But the biblical concept of truth is robustly objective and ontological. It refers to that which is real, genuine, and in accordance with actual fact as defined by God Himself. Jesus, in His high priestly prayer, defines it unequivocally: "Sanctify them in the truth; your word is truth" (John 17:17). Therefore, to think about what is *true* is, first and foremost, to saturate the mind with the propositions, narratives, and wisdom of Scripture. It is to measure every thought, every idea, and every piece of information we encounter against the plumb line of God's self-revelation. This demands a ruthless intellectual integrity and a courageous rejection of falsehood in all its forms—from the subtle self-deceptions we tell ourselves to the grand cultural lies and conspiracy theories that swirl around us. The psychological impact is one of profound stability. A mind anchored in objective truth is not tossed about by every new cultural trend or emotional storm. It possesses a cognitive anchor, a fixed point of reference that provides clarity and discernment. Cognitive Behavioral Therapy rightly identifies "distorted thinking" as a source of emotional distress; the biblical mandate goes deeper, calling us to ground our thinking not just in helpful patterns, but in the ultimate reality of God's Word. Stewardship of the mind begins here, with a relentless love for and pursuit of truth.

Second, we are to dwell on **Whatever is Honorable (*semnos*)**. This Greek word carries a sense of dignity, gravity, reverence, and moral weight. It describes something that is worthy of respect and veneration. To think about what is honorable is to cultivate a mind that is elevated, that considers things of substance and nobility. It is the conscious choice to direct our mental energy toward that which is dignified over that which is trivial, toward that which is reverent over that which is flippant, toward that which is weighty over that which is frivolous. This is the direct antithesis of the spirit of our age, which is often characterized by cynicism, gossip, sarcasm, and a crudity that degrades human dignity. When we fill our minds with the honorable—with biographies of noble saints, with literature that explores profound themes of sacrifice and courage, with music that lifts the soul heavenward—we are training our cognitive faculties to appreciate and aspire to greatness. Psychologically, this practice builds a mental immune system. A mind accustomed to the honorable will naturally recoil from the dishonorable, the crude, and the degrading. It fosters a sense of personal dignity and respect for others, as we begin to see people and ideas through a lens of God-given value and potential.

Third, the apostle commands us to dwell on **Whatever is Just (*dikaios*)**. This term pertains to righteousness, fairness, and right relationships. It is the principle of divine justice applied to our cognitive world. To think justly is to habitually consider the rights of others, to evaluate situations with fairness, and to align our internal judgments with God's moral law. It involves mentally championing the cause of the oppressed, evaluating our own motives with impartiality, and rejecting thoughts of prejudice, favoritism, or selfish advantage. A mind that dwells on justice is a mind that is actively engaged in the *Shalom* of God, which is fundamentally about right relationships. Psychologically, this protects us from the toxins of bitterness, envy, and a critical spirit. When we are wronged, the natural cognitive response is to dwell on the injustice, to rehearse the offense, and to nurse thoughts of vengeance. The discipline of dwelling on what is just calls us to a higher court—to entrust final judgment to God (Romans 12:19) while simultaneously filling our minds with thoughts of His perfect righteousness and His commands to act justly, love mercy, and walk humbly (Micah 6:8). This reorients our mental energy from being victims of injustice to being agents of God's justice in the world.

Fourth, and with piercing relevance to our hypersexualized culture, is the command to dwell on **Whatever is Pure (*hagnos*)**. This word denotes moral purity, chastity, holiness, and cleanliness. It calls for a rigorous custody of the eyes and the imagination. To think on what is pure is to actively guard the gates of the mind against any thought, image, or fantasy that would defile the temple of the Holy Spirit. This is a conscious war against lust, envy, greed, and any form of mental corruption. It is not merely the absence of dirty thoughts, but the active cultivation of a clean and holy imagination. This involves filling our minds with the purity of Christ, meditating on His spotless character, and consuming media that reflects moral integrity rather than exploiting brokenness. The psychological benefit is immense. Impure thoughts create cognitive dissonance, guilt, and shame, and they can forge powerful neural pathways of addiction. The discipline of purity, by contrast, brings mental clarity, integrity, and a profound sense of peace. It aligns our secret inner world with our public confession, creating a unified and integrated self that is not fractured by hidden sin.

Fifth, we are invited to dwell on **Whatever is Lovely (*prosphilēs*)**. This delightful term means pleasing, agreeable, amiable, or attractive. It is an invitation to appreciate beauty, grace, and kindness. God is the source of all beauty, and to dwell on the lovely is to trace the echoes of His character in His creation and in acts of human virtue. It is the cultivation of a disposition that actively looks for and finds delight in what is excellent and attractive—in a breathtaking landscape, a work of art that reflects divine glory, a gesture of kindness, or a melody that stirs the soul. This is the antidote to a critical, negative, and cynical spirit. A mind trained to see the lovely will find reasons for gratitude and joy even in a fallen world. Psychologically, this practice is a powerful combatant against depression and anxiety. It actively counters the brain's natural negativity bias by directing our attention to the evidence of God's goodness and grace that still permeates a groaning creation. It is the cognitive discipline of hope, teaching us to see the first rays of dawn while still in the night.

Finally, we are to dwell on **Whatever is Commendable (*euphēmos*)**. This word refers to that which is well-spoken of, of good report, or praiseworthy. It directs our mental attention to stories of virtue, acts of courage, examples of faith, and narratives of redemption. In a media ecosystem that is overwhelmingly drawn to scandal, conflict, and depravity, this is a radical act of cognitive resistance. It means deliberately seeking out and meditating on news of moral courage, selfless service, and artistic excellence. It involves sharing stories of God's faithfulness within the community of believers and reflecting on the testimonies of the saints throughout history.

Psychologically, this practice shapes our identity and our aspirations. We become what we behold. By filling our minds with the commendable, we are strengthening our connection to the great cloud of witnesses and building a mental repertoire of positive examples to guide our own choices. It fosters encouragement and builds faith, reminding us that God is at work and that virtue is possible, even in a dark world.

Together, these six virtues form a comprehensive cognitive diet. They are not a passive list but an active filter and a proactive pursuit. They provide the specific, concrete content for the renewed mind, outlining precisely what kinds of thoughts are worthy to occupy the sacred space between our ears, the very dwelling place of the Spirit of Christ.

10.4 The Cognitive-Behavioral Cycle in Pauline Theology

Beloved, as we delve deeper into the mechanics of cognitive stewardship, we discover a profound resonance between the inspired wisdom of the Apostle Paul and a core principle of modern psychology, yet Paul's framework is set upon a far more secure and transcendent foundation. The principle enshrined in Philippians 4:8 is not a static command to "think happy thoughts"; it is the linchpin in a dynamic, Spirit-empowered cognitive-behavioral cycle that is deeply embedded in Pauline theology. This cycle describes the process by which our thoughts, when brought into captivity to Christ, shape our beliefs, which in turn direct our actions, which then reinforce our thought patterns. It is the God-ordained process of sanctification applied to the very architecture of our minds.

The first and most critical phase of this cycle is the **Active Captivity of Thoughts**, as articulated with military precision in 2 Corinthians 10:5: "We destroy arguments and every lofty opinion raised against the knowledge of God, and take every thought captive to obey Christ." This verse unveils the reality of the mind as a spiritual battlefield. The "arguments" (*logismous*) and "lofty opinions" (*hypsōma*) represent sophisticated systems of thought, deeply entrenched worldviews, and high-minded speculations that are inherently hostile to the gospel. These are not mere intellectual disagreements; they are fortifications, strongholds (*ochyrōma*) erected by the enemy within our cognitive landscape.

The Pauline strategy is twofold: destruction and captivity. We are to *destroy* these strongholds, to tear down the lies and pretensions that have taken root. This is not a passive process. It is an act of violent, spiritual warfare, accomplished through the divine power of the Holy Spirit and the truth of God's Word. But Paul does not stop there. He commands us to *take every thought captive*. The Greek word *aichmalōtizō* means to lead away as a prisoner of war. This is the moment-by-moment discipline of cognitive stewardship. It is the practice of intercepting the constant stream of mental activity—the automatic negative thoughts (ANTs), the fearful speculations, the lustful imaginations, the bitter rehearsals—and subjecting them to immediate scrutiny and arrest.

In modern cognitive-behavioral therapy (CBT), this is akin to the practice of "thought catching" and "cognitive restructuring," where one learns to identify distorted thinking and challenge it with more realistic and balanced thoughts. But Paul's model is infinitely more robust. The standard for this captivity is not mere "realism" or "helpfulness," but obedience to Christ. Each thought is to be dragged before the throne of Christ and His Word and asked: "Do you align with the truth of God? Do you promote the honor of God? Are you consistent with the character of Christ?" A thought of self-condemnation must be held against the truth of "no condemnation for those in Christ Jesus" (Romans 8:1). A thought of anxiety about the future must be captive to the promise that "my God will supply every need of yours according to his riches in glory in Christ Jesus" (Philippians 4:19). This is not positive thinking; it is prophetic thinking. It is evaluating our internal narrative against the external, objective reality of God's revelation. This disciplined, active captivity is the necessary precondition for the positive cultivation commanded in Philippians 4:8. You cannot fill a mind that is already overflowing with captive, rebellious thoughts. You must first clear the ground through spiritual warfare.

Once the mind is being actively cleansed through this captivity, the second phase of the cycle can flourish: **The Renewed Mind Leading to Transformed Action.** This is the glorious outcome promised in Romans 12:2: "Do not be conformed to this world, but be transformed by the renewal of your mind. Then you will be able to test and approve what God's will is—his good, pleasing and perfect will." The transformation (*metamorphoō*) of our entire life—our habits, our relationships, our choices—is explicitly linked to the renewal of the mind. The mind is the control center. What is nurtured in the cognitive realm will inevitably manifest in the behavioral realm.

A mind that is consistently dwelling on what is true, honorable, just, pure, lovely, and commendable (Philippians 4:8) becomes a mind that is uniquely calibrated to "discern the will of God." This discernment is not a mystical feeling, but a rational, Spirit-led judgment. When a decision is to be made, the renewed mind, saturated with the categories of God's Kingdom, can instinctively recognize which path aligns with truth, which option promotes justice, which choice guards purity. For example, a person whose mind is habitually filled with God's truth will be less likely to believe the deceptive allure of a get-rich-quick scheme. A person whose mind dwells on what is just will be quick to recognize and oppose an unfair business practice. A person whose mind is trained on purity will instinctively turn away from a compromising situation.

This creates a powerful, self-reinforcing cycle. **Right thinking, according to the Philippians 4:8 standard, leads to right living.** And right living, in turn, produces experiential confirmation of God's goodness and faithfulness, which then reinforces the original right thinking. When you choose integrity over deceit because your mind is filled with the love of truth, you experience the peace and stability that comes from honesty. This peace then validates the initial cognitive choice, making it easier and more natural to choose truth the next time. Conversely, sinful behavior often begins with a tolerated sinful thought. A thought of envy, if not taken captive, can fester into a mindset of resentment, which may then erupt in gossip or slander, leading to broken relationships and a guilty conscience, which then pollutes the mind with further negative thoughts. The cognitive-behavioral cycle is inescapable; the only choice is whether it will be a virtuous cycle of renewal or a vicious cycle of corruption.

Therefore, the Pauline model presents a comprehensive and dynamic view of sanctification. It begins with the aggressive, disciplinary work of tearing down strongholds and taking every thought prisoner to Christ. It continues with the proactive, nurturing work of filling the liberated mind with the noble, virtuous, and praiseworthy things of God. And it culminates in a transformed life capable of discerning and delighting in the perfect will of God. This is not a self-help program; it is a Spirit-empowered cooperation with grace. We are called to the active duty of cognitive stewardship, trusting that as we work to capture and renew our thoughts, God Himself is at work within us, both to will and to work for His good pleasure (Philippians 2:13), thereby completing the glorious cycle from redeemed thought to redeemed action.

10.5 Practical Disciplines for Cognitive Stewardship

Beloved, having grasped the profound theology and strategic importance of the renewed mind, we now face the most pressing question: How, practically and daily, do we wage this war? How do we move from understanding Philippians 4:8 to living it? The transformation of our cognitive landscape does not happen by accident or by mere intention. It requires the same disciplined, regular, and intentional effort as training the body or learning a skilled trade. The Holy Spirit provides the power, but we are called to provide the disciplined cooperation. The following practices are not a new law, but time-tested, grace-empowered disciplines—spiritual exercises—that create the conditions for the mind to be renewed and for the peace of God to stand guard.

First and foremost is the foundational discipline of **Scripture Memorization and Meditation.** If the mind is to be filled with what is true, honorable, just, pure, lovely, and commendable, then it must have a source for this content. The ultimate and infallible source is the very Word of God. Memorization is the act of transferring the truth of Scripture from the pages of a book into the very circuitry of our brains. It is creating a sacred "database" within our own minds, a reservoir of God's thoughts that is instantly accessible by the Holy Spirit for guidance, comfort, conviction, and warfare. When a thought of fear arises, the Spirit can bring to remembrance, "God gave us a spirit not of fear but of power and love and self-control" (2 Timothy 1:7). When a thought of lust assaults, the memorized word declares, "How can a young man keep his way pure? By guarding it according to your word" (Psalm 119:9).

But memorization alone is not enough; it must be coupled with *meditation*. The Hebrew word for meditate, *hagah*, means to murmur, to mutter, to speak under one's breath. It implies a slow, repetitive, reflective chewing on the Word, much like a ruminant animal chews its cud. This is the practice described in Psalm 1, where the blessed man's "delight is in the law of the LORD, and on his law he meditates day and night." Meditation is the process of taking a memorized verse or passage and turning it over and over in the mind, asking questions of it, praying it back to God, applying it to specific situations, and allowing its truth to seep from the intellect down into the affections and the will. This is not transcendental meditation that seeks to empty the mind; it is biblical meditation that seeks to fill the mind with God. It is the active implementation of Philippians 4:8, where the content of our meditation is, by its divine nature, inherently true, honorable, just, pure, and commendable. This discipline systematically rewires our neural pathways, gradually replacing the world's default narratives with the story of God's redemption.

A second vital discipline is **The Prayer of Examen.** This ancient practice, refined in the Ignatian tradition, is a powerful tool for cultivating self-awareness and inviting the Holy Spirit's light into the hidden corners of our cognitive life. It is a structured, daily time of prayerful reflection, typically practiced at the end of the day, with the specific purpose of discerning God's presence and activity in the events of the day and in our internal responses to them. The Examen involves several steps, but for the purpose of cognitive stewardship, we focus on the review of thoughts and feelings.

In a quiet moment, we place ourselves in God's presence and ask Him for the light of His Spirit to see ourselves as He sees us. We then review the day, hour by hour or event by event, not to wallow in guilt, but to observe with curiosity and humility. We ask: *When did I feel the most peace today? What thought was I dwelling on? When did I feel the most anxiety, anger, or despondency? What specific thought triggered that feeling?* We invite the Lord to reveal patterns: "Lord, show me the recurring thoughts that do not align with Your truth. Reveal the 'lofty opinions' I have allowed to remain uncaptured." This is not narcissistic navel-gazing; it is a spiritual inventory conducted with a divine Partner. It allows us to catch the automatic negative thoughts (ANTs) we missed in the moment and to bring them to the cross for forgiveness and cleansing. It transforms our internal world from a chaotic, unexamined space into a sanctuary where God is invited to be the diagnostician and healer of our thought life.

Third, we must engage in the discipline of **Curated Media Consumption.** We live in an unprecedented age of information bombardment. Our minds are constantly being shaped by a torrent of input from news outlets, social media feeds, streaming services, and podcasts. The principle of "garbage in, garbage out" is a psychological and spiritual reality. We cannot naively consume a diet of cynicism, violence, sensuality, and fear-mongering and then wonder why our minds are filled with anxiety, lust, and despair. The practice of curated consumption is the active, prayerful application of the Philippians 4:8 grid to everything we allow into our minds.

This requires asking hard questions before we click, watch, or listen: *Is this source fundamentally committed to truth, or to sensationalism? Does this movie/TV show celebrate what is honorable and pure, or does it glamorize what is degrading and sinful? Does this social media feed promote what is lovely and commendable, or does it thrive on outrage, envy, and division?* This is not a call to a naive withdrawal from the world, but to a wise and discerning engagement with it. It means we may need to unfollow certain accounts, cancel certain subscriptions, or fast from certain forms of entertainment for a season. It means choosing to read literature that ennobles the human spirit, to listen to music that points toward transcendence, and to watch films that tell stories of redemption. This discipline acknowledges that our cognitive environment is a formative ecosystem, and we are called to be faithful stewards of that ecosystem, weeding out the toxic and planting the life-giving.

Finally, a profoundly simple yet transformative discipline is **Gratitude Journaling.** The command in 1 Thessalonians 5:18 to "give thanks in all circumstances" is, at its core, a cognitive command. It is a directive to actively seek out and acknowledge the evidence of God's grace, even in the midst of difficulty. Gratitude journaling is the practical, tangible outworking of this command. It is the daily discipline of writing down, by hand, three to five specific things for which one is grateful.

This practice is a powerful subset of dwelling on the "commendable" and the "lovely." It systematically forces a cognitive shift. Our brains have a natural negativity bias, a tendency to notice and remember threats and problems more easily than blessings. Gratitude journaling actively counteracts this bias. It trains the mind to scan the environment not for threats, but for gifts. It moves God from the periphery of our awareness to the center, as we recognize His hand in the small beauties and daily provisions of life. Neuroscientifically, this practice has been shown to activate the brain's reward centers and increase levels of dopamine and serotonin, the neurotransmitters associated with well-being. Theologically, it is an act of worship that acknowledges God as the source of every good and perfect gift (James 1:17). By ending each day by cataloging God's faithfulness, we are proactively filling our minds with commendable thoughts, reinforcing the guarding peace of God, and strengthening our faith for the challenges of tomorrow. It is a small, daily act of cognitive stewardship that, over time, can produce a seismic shift in our entire outlook on life, anchoring us ever more firmly in the goodness of our God.

10.6 Case Study: Applying the Filter

Beloved, let us now move from theory to the trenches. Let us witness the Philippians 4:8 filter in action, not as an abstract concept, but as a practical, moment-by-moment spiritual weapon in a common human struggle: a sudden, gripping thought of anxiety. Imagine the scenario: you are facing a significant professional challenge—a major presentation, a critical project deadline, a performance review. Without warning, a thought, sharp and invasive, pierces the peace of your mind: **"I am going to fail at this, and it will lead to my complete ruin."**

This is not a casual worry; it is a cognitive spear, laden with emotional poison. In the old, unrenewed pattern, this thought would be allowed to run rampant. It would trigger a cascade of physiological fear responses—racing heart, tense muscles—and spawn a host of related catastrophic thoughts about financial collapse, professional humiliation, and personal worthlessness. The mind, left undefended, becomes a theater for a horror movie of its own making. But for the cognitive steward, trained in the discipline of taking thoughts captive, this moment is not a defeat; it is the call to battle. The garrison peace of God has detected an intruder, and the sentinel of the will, empowered by the Spirit, now moves to intercept it.

The first and most critical action is to **arrest the thought.** Instead of allowing it to morph into a full-blown narrative of despair, the steward consciously halts its progress. This is the application of 2 Corinthians 10:5. The thought is identified, named, and isolated: "This is a thought of catastrophic anxiety. I am now going to take it captive." It is dragged from the shadowy recesses of passive fear into the bright light of conscious, critical examination. The Philippians 4:8 filter becomes the divine interrogation protocol.

The steward begins the interrogation, systematically applying each criterion:

Is this thought TRUE (*alēthē*)? This is the foundational question. The steward confronts the thought's core assertion: "Is failure an absolute, foregone certainty?" The answer, rationally, is no. It is a possibility, but not a certainty. The thought presents a feared future as an unalterable fact, which is a classic cognitive distortion known as "fortune-telling." The steward then counteracts with a higher truth from the database of Scripture: "What is God's promise in this situation?" A verse like Philippians 4:19 comes to mind: "And my God will supply every need of yours according to his riches in glory in Christ Jesus." The promise is not for success as the world defines it, but for provision. The truthful reality is that my ultimate security does not rest on this outcome, but on the covenant faithfulness of my God. The thought of ruin is exposed as a lie, because it ignores the overarching providence and provision of God.

Is this thought HONORABLE (*semnos*)? The steward now evaluates the thought's dignity. "Does this thought, 'I am a failure headed for ruin,' dignify my status as a redeemed child of the King of the universe?" The answer is a resounding no. It is a degrading, dishonorable thought that reduces a person made in the image of God, indwelt by the Holy Spirit, and destined for eternal glory to a mere victim of circumstance. It is a thought utterly devoid of the nobility and gravity that should characterize the inner life of a saint. To dwell on it is to engage in cognitive self-degradation.

Is this thought JUST (*dikaios*)? Here, the steward assesses the thought's fairness, particularly toward God. "Is it fair, is it right, to entertain a thought that functionally accuses God of abandonment? Given His track record of faithfulness throughout my life and throughout salvation history, is it just to assume He will fail me now?" This thought puts God on trial and finds Him guilty of negligence before the evidence has even been presented. It is a profound injustice against the character of a faithful God. It violates the principle of right relationship with a Father who has proven His love definitively on the cross.

Is this thought PURE (*hagnos*)? The steward examines the thought's moral quality. "Is this thought pure, or is it mixed with the contaminating impurity of unbelief?" Anxiety, at its root, is often a form of practical unbelief—a failure to trust God's goodness, power, and wisdom in a given situation. The thought "I will be ruined" is saturated with the impurity of distrust. It defiles the mind by introducing the toxic element of doubt regarding God's sovereign care. It is a foreign substance that pollutes the temple of the Spirit.

Is this thought LOVELY (*prosphilēs*)? The steward considers the thought's aesthetic quality. "Is this a beautiful, agreeable, or pleasing thought? Does it bring a sense of peace or a sense of dread?" The thought of ruin is intrinsically ugly. It is dissonant, jarring, and destructive to inner harmony. It is the opposite of the lovely peace that Christ offers. A mind filled with such thoughts cannot be a place of beauty or rest.

Is this thought COMMENDABLE (*euphēmos*)? Finally, the steward evaluates the thought's edifying potential. "Is this a thought worth sharing? If I were to voice this to a struggling brother or sister in Christ, would it build them up in faith, or would it drag them down into fear? Is it of good report?" The thought of imminent ruin is not commendable. It is a narrative of despair that, if shared, would spread anxiety rather than faith. It fails the test of corporate usefulness.

Having exposed the anxious thought as a false, dishonorable, unjust, impure, ugly, and unhelpful intruder, the steward does not merely reject it. Nature abhors a vacuum, and so does the mind. **The final, crucial step is active replacement.** The captive thought is evicted, and a truthful, God-honoring counterpart is deliberately installed in its place. The steward, drawing on the memorized Word, might consciously choose to dwell on a new thought: **"My God is in control, and He will provide for all my needs according to His glorious riches in**

Christ Jesus. My identity and security are in Him, not in this outcome."

This new thought is then run through the same filter: It is *true* (based on Scripture). It is *honorable* (it dignifies God's sovereignty and my identity in Christ). It is *just* (it gives God the trust He is due). It is *pure* (it is rooted in faith). It is *lovely* (it brings a sense of peace and order). It is *commendable* (it is a testimony of faith that would encourage others). This is the practice of cognitive stewardship in its fullest expression—not just a defensive battle against lies, but an offensive campaign to occupy the mind with the liberating truth of the Gospel. Each time this process is undertaken, a stronghold is weakened, a neural pathway is rerouted, and the mind is progressively renewed into the likeness of Christ, who, in the face of the ultimate trial, entrusted Himself to Him who judges justly.

10.7 Conclusion: The Guarded Mind and the God of Peace

Beloved, as we culminate our deep excavation of the Philippians 4:8 principle, we arrive at the glorious synthesis of its promise and its purpose. This disciplined practice of cognitive stewardship is revealed to be nothing less than the God-ordained, Spirit-empowered methodology for maintaining and cultivating the very "peace of God" promised in the preceding verses. It is the active, human response that cooperates with the divine grace which stands guard over our inner being. We must be utterly clear: this is not, as the world practices, a technique of "positive thinking." Positive thinking is a subjective and often fragile endeavor to manipulate one's emotional state by focusing on pleasant but potentially unfounded optimism. It is a house built on the sand of personal sentiment. The Philippians

4:8 mandate, by stark contrast, is the rigorous discipline of **truth-based thinking**. Its foundation is not the shifting sands of how we feel, but the unshakable bedrock of who God is, what He has declared, and the inherent nature of His creation and His Kingdom. We are not called to think positively about a situation; we are called to think truly about it, viewing it through the transcendent, objective realities of God's truth, justice, purity, and beauty.

This truth-based cognitive stewardship is the practical engine of the mind's renewal that Paul commands in Romans 12:2. It is the "how" of that transformation. The mind is not renewed by a passive, mystical osmosis. It is renewed through the active, deliberate, and repeated choice to dwell upon, to marinate in, to analyze and appreciate the things of God. Every time a believer, empowered by the Spirit, intercepts a lie and replaces it with God's truth, a small but significant renovation occurs in the cognitive structure. Every moment spent meditating on what is honorable and just, rather than on what is cynical and corrupt, is a moment spent scrubbing the mind clean of the world's grime and restoring the luster of the *Imago Dei*. This is not a one-time event but a lifelong process of cultivation. It is the mental equivalent of tending a garden. We cannot merely pray for a beautiful garden; we must pull the weeds of falsehood and plant the seeds of virtue. The Philippians 4:8 virtues are the divine seed packets, and the discipline of dwelling on them is the faithful act of planting and watering, trusting that God Himself will give the growth (1 Corinthians 3:7).

The outcome of this diligent cultivation is a transformed cognitive environment. A mind consistently nourished on truth, honor, justice, purity, loveliness, and excellence becomes a habitat where faith naturally flourishes. Faith, as Hebrews 11:1

tells us, is the assurance of things hoped for, the conviction of things not seen. This assurance and conviction are cognitive acts. They are firm beliefs held in the mind against contrary evidence. A mind saturated with the reality of God's character and promises is a mind that finds it increasingly natural to trust Him. The "substance" of faith becomes more real to the mind than the visible circumstances. Conversely, in this well-tended mental environment, anxiety withers. Anxiety is a parasite that feeds on uncertainty, falsehood, and catastrophic imagination. When the mind is fortified with truth, the food source for anxiety is cut off. When the imagination is filled with what is lovely and commendable, there is less room for the grotesque caricatures of fear to take root. The peace of God, which acts as a garrison, finds its task immeasurably easier when the city it guards is not in a state of constant internal rebellion and chaos, but is ordered, supplied, and aligned with the Kingdom of light.

This leads us to the ultimate, breathtaking promise that frames this entire discourse. The culmination of this practice is not merely a well-ordered mind or a peaceful emotional state, as desirable as those are. The culmination is the manifest presence of God Himself. Paul concludes this section not by saying "and the peace of God will be with you," but by making a profound theological declaration: **"and the God of peace will be with you" (Philippians 4:9).** This is a staggering escalation. We are promised not just a gift from God, but the Giver Himself. The "God of peace" is not a distant deity who sends a tranquil feeling from heaven. He is a Person who draws near, who takes up residence, who makes His home in the cognitive and emotional space that has been prepared for Him through obedience. The God of peace inhabits the environment of peace. When we, through the disciplined stewardship of our thoughts, create a mental sanctuary characterized by truth, honor, justice, purity, loveliness, and excellence, we are, in effect, preparing a throne room for the King. We are sweeping out the clutter of lies, fear, and impurity and furnishing the room with the beautiful furniture of His own character. And He, in His faithfulness, comes to dwell in that prepared place. His presence then becomes the ultimate source of our peace, the final guardian of our hearts and minds. The guarded mind and the God of peace are thus inextricably linked in a divine symbiosis: our cognitive obedience creates a habitat for His presence, and His presence consummates and perpetuates our peace. This is the glorious end of all true cognitive stewardship—not just a well-managed mind, but a mind inhabited by, and enthralled with, the God of peace.

CHAPTER 11

Spiritual Disciplines for Mental Resilience: Prayer, Meditation, and Contemplation

Beloved, we have now journeyed through the critical terrain of cognitive stewardship, learning to take every thought captive and to cultivate a mind fortified by the truth, beauty, and goodness of God's character. Yet, if our spiritual warfare were confined solely to the realm of conscious thought, we would be engaged in a battle of endless, exhausting mental effort. The mind, while a command center, is not an island. It is intimately connected to the deeper, often subconscious, currents of the soul—the wellspring of our affections, our fears, our longings, and our fundamental sense of identity and security. To build a truly resilient inner life, one capable of withstanding the relentless pressures of a fallen world, we must move beyond managing the *content* of our thoughts to shaping the very *posture* and *orientation* of our entire inner being. This sacred work is the domain of the ancient, often misunderstood, but profoundly essential spiritual disciplines of prayer, meditation, and contemplation.

11.1 Introduction: Fortifying the Inner Man

The modern approach to mental health often focuses on symptom management: techniques to reduce anxiety, strategies to counter depressive thoughts, and behaviors to improve mood. While these can be valuable tools of general grace, they often operate on a superficial level, like rearranging the furniture in a house with a crumbling foundation. The biblical vision for human flourishing is far more comprehensive and robust. It calls for the fortification of the entire "inner man," a Pauline phrase that encompasses the deepest core of our personhood—our spirit, our heart, our mind, and our will, all understood as an integrated whole (Ephesians 3:16). This inner man is the citadel of the soul, and its strength determines our capacity to endure suffering, to resist temptation, and to maintain joy and peace irrespective of external circumstances.

The spiritual disciplines of prayer, meditation, and contemplation are the God-ordained means for this fortification. To view them as esoteric exercises reserved for monks and mystics is to commit a grave error and to deprive oneself of essential spiritual nutrients. They are, in reality, intensely practical means of grace—channels through which God Himself, by His Spirit, strengthens, stabilizes, and secures our inner being. They are not about achieving a mystical state of bliss, but about realigning the fundamental orientation of our soul Godward, grounding our entire existence in the bedrock reality of His presence.

Consider the analogy of a tree. Cognitive stewardship is like carefully pruning the branches and ensuring the leaves are healthy—it deals with the visible, outward expressions. But the disciplines of prayer, meditation, and contemplation are about sinking the roots deep into the soil, drawing up water from hidden springs, and anchoring the tree so that when the storms of life—the winds of adversity, the droughts of despair, the floods of anxiety—come, it will not be toppled. They work at the level of our fundamental trust, our core identity, and our subconscious reliance.

Prayer, in its fullest sense, is more than a laundry list of requests; it is the lifeblood of relationship, the ongoing conversation that reorients our perspective from our problems to God's sovereignty. Meditation, distinct from its Eastern counterparts, is the deep, ruminative engagement with Scripture that allows truth to migrate from the head to the heart, transforming dogma into delight. Contemplation is the prayerful, wordless resting in the presence of God, the stilling of the soul to simply "behold" Him, allowing His beauty and majesty to recalibrate our affections and quiet our fears.

Together, these practices form a triad of resilience. They train the soul to find its rest not in the absence of trouble, but in the presence of God. They build what the old theologians called "habits of the heart"—ingrained patterns of dependence, trust, and worship that become our default setting in times of crisis. When anxiety arises, a soul trained in these disciplines does not merely try to counter a thought; it knows, from practiced experience, how to turn in dependent prayer, to recall a meditated-upon promise, and to rest in the contemplative awareness of a loving Father. This is not a quick fix; it is the slow, steady, and supernatural work of grace that fortifies the inner man, making him impervious to the superficial assaults of a transient world and grounding him in the eternal reality of the God who is our refuge and strength, an ever-present help in trouble (Psalm 46:1).

11.2 The Taxonomy of Prayer: Beyond Petition

Beloved, we must now expand our vision of prayer beyond the narrow confines of petition. While asking God for our needs is a vital and scriptural practice—commanded by Christ Himself in the Lord's Prayer—to limit our communion with the Divine to a list of requests is to reduce a symphonic relationship to a single, repetitive note. A robust and resilient inner life is cultivated through a full-orbed prayer life that engages every facet of our being with every facet of God's character. This is a taxonomy of prayer, a classification of different forms of divine communication, each designed by God to fortify a specific dimension of our soul and to build mental and emotional endurance. Let us explore these profound modalities, understanding that each is a unique means of grace for the weary and war-torn soul.

First, we return to **The Prayer of Examen (Review of the Day)**, a discipline we introduced in the context of cognitive stewardship, but whose depths we have not yet fully plumbed for emotional and psychological resilience. Developed by St. Ignatius of Loyola, the Examen is far more than a simple review of sins. It is a structured practice of prayerful awareness, a daily pilgrimage through the landscape of one's own heart in the compassionate light of the Holy Spirit. The classic Examen involves five movements: giving thanks for the day's gifts, petitioning for the light to see oneself as God sees, reviewing the day with curiosity and honesty, expressing sorrow for sin and gratitude for grace, and looking with hope toward the next day.

The psychological power of this discipline is immense. It is a divinely-sanctioned practice of emotional intelligence and integration. By systematically bringing the full spectrum of our daily experiences—the sudden joy, the flash of irritation, the quiet consolation, the subtle temptation, the sense of accomplishment, the pang of failure—into the safe and forgiving presence of God, we prevent the repression or denial of our emotional life. Repressed emotions do not disappear; they fester in the subconscious, emerging later as anxiety, depression, or unexplained outbursts of anger. The Examen provides a holy container for these experiences. It allows us to say, "Lord, I felt a surge of envy when my colleague was praised. I bring this to You. Show me the wound in my heart that this touches, and heal me with Your love." This process fosters psychosomatic integration, where the soul, the mind, and the emotions are brought into harmony under the lordship of Christ. It transforms the inner world from a chaotic battlefield of conflicting impulses into a ordered kingdom where the Prince of Peace reigns, bringing a profound sense of coherence and peace that is the very antithesis of mental fragmentation.

Second, we encounter **The Prayer of Recollection (Practicing the Presence)**, a discipline immortalized by Brother Lawrence, a 17th-century Carmelite lay brother. His profound insight was that our communion with God need not be confined to set times of formal prayer, but could become a continuous, living reality. The Prayer of Recollection is the conscious, habitual discipline of redirecting one's attention from the distractions of the task at hand to the reality of God's immediate presence. It is the mental and spiritual practice of "setting the LORD always before me" (Psalm 16:8).

In modern psychological terms, this is a form of "mindfulness," but with a crucial, transcendent object: the ever-present "I AM." The frantic, scattered nature of modern life, with its constant demands and digital interruptions, is a primary generator of anxiety. The mind, pulled in a dozen directions, loses its center and becomes a vortex of stress. The Prayer of Recollection is the spiritual technology that counters this fragmentation. By developing the habit of pausing, even for a second, amidst washing dishes, answering an email, or sitting in traffic, to acknowledge, "Lord, You are here with me in this moment," we perform a cognitive and spiritual reset. We are anchoring the soul not in the churning chaos of circumstance, but in the eternal, unchanging, and loving presence of God. This practice breaks the tyrannical power of anxiety by repeatedly asserting a greater reality than the presenting problem. It transforms mundane stress from a cause of distress into an opportunity for communion, sanctifying the ordinary and building a bedrock of stability that can withstand the tremors of daily life.

Third, we must embrace the often-neglected but biblically-rich practice of **Lament Prayer (Psalmic Expression)**. Nearly a third of the Psalter is comprised of laments, providing a God-given grammar for grief, anger, confusion, and despair. Lament is not a failure of faith; it is an act of faith—the faith that continues to address God even from the depths of the pit. A formal lament, as modeled in Psalms like 13, 22, and 88, typically follows a movement: an address to God, a passionate complaint, a request for help, an expression of trust, and a vow to praise.

This structure is profoundly therapeutic. It provides a sacred and structured outlet for the most powerful and potentially destructive human emotions. When grief or rage is left unexpressed, it turns inward, metastasizing into bitterness, cynicism, or clinical depression. Lament prayer externalizes this pain, directing it toward the only One who can ultimately bear it. It moves the soul from disorientation—the feeling that the world has come off its axis—to reorientation around the fixed point of God's covenant faithfulness. The act of vocalizing the complaint, of "arguing your case" before the Lord, as the prophets did, is a form of emotional and cognitive processing that prevents these energies from festering. It is the spiritual equivalent of lancing a wound to let the infection drain. By giving us permission to shout our "Why?" at heaven, God invites us into an honest relationship where our deepest pain can be met by His deeper grace, preventing the emotional paralysis that so often accompanies unprocessed suffering.

Finally, we ascend to the quiet heights of **Contemplative Prayer (Wordless Adoration)**. This is the prayer that moves beyond words, images, and even specific thoughts. It is the prayer of quiet, the restful gaze upon God, the simple "beholding" of the Divine. It is the practice of "ceasing" (Psalm 46:10) and of stilling and quieting the soul "like a weaned child with its mother" (Psalm 131:2). This is not a state of blank-mindedness, but a focused resting in the awareness of God's loving presence.

In a world saturated with noise, information, and stimulation, the soul's inner world often mirrors the external chaos. This hyper-stimulation is a primary driver of the modern anxiety epidemic. Contemplative prayer is the direct and powerful antidote. It is a mental discipline of voluntarily withdrawing from the cacophony to attend to the "still, small voice" (1 Kings 19:12). By sitting in silence before God, perhaps simply repeating a sacred word or phrase like "Abba" or "Jesus" to focus a wandering mind, we actively calm the central nervous system and retrain the brain to exist in a state of restful alertness. This practice counters the "fight or flight" response at a physiological level, lowering cortisol and promoting a state of peace. Theologically, it is an act of supreme trust and love—a wordless surrender to the reality that before Him, we are known, and that is enough. It is in this silent, loving attention that the soul is most deeply reconfigured, its frantic striving replaced by a received peace, its fragmented identity unified in the simple reality of being a beloved child in the presence of a loving Father. This is the ultimate fortification, a peace that is not of this world and therefore cannot be taken from it.

11.3 Biblical Meditation vs. Secular Mindfulness: A Critical Distinction

Beloved, in our therapeutic age, the practice of "mindfulness" has surged to the forefront of popular psychology, hailed as a panacea for stress, anxiety, and the distractions of modern life. Its techniques are taught in corporate boardrooms, schools, and clinics, promising a path to inner calm and self-mastery. For the Christian seeking mental resilience, this cultural moment demands a careful, theologically rigorous critique. We must ask: Is this practice a neutral tool we can baptize for our use, or does it contain a worldview that is fundamentally at odds with a biblical understanding of the human person and the path to true peace? To answer this, we must draw a critical and clear distinction between the secular practice of mindfulness and the ancient, biblical discipline of meditation. They may appear similar on the surface as practices of attention, but they differ in their fundamental goal, their methodology, and most importantly, their object. This distinction is not a matter of mere semantics; it is a matter of spiritual direction and ultimate destination.

Let us first define **Secular Mindfulness.** Rooted in Buddhist and Hindu contemplative traditions but often stripped of their explicit metaphysical beliefs in its modern therapeutic application, mindfulness is typically defined as "paying attention to the present moment, on purpose, non-judgmentally." The practitioner is instructed to sit quietly and bring their awareness to a neutral anchor, most commonly the sensation of the breath. As thoughts, emotions, or bodily sensations arise, the goal is not to engage with them, but to simply observe them as passing mental events, like clouds drifting across the sky, and then to gently return the attention to the breath. The overarching aims are stress reduction, emotional self-regulation, and a detachment from the "monkey mind" and its turbulent contents. The underlying philosophy is often one of immanence and non-attachment, where the self is the ultimate reference point and the goal is to achieve a state of equanimity by realizing the transient, and therefore ultimately illusory, nature of one's own thoughts and feelings.

Now, contrast this with **Biblical Meditation (*Hagah*).** The Hebrew word *hagah*, which is translated as "meditate" in key texts like Joshua 1:8 ("This Book of the Law shall not depart from your mouth, but you shall *meditate* on it day and night") and Psalm 1:2 ("but his delight is in the law of the LORD, and on his law he *meditates* day and night"), carries a completely different connotation. *Hagah* means to murmur, to mutter, to speak under one's breath. It is an active, vocal, and engaged process. It brings to mind the image of a person slowly reading the

Scriptures aloud to themselves, chewing on a phrase, turning it over in their mind, and whispering it repeatedly, allowing its sound and meaning to penetrate their consciousness. This is not the practice of emptying the mind, but of *filling* it. It is not about detached observation, but about deep, relational *rumination*. Just as a cow chews its cud—slowly, methodically, and repeatedly breaking down the raw material to extract all its nourishing potential—so the believer *hagahs* on the Word of God, breaking it down, digesting it, and internalizing its life-giving truth. The goal is not detachment, but profound attachment—a deeper union with the God who has spoken.

This leads us to the most critical distinction of all: **The Object of Focus.** This is the theological fault line that separates these two practices. In secular mindfulness, the object of focus is ultimately the self. The breath is a biological function of the self. The thoughts and feelings observed are the products of the self. The entire exercise, however beneficial for stress reduction, circles back to the autonomous individual. It is a closed system. The practitioner is both the observer and the observed, trapped within the confines of their own consciousness.

Biblical meditation, by its very nature, shatters this closed system. Its object is emphatically and exclusively *external* to the self. The object is the character, the works, and the spoken Word of the transcendent, personal God. The Psalmist does not meditate on his breath; he meditates on God's "precepts" and "ways" (Psalm 119:15), on His "mighty deeds" (Psalm 77:12), and on His "faithfulness" (Psalm 119:148). The focus is pulled out of the subjective, internal whirlpool and anchored in the objective, external reality of who God is and what He has done. This is not a technique for self-improvement; it is an act of worshipful inquiry.

The result of this fundamental difference in object is a profound difference in outcome. The result of secular mindfulness is, at its best, a physiological calm—a quieting of the nervous system, a reduction in the stress hormone cortisol. It is a valuable tool for managing the symptoms of a disordered inner world. But it does not and cannot address the root cause of that disorder, which is a broken relationship with God and a mind at war with its Creator.

The result of biblical meditation, however, is not merely physiological calm, though that may be a blessed byproduct. The result is a *transformed perspective and a deepened faith*. As we actively *hagah* on the truth of God's sovereignty, our anxieties about the future shrink in perspective. As we ruminate on His goodness, our resentment and fear begin to dissolve. As we murmur His promises, our faith is strengthened to believe them. The mind is not just quieted; it is *renewed* (Romans 12:2). The soul is not just regulated; it is *restored* (Psalm 23:3). We are not simply observing our thoughts from a detached distance; we are actively replacing the lies of the enemy and the flesh with the liberating truth of God. We are not seeking to empty ourselves, but to be filled with the very mind of Christ (1 Corinthians 2:16). Therefore, while the world offers a technique to manage the symptoms of a fallen psyche, God offers a transformative discipline that strikes at the root, reorienting our entire being—heart, soul, and mind—away from the fragile self and toward the rock-solid reality of the eternal, triune God.

11.4 The Practice of Contemplation: Gazing Upon the Divine

Beloved, we now arrive at the quiet epicenter, the still point of the turning world of spiritual discipline—the practice of contemplation. If meditation, which we have previously explored, is the diligent, focused, and often laborious process of chewing upon the Word of God, of turning it over in the mind and heart with the intensity of one searching for hidden treasure, then contemplation is the serene, wordless enjoyment of the treasure once it has been found. It is the soul's Sabbath rest from its striving. It is the transition from *doing* to *being*, from *seeking* to *dwelling*, from the active intellect to the receptive spirit. It is, in the most profound sense, the loving, steady, and adoring gaze of the soul upon the beauty, majesty, and sheer goodness of God. It is the fulfillment of the Lord's staggering promise in the Beatitudes: **"Blessed are the pure in heart, for they shall see God"** (Matthew 5:8).

Let us be clear from the outset: this "seeing" is not a physical vision, nor is it primarily an intellectual comprehension. It is a spiritual perception, a noetic faculty awakened and purified by the Holy Spirit. It is an apperception—a knowing by being in relation—that transcends the subject-object dichotomy of our ordinary cognition. In contemplation, we do not so much *think about* God as we *rest in* His presence. We do not analyze His attributes as a scientist dissects a specimen; we apprehend His glory as a child absorbs the love of a parent, or as a lover rests in the silent, knowing gaze of the beloved. This is not an esoteric practice reserved for a spiritual elite, for mystical specialists in cloistered monasteries. No, this is the birthright of every believer indwelt by the Spirit of Christ. It is the logical and glorious culmination of the renewal of the mind, for a mind that has been washed by the water of the Word and is being progressively conformed to the mind of Christ will naturally, and even irresistibly, begin to long for the direct, unmediated communion that contemplation offers.

To understand the mechanics and the theological underpinnings of this sacred gaze, we must first immerse ourselves in the ancient and time-tested pathway that the Church has used for centuries to train the soul in this art: the practice of **Lectio Divina**, or "Divine Reading." This is not a Bible study method in the modern, academic sense. It is a holistic, spiritual practice that engages the whole person—body, soul, and spirit—in a dynamic dialogue with the living God through His living Word. Lectio Divina is a river with four distinct, yet flowing and interpenetrating, currents: Lectio (reading), Meditatio (meditation), Oratio (prayer), and Contemplatio (contemplation). It is a ladder of ascent from the printed page to the heart of the Divine. The first movement, ***Lectio***, is the foundational act of slow, receptive, and reverent reading. Here, we are not reading for information, nor are we scanning the text for a sermon point or a theological argument. We are reading for *formation*. We approach the Scripture as if it were a love letter, reading it aloud, slowly, savoring each word, each phrase, as a connoisseur savors a fine wine. We are listening for the still, small voice, the particular word or phrase that the Holy Spirit seems to illuminate, that seems to "shimmer" or resonate with a peculiar weight and significance for us in that moment. We read not to master the text, but to be mastered by it. We are like Mary, sitting at the feet of Jesus, listening to His word (Luke 10:39), in a posture of humble, attentive submission. This is the stage of simplicity, of receiving the Word in its literal sense, allowing it to enter the ear gate and the eye gate without immediate analysis or judgment.

From this receptive reading, we naturally flow into the second movement, ***Meditatio***, or meditation. If Lectio is taking a single, small morsel of the divine banquet into our hands, Meditatio is the process of chewing it thoroughly. This is where we engage the cognitive faculties that we have been diligently renewing. We ponder the selected word or phrase. We ruminate on it. We ask questions of it: What does this reveal about the character of God? What does it reveal about the human condition? How does this connect with the great narrative of Scripture? We might use our knowledge of the original languages, of the historical context, of the wider canonical witness, but all in the service of *savoring* the truth, not just dissecting it. We are like the blessed man of Psalm 1, whose "delight is in the law of the LORD, and on his law he meditates day and night." This meditation is not a cold, intellectual exercise; it is a warm, personal engagement. We are seeking to implant the Word deep within the soil of our inner being, so that it might take root and bear fruit. We are, in a sense, seeking to memorize it with our hearts, not just our minds.

As we meditate, the Word, now active and sharp (Hebrews 4:12), begins to do its surgical work. It confronts us, comforts us, corrects us, and calls us. This encounter inevitably provokes a response from the depths of our spirit, which is the third movement: ***Oratio***, or prayer. Oratio is our heartfelt response to the God who has spoken to us through His Word. It is the dialogue becoming a conversation. This prayer is not a formal, pre-written petition; it is spontaneous, authentic, and varied. It may be a prayer of thanksgiving for a truth revealed, a prayer of confession for a sin exposed, a prayer of supplication for the grace to obey a command, or a prayer of lament when the Word stirs up our pain or confusion. It is the cry of the creature to the Creator, the child to the Father, the beloved to the Lover. It is

David in the Psalms, pouring out his soul—his anguish, his joy, his doubt, his trust. In Oratio, the truth that was first received objectively in Lectio and then internalized subjectively in Meditatio now becomes personal and relational. We are no longer just thinking about God; we are talking *with* Him. The monologue of divine revelation has sparked the dialogue of relationship.

And then, something mysterious and glorious can happen. The conversation, having reached a point of deep intimacy and trust, can fall into a sacred silence. This is the fourth and ultimate movement: ***Contemplatio***, contemplation. In this stage, words cease. The effort of reading, the activity of meditating, and even the volition of praying subside into a still, quiet, and receptive rest in the presence of God. It is the "be still, and know that I am God" of Psalm 46:10. In contemplation, we move from *doing* to *being*. We stop talking *to* God or *about* God, and we simply rest *in* God. We are like the disciple John, leaning on Jesus' breast at the Last Supper (John 13:23), secure in a love that needs no words. This is not emptiness; it is fullness. It is not the absence of thought, but the presence of a Knowledge that surpasses thought. It is a knowing by love, an intuitive apprehension of the Divine Reality that is granted as a gift of grace. In this silent gaze, the distinctions between Lectio, Meditatio, and Oratio blur. The Word we read, the truth we meditated upon, and the prayer we offered all converge into a single, luminous encounter with the Living Word, Jesus Christ. We have moved from the text as a pointer to God, to God Himself.

This transformative process of Lectio Divina finds its ultimate theological validation and explains its profound psychological effect in the apostle Paul's magnificent declaration in **2**

Corinthians 3:18: **"And we all, with unveiled face, beholding the glory of the Lord, are being transformed into the same image from one degree of glory to another. For this comes from the Lord who is the Spirit."** This single verse is the cornerstone of a theology of contemplation and the key to understanding its role in building psycho-spiritual resilience.

Let us unpack this dense and glorious truth. First, Paul states that we behold **"with unveiled face."** This is a direct contrast to Moses, who had to veil his face after being in the presence of God because the glory was fading, and the people could not bear to look upon it (2 Corinthians 3:13). But in Christ, the veil has been removed (2 Corinthians 3:14-16). Through His atoning work and the indwelling Spirit, we have bold and direct access to the very glory of God. We are invited to gaze, not at a reflection, but at the reality itself. The veil of sin, shame, and separation has been torn in two, from top to bottom.

What is it we are beholding? **"The glory of the Lord."** The Greek word for "beholding" here is *katoptrizō*, which can mean to mirror, or to look into a mirror. It suggests a direct, attentive, and reflective gaze. We are looking into the glory of the Lord as into a mirror. And what is that glory? It is the glory of God in the face of Jesus Christ (2 Corinthians 4:6). In contemplation, we are not gazing upon an abstract concept or a blinding, formless light. We are gazing upon the person of Jesus Christ as He is revealed in the Scriptures—His compassion, His righteousness, His humility, His obedience, His suffering, His exaltation. We behold the glory of a God who is love, a God who is sovereign, a God who is with us. This is a personal, relational gaze.

Now, the staggering result of this beholding: **"we are being transformed into the same image."** The Greek word for "transformed" is *metamorphoō*, from which we get our word "metamorphosis." It denotes a profound, fundamental, and comprehensive change of form and essence. This is the same word used to describe Jesus' transfiguration (Matthew 17:2). This is not mere behavior modification or positive thinking. This is a ontological renovation of the deepest structures of our personhood. And notice the passive voice: "we *are being* transformed." This is not something we achieve through strenuous self-effort. It is something that is *done to us*. It is a work of grace.

How does this transformation happen? Precisely **through the act of beholding.** The means of this metamorphosis is the steady, faithful, contemplative gaze upon the glory of the Lord. This is the central mystery and power of contemplation. We become what we behold. The soul, in its fundamental nature, is *assimilative*. It internalizes and takes on the qualities of that upon which it focuses its deepest attention. Just as a person who spends years gazing at and studying great art begins to internalize its beauty and proportion, or just as a couple married for decades begins to resemble each other in mannerism and expression, so the soul that gazes upon the glory of God in Christ is gradually, inexorably, reconfigured according to that glory. The patterns of thought, the dispositions of the heart, the very architecture of the unconscious mind, are all slowly and surely aligned with the "image" of the Son (Romans 8:29).

This process happens **"from one degree of glory to another."** The transformation is progressive and gradual. It is not an instantaneous zap that perfects us. It is a lifelong pilgrimage of deepening conformity. Each moment of true contemplation, each faithful gaze, adds another "degree" of glory, another layer of Christlikeness. It is a cumulative process, like the slow, imperceptible growth of a tree or the gradual brightening of the dawn. We may not feel it happening in the moment, but over time, the change is undeniable.

And Paul leaves no doubt as to the divine Agent of this entire process: **"For this comes from the Lord who is the Spirit."** The entire cycle—the unveiled access, the capacity to behold, the transformative power of the gaze—is the sovereign work of the Holy Spirit. Contemplation is not a technique we master; it is a grace we receive. The Spirit removes the veil, illuminates the glory of Christ in the Word, draws us into the gaze, and then performs the miracle of transfiguration within the inner person. Our part is to show up, to be present, to offer our attention, to consent to the process. The Spirit's part is to accomplish the miracle.

Now, what are the profound psycho-spiritual implications of this transformative contemplation for the building of resilience? The connection is direct and powerful. Resilience—the capacity to withstand trauma, to adapt to adversity, to bounce back from disappointment, and to endure prolonged suffering without disintegrating—is not primarily a matter of technique or grit. It is a function of *secure identity*. When a person's sense of self is fragile, fragmented, and dependent on external validation, performance, or circumstances, they are psychologically brittle. The slightest criticism, the smallest failure, the inevitable loss, can shatter them. But when a person's identity is solid, integrated, and rooted in something unchanging, eternal, and loving, they possess a core stability that can withstand the hurricanes of life.

Contemplation is the supreme means by which this secure identity is forged. As we steadfastly behold the glory of the Lord, our identity is progressively and relentlessly re-anchored *outside of ourselves*. We are no longer defined by our successes or failures, our possessions or our poverty, our health or our sickness, the praise or the condemnation of others. We are defined by the One upon whom we gaze. We discover that our true self is the self that is hidden with Christ in God (Colossians 3:3). Our worth is grounded in His unchanging valuation of us in the Beloved. Our security is found in His omnipotent grip that will never let us go. Our future is guaranteed by His resurrection power.

This is the bedrock of resilience. When the storm hits, the contemplative soul has a place to stand. It can look at the raging waves and the howling wind and, because its gaze is fixed on the glory of Christ, it can say, "None of this changes who I am. I am His. His glory is my destiny. This suffering is temporary, but my transformation into His image is eternal." The contemplative gaze creates an inner citadel, a fortified place in the spirit, that cannot be breached by the vicissitudes of fate. The soul learns to dwell in the "secret place of the Most High" (Psalm 91:1), and from that place of unassailable peace, it can face anything.

Furthermore, this transformation "from one degree of glory to another" specifically builds resilience by reconfigured our emotional and cognitive responses to suffering. As we behold the glory of Christ in His *humility*, we are slowly freed from the need to be right, to defend our honor, to cling to our rights. This makes us resilient against the wounds of insult and injustice. As we behold His *obedience*, even to death on a cross, we are given a paradigm for our own suffering, seeing it not as meaningless punishment but as a participation in His redemptive purposes. As we behold His *compassion*, our own hearts are softened, making us resilient against the hardening effects of bitterness and cynicism. As we behold His *sovereignty*, we are enabled to trust that even the most chaotic and evil events are held within His ultimate control, thus building resilience against the terror of randomness and chaos. Every facet of Christ's glory, when beheld contemplatively, becomes a source of strength, a resource for endurance, a wellspring of life in the midst of death.

Therefore, the practice of contemplation is not a spiritual luxury for the few. It is a psychological and spiritual necessity for every believer who wishes to navigate the trials of this life with faith, hope, and love. It is the means God has ordained for our deepest healing and our most profound strengthening. It is in the silent, loving gaze upon His glory that our fragmented selves are integrated, our anxious hearts are stilled, and our weary souls are renewed. We are transformed, not by our own frantic striving, but by His glorious being. We are made resilient, not by building thicker walls around our ego, but by losing ourselves in the infinite, unshakable reality of God.

11.5 The Neuro-Theology of Spiritual Disciplines

Beloved, we now stand at a fascinating and profoundly significant intersection—the crossroads where the ancient paths of spiritual discipline meet the modern frontiers of neuroscience. For too long, a false dichotomy has persisted in the minds of many believers: the sacred realm of the spirit versus the secular realm of science. This is a vestige of the very Gnostic dualism our entire treatise has sought to dismantle. If we truly believe in the doctrine of Creation—that God is the author of all reality, both visible and invisible—and if we hold to the psychosomatic unity of the human person as an integrated *nephesh*, then we must affirm that all truth is God's truth. General Revelation—the book of nature—and Special

Revelation—the book of Scripture—when read rightly, will never ultimately conflict. They are two chapters of the same divine narrative. Therefore, when modern neuroscience, through its sophisticated tools of fMRI and EEG, begins to map the brain activity of praying saints and meditating contemplatives, we should not be alarmed or dismissive. We should lean in with expectant curiosity, for we are being given a glimpse into the divine engineering of the human person. We are seeing, at a physiological level, how the God who formed our neural pathways has designed the spiritual disciplines to have tangible, healing, and transformative effects on the very physical substrate of our minds.

This emerging field, often termed **Neuro-Theology**, is not an attempt to reduce spiritual experience to mere biochemistry. That would be the error of reductionist materialism, a heresy against the biblical vision of the human person. Rather, neuro-theology offers a complementary perspective. It explores the neural *correlates* of spiritual states and practices. It shows us how the soul, in its communion with God, interfaces with and influences the brain, and vice-versa. This is a glorious confirmation of our holistic anthropology. The spiritual disciplines are not disembodied, ghostly exercises. They are whole-person activities that engage the body, which includes the brain, and through this engagement, they facilitate the renewal of the mind (Romans 12:2) and the transformation of the entire person.

Let us delve into three key areas where modern neuroscience provides striking corroboration for the wisdom and efficacy of the spiritual practices we have been exploring, particularly those of prayer, meditation, and contemplation.

First, consider the finding regarding the **Reduced Activity in the Default Mode Network (DMN)**. The Default Mode Network is a recently discovered, large-scale brain network that is most active when we are *not* focused on the outside world. It is the neurological seat of the self-referential, autobiographical, and narrative-making aspects of our mind. When you are daydreaming, worrying about the future, ruminating on a past offense, constructing your self-image, or generally lost in a stream of consciousness about *yourself*—your DMN is highly active. For this reason, it has been nicknamed the "me-network." While it is essential for self-awareness and introspection, its hyperactivity is strongly correlated with a host of psycho-spiritual maladies. It is the neural engine of anxiety, depression, and what the spiritual masters called "accidie" or acedia—that restless, dissipated state of soul where the mind flits from one worry to another, unable to find rest.

Now, observe the profound spiritual and neurological significance of what happens during deep, focused prayer and contemplative meditation. Neuroimaging studies on experienced Christian contemplatives, as well as seasoned practitioners of other meditative traditions, consistently show a marked *decrease* in activity within this Default Mode Network. When the mind is steadily focused on a sacred word, a passage of Scripture, or the loving presence of God, the chaotic chatter of the self-referential mind begins to quiet. The relentless inner monologue—the "chattering monkey" of the mind—subsides.

This is a stunning scientific validation of biblical commands. The Apostle Paul instructs us in 2 Corinthians 10:5 to "take every thought captive to obey Christ." What is the neurological correlate of this spiritual warfare? It is the conscious, willful redirection of cognitive resources *away* from the self-generating, often sinful, narratives of the DMN and *toward* the objective reality of Christ and His truth. The practice of contemplation, of "beholding the glory of the Lord," directly calms the neurological center of our egoic anxiety. It is the physiological manifestation of Jesus' invitation: "Come to me, all who labor and are heavy laden, and I will give you *rest*" (Matthew 11:28). The "labor" and "heavy burden" often exist as a hyperactive DMN—a mind that cannot stop working, worrying, and justifying itself. The "rest" that Christ offers is experienced, in part, as the blessed quieting of this network. We are, quite literally, giving our brains a rest from ourselves. This is not self-annihilation; it is the re-centering of the self upon its true foundation in God, which brings a profound peace that surpasses all understanding (Philippians 4:7) and guards our hearts and minds—our very neurophysiology—in Christ Jesus.

Secondly, neuroscience reveals **Increased Grey Matter in the Prefrontal Cortex** among long-term practitioners of meditation and prayer. Grey matter refers to the tissue in the brain that contains most of the brain's neuronal cell bodies. It is fundamental to processing information, and its density is linked to cognitive ability. The Prefrontal Cortex (PFC) is the most highly evolved part of the human brain, often called the "executive center." It is responsible for a suite of higher-order functions that are absolutely essential for a life of discipleship and embodied stewardship: focused attention, complex decision-making, long-term planning, impulse control, and—crucially—emotional regulation.

What does it mean, theologically and psychologically, that spiritual disciplines like prayer and meditation can physically thicken and strengthen this part of the brain? It means that these practices are a form of *cognitive and emotional training*. They are the gymnasium for the mind. When we discipline ourselves to sit in silence, to focus our attention on God in the face of a thousand distractions, to return our wandering mind to the anchor of a Scripture verse again and again, we are not just having a "spiritual" experience. We are performing reps for our Prefrontal Cortex. We are strengthening the neural pathways that govern self-control, focus, and emotional stability.

This has direct and powerful implications for our sanctification. The fruit of the Spirit includes "self-control" (Galatians 5:23). Neuroscience shows us that this spiritual fruit has a physical dimension. As we cooperate with the Holy Spirit through the discipline of prayer, He facilitates a neurological renovation that enhances our capacity for that very self-control. The ability to "be quick to hear, slow to speak, slow to anger" (James 1:19) is not just a matter of trying harder; it is a function of a well-regulated brain, a brain whose executive center has been trained and strengthened through spiritual practice. The increased grey matter in the PFC is the General Revelation counterpart to the Special Revelation promise that God is at work in us, "both to will and to work for his good pleasure" (Philippians 2:13). His working encompasses our very neuroplasticity—the brain's God-given ability to reorganize itself by forming new neural connections throughout life. The spiritual disciplines are the means by which we actively, willingly participate in this divinely orchestrated process of mental renewal.

Finally, consider the well-documented effect of these practices on **Lowered Cortisol Levels**. Cortisol is the body's primary stress hormone. It is a key component of the "fight-or-flight" response, essential for survival in acute danger. However, in our modern world, chronic psychological stress leads to chronically elevated cortisol levels, which have a devastating effect on the entire psychosomatic system. High cortisol contributes to anxiety, depression, digestive problems, headaches, heart disease, sleep disturbances, weight gain, and memory and concentration impairment. It is, in a very real sense, the biochemical signature of a life lived in a state of fear, urgency, and alienation from the peace of God.

The finding that contemplative prayer and meditation significantly reduce cortisol levels is nothing short of a scientific demonstration of the gospel's power to heal the wounds of the Fall at a physiological level. It is the hormonal embodiment of the peace of Christ. When we enter into the secret place of prayer, when we practice the presence of God, when we cast our anxieties upon Him because He cares for us (1 Peter 5:7), we are not just reciting pious words. We are initiating a cascade of neuroendocrine events that counteracts the very curse of toil and strife pronounced in Genesis 3. The "sweat of your face" (Genesis 3:19) is paralleled by the cortisol of your adrenal glands. The rest of God, found in Christ, directly opposes this.

This is a powerful affirmation of the holistic nature of salvation. The redemption we have in Jesus is not merely a legal transaction recorded in a heavenly ledger; it is a therapeutic, restorative process that begins to heal the psychosomatic damage of sin here and now. When the Psalmist declares, "I lie down and sleep; I wake again, because the LORD sustains me" (Psalm 3:5), he is testifying to a state of trust that has direct physiological consequences—lowered cortisol, a relaxed nervous system, and restorative sleep. The spiritual discipline of trust, enacted through prayer, becomes a means of grace for the body. It reinforces the glorious truth that our bodies are temples of the Holy Spirit (1 Corinthians 6:19), and that the same God who indwells us has designed practices for our care that bring every system, including our neuroendocrine system, into a greater state of harmony and health.

Therefore, the findings of modern neuroscience do not explain away the mystery of prayer; they illuminate the wisdom of the Creator. They show us that God, in His infinite kindness, has designed the spiritual life to be the most integrated and holistic path to human flourishing. The commands to "pray without ceasing" (1 Thessalonians 5:17), to "set your minds on things that are above" (Colossians 3:2), and to "be transformed by the renewal of your mind" (Romans 12:2) are not arbitrary religious duties. They are the Manufacturer's instructions for the optimal operation of the most complex creation in the universe—the human person, fearfully and wonderfully made. The quieting of the Default Mode Network, the strengthening of the Prefrontal Cortex, and the lowering of cortisol are not the *goal* of spiritual discipline; they are blessed, tangible byproducts of a soul turning its gaze upon its Creator and finding, in Him, the rest, order, and peace for which it was eternally designed.

11.6 Integrating the Disciplines: A Rule of Life for Mental Resilience

Beloved, we have now surveyed, with both theological depth and neuroscientific corroboration, the individual disciplines that constitute the sacred architecture of a renewed mind. We have explored the critical work of capturing thoughts, the transformative power of meditation upon Scripture, the grounding practice of thanksgiving, the intimate dialogue of prayer, and the sublime rest of contemplation. Yet, to view these disciplines as isolated techniques, as spiritual tools we pull out only in moments of crisis, is to fundamentally misunderstand their God-ordained purpose. A tool used only in an emergency remains a stranger in our hand; it lacks the familiar, worn-in feel that comes from daily, habitual use. The spiritual disciplines are not meant to be emergency flares launched from a sinking ship; they are meant to be the very timbers and rigging of the ship itself, the constitutive elements of a seaworthy vessel, capable of navigating both calm seas and violent storms. To move from a reactive spirituality, which frantically seeks God only when the waves are already crashing over the bow, to a proactive and resilient spirituality, we must move from practicing disciplines to inhabiting a *discipleship*. This is where the ancient and wise Christian concept of a **"Rule of Life"** becomes not merely helpful, but essential for the modern steward of mental and emotional health.

A Rule of Life, from the Latin *regula*, meaning a guide or a pattern, is not a set of restrictive, legalistic rules designed to crush the spirit. Quite the opposite. It is a trellis upon which the vine of a God-oriented life can grow and flourish. It is the intentional, prayerful structuring of our time and habits to create a sustainable rhythm of grace, a divine ecology in which the soul can naturally and consistently turn toward God. In a world characterized by chaos, fragmentation, and the tyranny of the urgent, a Rule of Life is a proactive act of resistance. It is the practical outworking of Paul's command in 1 Corinthians 14:40: "But all things should be done decently and in order." The order he speaks of is not merely for corporate worship, but for the whole of the Christian life. It is the *kosmos*—the beautiful, harmonious order—that stands against the *chaos* of a mind and life untethered from its Creator.

Theologically, the foundation for a personal Rule of Life rests upon the very character of God, who is not a God of disorder but of peace (1 Corinthians 14:33). His creation reflects His orderly nature: the planets move in their appointed orbits, the seasons follow their reliable cycle, the human body operates with breathtaking biological rhythms. Our own psychosomatic unity, as we have seen, thrives on rhythm and regularity—from circadian sleep-wake cycles to the neural pathways strengthened by repetition. A Rule of Life is, therefore, our conscious cooperation with the grain of the universe. It is our attempt to align the microcosm of our personal daily existence with the macrocosm of God's created and redemptive order. It is a form of *imitatio Dei*—the imitation of God—reflecting His faithfulness and constancy through our own faithful and constant practices.

For the steward specifically tasked with the cultivation of mental resilience, a Rule of Life is the indispensable framework that transforms sporadic moments of peace into an abiding state of shalom. Resilience is not built in a day; it is forged in the countless, small, daily choices to turn our attention Godward. It is the cumulative effect of a thousand tiny acts of surrender, a million minor moments of recentering. Without a structure, these acts are left to chance, vulnerable to the whims of our fluctuating moods and the relentless demands of a distracting world. A Rule of Life provides the structure. It is the strategy that ensures the tactics of the spiritual disciplines are deployed consistently across the theater of our daily lives.

Let us then construct, in principle, what such a Rule of Life for mental resilience might entail. This is not a one-size-fits-all prescription, for the Spirit distributes gifts and calls according to His will, and our life circumstances vary greatly. But the principles are universal, and they can be adapted to the unique vocation and season of each believer.

First and foremost, a resilient Rule of Life must be anchored in **Set Times for Lectio Divina**. This is the non-negotiable core, the daily immersion in the life-giving Word. This is not a hurried, checkbox-oriented "devotional minute." It is a scheduled, protected appointment with the Divine Physician. For many, this finds its natural home in the morning, setting the tone for the day, filling the mind with truth before it is assailed by the world's false narratives. The practice of *Lectio*—slow, receptive reading—followed by *Meditatio*—rumination on a key phrase—and flowing into *Oratio*—heartfelt response—and culminating in *Contemplatio*—silent rest—becomes the daily recalibration of the soul's compass. It is the implementation of Joshua 1:8: "This Book of the Law shall not depart from your mouth, but you shall meditate on it day and night, so that you may be careful to do according to all that is written in it. For then you will make your way prosperous, and then you will have good success." The "prosperity" and "success" here are, in no small part, the prosperity of a mind at peace and the success of a life resiliently oriented toward its true North.

But the spiritual life cannot be sustained on a single daily feeding. The pressures of the day are relentless. Therefore, a robust Rule of Life incorporates **Moments of Recollection on the Hour**. This is the practice, often associated with the ancient monastic "Divine Office" or the Orthodox "Jesus Prayer," of punctuating the day with brief moments of recentering. It is the practical application of 1 Thessalonians 5:17 to "pray without ceasing." This does not mean being in a state of formal prayer every second, but rather cultivating a God-consciousness that runs like a subterranean river beneath all our activities. A simple way to practice this is to let the chime of a clock on the hour, or the transition between tasks, serve as a trigger. In that moment, one pauses for just thirty seconds. One closes their eyes, takes a deep, conscious breath, and offers a short, pre-selected Scripture anchor: "Lord Jesus Christ, Son of God, have mercy on me, a sinner." Or perhaps, "The Lord is my shepherd, I shall not want." Or simply, "Thy will be done." This momentary recollection is a spiritual reset button. It pulls the mind back from the brink of anxiety, it interrupts the spiral of negative self-talk, and it re-anchors the soul in the present moment and in the presence of God. Neurologically, it is a deliberate intervention in the Default Mode Network, a brief but powerful cessation of its self-referential chatter. Over time, these hourly moments create a web of mindfulness that holds the day together, preventing the fragmentation that leads to mental and emotional exhaustion.

Furthermore, a Rule of Life for resilience must include a **Weekly Examen**. This is a more extended, reflective practice, ideally performed at the end of each day, but which can be adapted for a weekly review. Rooted in the Ignatian tradition, the Examen is a prayerful review of the day in God's presence. It is not a morbid introspection or a scrupulous cataloging of failures. It is a dialogue with the Holy Spirit, asking for His light to see the day as He sees it. A simple structure involves five movements:

1. **Thanksgiving:** Beginning with gratitude for the specific gifts and graces of the day.
2. **Petition for Light:** Asking the Holy Spirit to illuminate the events, interactions, and interior movements of the day.
3. **Review with Gratitude:** Walking through the hours of the day, noticing where one was conscious of God's presence and where one felt life, peace, and consolation.

4. **Review with Contrition:** Noticing with honesty, but without self-flagellation, the moments of failure, anxiety, or turning away from God's presence—the moments of desolation.
5. **Resolution and Looking Forward:** Seeking God's forgiveness where needed, and asking for grace for the next day, perhaps focusing on one particular area where one desires to grow.

The psycho-spiritual power of the Examen is immense. It is a form of *therapeutic memory reconsolidation*. It takes the raw, often chaotic data of our daily experience and, in the presence of the Healer, processes it, integrates it, and extracts meaning from it. It prevents the accumulation of unprocessed emotional residue that can lead to chronic stress, bitterness, and depression. It trains the mind to look for God in all things, fostering a sense of divine providence and purpose that is the bedrock of resilience.

Finally, and perhaps most critically for our over-stimulated age, a resilient Rule of Life must carve out a **Dedicated Period for Contemplative Silence**. This is beyond the quiet that concludes a Lectio Divina session. This is a substantial block of time—twenty, thirty, or sixty minutes—set aside weekly or even daily, for the sole purpose of being silent before God. This is the practice of "Be still, and know that I am God" (Psalm 46:10). In this dedicated silence, we lay aside all words, all intercessions, all intellectual activity. We simply sit in the loving, affirming presence of our Heavenly Father. We practice the "prayer of quiet" where the soul rests in the awareness that it is loved, held, and known.

This discipline is the ultimate antidote to the performance-driven anxiety that plagues so many believers. In the silence, we are not *doing* anything for God. We are simply *being* His child. This is where the deep, non-contingent identity we spoke of is solidified. It is in this silence that the transformative beholding of 2 Corinthians 3:18 occurs most powerfully. The mind, stripped of its usual props and activities, learns to find its satisfaction in God alone. The resilience forged here is not the resilience of a stronger ego, but the resilience of a soul that has learned to draw life directly from the Vine, apart from any fruit it may or may not produce (John 15:5).

Integrating these elements—daily Lectio, hourly recollection, a weekly Examen, and dedicated contemplative silence—creates a comprehensive rhythm of grace. This Rule becomes the trellis. The daily Lectio is the deep watering at the root. The hourly recollections are the frequent tendings that keep the plant oriented toward the sun. The weekly Examen is the careful pruning that removes dead growth and encourages healthy development. The contemplative silence is the patient allowing of the plant to simply *be* in the sunlight, receiving its life without effort.

This structured, intentional life is the path to a resilient and peaceful mind. It is the practical, lived-out reality of offering our bodies as a living sacrifice, and being transformed by the *renewal of our mind* (Romans 12:1-2). It is how we move from a state of being constantly shaped by the world's chaos to a state of being progressively conformed to the peaceful order of Christ's kingdom. It is, in the end, the most faithful way to steward the magnificent, God-given, but fallen, instrument of our minds, restoring them to their original purpose: to know

God, and in knowing Him, to find a peace that the world can neither give nor take away.

11.7 The Fortified Soul

Beloved, as we draw our extensive exploration of the renewed mind to its culmination, we arrive at a pivotal and sobering truth, one that stands as both a bulwark against despair and a clarion call to disciplined faithfulness. The spiritual disciplines of prayer, meditation, and contemplation, which we have examined with such exegetical care and scientific corroboration, are not, in their ultimate essence, self-help techniques for achieving a state of personal tranquility. They are not spiritualized versions of secular mindfulness, co-opted for a Christian audience. No, they are something far more profound, far more potent, and far more demanding. They are, in the economy of God's grace, His divinely prescribed and sovereignly ordained means for fortifying the human soul against the relentless, corrosive, and disintegrating onslaught of a world that lies in the power of the evil one (1 John 5:19). They are the construction materials for an inner citadel, the divine architecture for a psyche that can withstand the siege.

This fortification is not a magical shield that renders the believer impervious to the slings and arrows of outrageous fortune. The promise of the gospel, contrary to the heresies of the prosperity movement, is not an exemption from suffering. Our Lord Himself told us with stark clarity, "In the world you will have tribulation" (John 16:33a). The spiritual disciplines are not a guarantee against suffering; they are the God-given instruments that prepare us to endure suffering, to navigate it, and even to find within its crucible a deeper participation in the sufferings of Christ (Philippians 3:10). They do not build a moat around our lives to keep the dragons out; they forge the armor and the sword with which we face the dragons, ensuring that when they breathe their fire, we are not consumed but refined.

The resilience that is cultivated through this faithful, daily practice is of a unique and supernatural character. It is fundamentally different from the stoic resilience of the ancient philosophers, who taught a detachment from emotion and a grim endurance of fate. It is equally distinct from the modern therapeutic resilience, which often centers on building self-esteem, fostering a positive self-narrative, and enhancing personal coping mechanisms. While these may have a temporal, limited value, the resilience forged in the crucible of spiritual discipline is of an entirely different order. It is a resilience grounded not in the shifting sands of subjective feeling or positive thinking, but in the eternal, objective, and unassailable reality of God Himself—His character, His promises, His covenant faithfulness, and His sovereign rule over every atom and every angel in the universe.

Consider the profound implications of this distinction. When a soul's stability is dependent on its ability to maintain a positive self-image, what happens when that image is shattered by moral failure? When resilience is built upon the foundation of "coping skills," what occurs when the suffering exceeds any human capacity to cope? When one's peace is contingent upon favorable circumstances, where is the anchor when the storm rages uncontrollably? Such foundations are destined to crumble, for they are built upon the self, which is itself fallen, fragile, and mutable. But the resilience cultivated through the disciplines is built upon the Rock of Ages. It is an external stability that is internalized through faithful practice. It is the slow, steady process of having our inner being—our *nephesh*—

re-anchored outside of itself in the One who is the same yesterday, today, and forever (Hebrews 13:8).

This is the work of fortification. Through the discipline of prayer, we are not merely listing our requests; we are actively practicing dependence. We are strengthening the neural and spiritual pathways of trust, rehearsing the foundational truth that we are not autonomous beings but creatures in constant need of our Creator's grace. In the heat of trial, the soul trained in prayer does not first ask, "How can I fix this?" but rather, "Father, into your hands I commit my spirit" (Luke 23:46). This is a learned response, a habit of the heart forged in the countless quiet moments of daily surrender.

Through the discipline of meditation upon Scripture, we are not merely memorizing data; we are marinating our consciousness in a reality more true than our temporary afflictions. We are, as the Psalmist says, hiding God's word in our heart that we might not sin against Him (Psalm 119:11), but also that we might not despair in the darkness. When the diagnosis comes, the mind saturated with the truth of God's sovereignty and goodness has a pre-existing framework into which to place the terrifying new information. It does not default to "This is meaningless chaos," but rather to "Even here, Your right hand will hold me fast" (cf. Psalm 139:10). The promises of God, diligently meditated upon, become more real to the fortified soul than the grim prognosis on the doctor's chart. They become the lenses through which all of reality is interpreted.

And through the supreme discipline of contemplation, we are engaging in the most direct form of fortification. We are, as we have seen, "beholding the glory of the Lord" and "are being transformed into the same image from one degree of glory to another" (2 Corinthians 3:18). This is the ultimate psycho-spiritual defense. As we gaze upon His glory, our identity is progressively and irrevocably fused with His. The insults of the world, the accusations of the devil, and the condemnations of our own fallen conscience lose their power because our sense of self is no longer derived from those sources. It is derived from the affirming, loving gaze of the Father, who declares us His beloved children in the Son. A soul that knows itself to be the object of such divine delight is a soul that can withstand any earthly humiliation. A mind that is being reconfigured according to the self-giving love of Christ is a mind that can face persecution, loss, and even death without being conquered by hatred or despair.

Therefore, the believer who diligently practices these disciplines does not escape their circumstances. The notion of a flight from the world is a Gnostic fantasy, not a biblical mandate. We are called to be in the world, though not of it (John 17:15-16). The fortified soul meets its circumstances—all of them, from the mundane irritations to the catastrophic losses—with a fundamentally different internal posture. It meets them with a *mind anchored in peace*. This is the peace of Christ, which He explicitly gives to us, a peace that is categorically different from the world's fleeting sense of calm (John 14:27). It is a peace that rules as an umpire in our hearts (Colossians 3:15), making calls based on the objective truth of the gospel, not on the subjective turmoil of our emotions.

It meets them with a *heart saturated with truth*. The heart, in the Hebrew conception, is the center of the will, intellect, and emotions. A heart saturated with truth is one where the divine logos has taken root so deeply that it governs the volitional, cognitive, and affective domains. The decisions made from this heart are wise, the thoughts that emerge from it are pure, and the emotions that flow from it, while perhaps anguished, are ultimately ordered by a deeper trust. This saturation is the antidote to the poisonous lies of the enemy, who is the father of lies (John 8:44), and who seeks to shipwreck our faith by distorting our perception of God, ourselves, and our situation.

And finally, the fortified soul meets all circumstances with a *soul resting in the loving presence of the Divine*. This is the culmination of all the disciplines: a state of being, a settled orientation of the entire person toward God as the ultimate reality and the ultimate good. It is the experiential knowledge of the love of Christ that surpasses knowledge, leading to being "filled with all the fullness of God" (Ephesians 3:19). From this place of rest, activity flows not from a place of frantic striving to earn favor or avert disaster, but from the overflow of a secure relationship. The soul at rest in God is like a tree planted by streams of water, and it does not fear when heat comes, for its leaves remain green, and it is not anxious in the year of drought, for it does not cease to bear fruit (Jeremiah 17:7-8).

This, then, is the fortified soul. It is not a soul that has all the answers. It is not a soul that never feels pain. It is not a soul that is immune to doubt or confusion. It is, rather, a soul that has been so thoroughly re-oriented toward the Reality of God that, like a well-built ship, it can be tossed by the fiercest waves and yet not be capsized, because its ballast is deep and its keel is true. The disciplines are the means by which we, in cooperation with the Holy Spirit, build that ballast and shape that keel. They are the patient, often unglamorous, daily work of taking our disordered, anxious, and fragile minds and submitting them to the gracious, surgical, and transformative work of the Master Architect, who is building within us a fortress of faith, a sanctuary of shalom, capable of standing firm until the day of His glorious appearing.

CHAPTER 12

Addressing Affliction: A Pastoral and Theological Approach to Anxiety, Depression, and Despair

Beloved, we now turn our attention from the proactive fortification of the soul to the critical, compassionate task of ministering to those whose inner defenses have been breached, whose minds are under a state of siege, and whose souls are shrouded in a darkness that feels, to them, absolute and impenetrable. We move from the gymnasium of spiritual discipline to the field hospital of the church, where the wounded in spirit are brought for triage, healing, and restoration. The subject before us is one of immense pastoral urgency and profound theological complexity: the reality of severe mental and emotional affliction—clinical-level anxiety, debilitating depression, and the soul's dark night of despair. This is not a discussion about occasional sadness or situational worry; this is an exploration of the abyss, a mapping of the terrain where the *nephesh*—the integrated whole person—experiences a profound and often terrifying dis-integration.

The church of Jesus Christ, the very body of the One who was "a man of sorrows and acquainted with grief" (Isaiah 53:3), is called by its very nature to be a sanctuary for the broken, a refuge for the weary, and a place where the bruised reed is not broken and the smoldering wick is not quenched (Matthew 12:20). Yet, we must confess with humility and grief that the modern church has often struggled, and at times failed catastrophically, to minister with wisdom, compassion, and efficacy to those suffering from these profound psycho-spiritual maladies. Our history is marred by two devastating and equally unbiblical ditches on either side of the narrow road of truth.

On one side lies the ditch of **simplistic spiritualization**. This is the error of Job's comforters, dressed in modern evangelical garb. It operates from a flawed, often subconscious, causal assumption: deep, persistent mental suffering must be the direct and immediate fruit of personal, unconfessed sin, a demonic stronghold born out of willful disobedience, or a simple, culpable lack of faith. The pastoral response that flows from this framework is one of suspicion, interrogation, and exhortation. The suffering one is subtly or overtly encouraged to "pray more," "have more faith," "repent of a specific sin," or "renounce a demonic influence." When these prescriptions fail to produce a cure, as they often do when the affliction has complex physiological or deeply embedded psychological roots, the sufferer is left with a double burden: their original anguish, now compounded by the crushing weight of spiritual failure and shame. They are led to believe that their inability to "snap out of it" through spiritual effort is itself a testament to their defective faith. This approach is not only pastorally cruel but also a profound theological error, a misreading of the Fall and its multifaceted impact on human existence, and a denial of the complex channels of affliction we have previously explored.

On the other side of the road lies the equally perilous ditch of **secular reductionism**. In a well-intentioned effort to avoid the blame and shame of the first approach, the church sometimes capitulates entirely to a secular, medicalized model of mental illness. In this framework, conditions like major depressive disorder or generalized anxiety disorder are viewed *solely* as brain diseases, chemical imbalances, or maladaptive cognitive patterns. The spiritual dimension of the person is politely ignored or relegated to a secondary, almost irrelevant, concern. The sufferer is swiftly referred to a therapist or a psychiatrist, and the community of faith, feeling out of its depth, abdicates its God-given role as a agent of holistic healing. While competent medical and psychological care is an essential, God-honoring component of treatment—a point we will strongly affirm—to see it as the *only* component is to deny the reality of the human as a spiritual being, to fragment the psychosomatic unity, and to rob the sufferer of the unique comforts and resources of the gospel. It is to treat the symptom while ignoring the state of the soul that inhabits the malfunctioning brain.

This chapter, therefore, constitutes a robust argument for a *via media*, a third way that is both biblically faithful and scientifically informed. We will argue unapologetically for a **multi-faceted, integrative approach** that holds in delicate, pastoral tension the irreducible spiritual nature of the human person with the undeniable physical and psychological realities of their affliction. This approach refuses to choose between prayer and Prozac, between exorcism and therapy, between the sanctuary and the counselor's office. It recognizes that because the human person is a complex, integrated whole—a *nephesh*—their healing must address the whole person: the spirit, the soul (*psyche*), and the body (*soma*).

This integrated model is not a mere pragmatic compromise; it is a direct implication of our core theological commitments. If we believe in the doctrine of Creation, then we must honor the structures of the brain and the body as God's good design, albeit now fallen, and we must embrace the legitimate insights of sciences like neurobiology and psychology as part of God's General Revelation. If we believe in the pervasive, cosmic impact of the Fall, then we must acknowledge that mental affliction can arise from a tangled web of sources: genetic predispositions (the brokenness of creation), traumatic experiences (the brokenness of relationship), personal sin (the brokenness of will), and demonic oppression (the brokenness of the spiritual realm). And if we believe in the comprehensive scope of Redemption in Christ, then we must proclaim a gospel that promises the ultimate healing of *all* things—including our minds and emotions—and that provides resources for healing in the present age through the ministry of the Spirit, the truth of the Word, and the love of the community.

This chapter will, therefore, seek to equip you—pastors, counselors, small group leaders, and every member of the body of Christ—to become a more effective and compassionate shepherd to the wounded soul. We will delve into a theological understanding of anxiety and depression that is neither dismissive nor despairing. We will explore the vital role of professional intervention—psychotherapy and psychiatry—as a legitimate and often necessary means of common grace, and we will provide a theological framework for understanding and utilizing these tools without capitulating to a secular worldview. We will examine the essential, non-negotiable role of the community of faith—the *koinonia*—as a tangible embodiment of God's presence and patience. And we will consider the specific spiritual disciplines and pastoral practices that can serve as lifelines for those drowning in despair, while always acknowledging the mysterious reality that some afflictions, like Paul's thorn, are not removed in this life, and must be endured through the sufficient grace of Christ.

Our goal is to move the church from a place of fearful ignorance or simplistic judgment to a place of confident, wise, and tender ministry. We seek to create communities that are truly safe for the broken, where a person can speak of their suicidal thoughts without triggering a panic of amateur demonology, and where they can share their struggle with medication without being made to feel second-class in the kingdom of God. We are called to be the hands and feet of the Great Physician, and that requires us to understand the whole person He came to heal. Let us then begin this solemn and sacred task, with Bibles open, minds engaged, and hearts full of the compassion of Christ.

12.1 Shepherding the Wounded Soul

Beloved, before we can even begin to discuss protocols, therapies, or interventions, we must first establish the fundamental pastoral posture required for this sacred work. Shepherding the wounded soul is an act of profound spiritual and emotional hospitality. It demands that we lay aside our preconceived solutions, our hurried diagnoses, and our own discomfort with another's pain, and simply learn to *be present*. The initial and often most powerful ministry we can offer to a person gripped by anxiety or lost in the bleak landscape of depression is not a word of exhortation, but the ministry of *attentive, non-anxious presence*. This is an incarnational ministry. Just as the Word became flesh and *dwelt among us* (John 1:14), pitching His tent in the midst of our brokenness, so we are called to pitch our tent of presence beside the suffering one.

This runs utterly counter to the impulse to fix, to solve, to explain away. A soul in despair does not need a lecture; it needs a witness. It does not need a formula; it needs a friend who is willing to sit in the ashes with them, as Job's friends did for seven days and seven nights before they fatally opened their mouths (Job 2:13). Their silent presence was, in fact, their only truly helpful act. This pastoral presence is a tangible reflection of God's own character. The Psalmist does not say, "God explains all things," but rather, "God is our refuge and strength, a very *present* help in trouble" (Psalm 46:1, emphasis added). The Hebrew word for "present help" (*matsa'*) implies one who is found, who is *there*, readily available. Our first task is to be there, to be found by the suffering one as a safe harbor in their storm.

This presence must be undergirded by a radical deconstruction of the stigma that so often surrounds mental affliction within the church. We must actively, from the pulpit and in our small groups, dismantle the false notion that anxiety and depression are somehow less "spiritual" or more shameful than physical illnesses like cancer or diabetes. Would we ever tell a diabetic that their condition is due to a lack of faith? Would we accuse a cancer patient of harboring unconfessed sin as the sole cause of their tumor? Such a response would be rightfully seen as barbaric and theologically ignorant. Yet, we routinely subject those with mental afflictions to this very standard. This is a failure of our theological imagination and a denial of the psychosomatic unity we profess.

We must reclaim a robust theology of suffering that makes room for the mystery of affliction that is not directly tied to personal sin. The man born blind in John 9 stands as an eternal testament against this simplistic causality. The disciples' question, "Rabbi, who sinned, this man or his parents, that he was born blind?" (John 9:2), is the quintessential expression of this destructive theology. Jesus' response is liberating and definitive: "It was not that this man sinned, or his parents, but that the works of God might be displayed in him" (John 9:3). The affliction existed within the broader context of a fallen creation, but its purpose was to become a platform for divine revelation and glory. Similarly, the Apostle Paul's "thorn in the flesh" (2 Corinthians 12:7), which many patristic and modern commentators believe was a chronic, debilitating physical ailment, was not given as a punishment for sin, but as a preventative against pride, and its purpose was to showcase the perfection of God's power in the midst of human weakness. By applying this broader theological framework to mental suffering, we can begin to remove the crushing burden of guilt and shame that so often paralyzes the afflicted and silences them within the community.

Furthermore, the shepherding pastor or friend must become a student of lament. A significant portion of the Psalter—the very prayer book of God's people—is comprised of laments. These are raw, unfiltered cries of anguish, confusion, and despair directed toward God. Psalms like Psalm 22 ("My God, my God, why have you forsaken me?"), Psalm 42 ("Why are you cast down, O my soul, and why are you in turmoil within me?"), and Psalm 88 (which ends in unrelieved darkness) give divine permission for the expression of deep pain. They provide a grammar for suffering that is both honest and faithful. The lament psalms teach us that true faith is not the absence of struggle, but the stubborn decision to bring our struggle *to* God, even when He seems absent. Shepherding the wounded soul often means giving them permission to voice their own lament, to scream their "why?" into the seeming void, and to assure them that such cries are not a sign of faithlessness, but are in fact a profound act of faith, a desperate clinging to a God who they believe is there, even when all sensory and emotional evidence suggests otherwise. We must create spaces in our worship and our community life where it is safe to not be okay, where the language of lament is as welcome as the language of praise, for both are found on the lips of the faithful in the Scriptures.

12.2 A Theological Taxonomy of Mental Affliction

Beloved, having established the essential pastoral posture of presence and destigmatization, we must now equip ourselves with a more refined set of diagnostic lenses. To shepherd effectively, we must learn to discern, with humility and wisdom, the complex, often interwoven, threads that form the tapestry of a person's suffering. A one-size-fits-all approach is not only ineffective but can be actively harmful. To treat a profound biochemical depression as if it were solely a demonic stronghold is to commit spiritual malpractice. Conversely, to address a soul-crushing crisis of meaning and faith as a simple matter of serotonin reuptake inhibition is to offer a stone when the sufferer is pleading for the living bread. Therefore, we must build upon the foundational framework of the four channels of affliction from Chapter 4 and develop a more detailed **theological taxonomy of mental affliction**. This taxonomy is not a tool for amateur diagnosis, but a pastoral map to guide our compassion, our questions, and our prayers, always leading us toward a multi-faceted, holistic response.

The first domain of this taxonomy encompasses the **Somatic Causes**. We must begin here, at the level of the physical body, for we are *nephesh*, psychosomatic unities, and the state of the *soma* profoundly influences the state of the *psyche*. This category acknowledges that our fallen biology, subject to the curse of entropy and decay, is a primary theater for affliction. Here we find:

- **Brain Chemistry Imbalances:** The intricate symphony of neurotransmitters—serotonin, dopamine, norepinephrine, and others—can fall into dissonance. This is not a moral failing; it is a physiological reality, a manifestation of the creation "subjected to futility" (Romans 8:20). To dismiss a major depressive episode as "all in your head" is to state a biological truth while utterly missing the theological point: the "head," the brain, is a physical organ, and like the pancreas or the heart, it can malfunction.
- **Hormonal Disorders:** The thyroid gland, the adrenal system, the reproductive hormones—these powerful regulatory systems, when dysregulated, can cast a long shadow over the mind. Postpartum depression, for instance, has clear hormonal components intertwined with massive psychological and spiritual adjustment. The book of Lamentations gives voice to a feeling that resonates with many in such states: "He has made my flesh and my skin waste away; he has broken my bones... He has made my soul bereft of peace; I have forgotten what happiness is" (Lamentations 3:4, 17).
- **Genetic Predispositions:** Just as some families have a predisposition to hypertension or diabetes, research clearly shows heritable factors for conditions like bipolar disorder or schizophrenia. This is the sobering reality of generational brokenness and the corporate nature of the Fall, where "the iniquity of the fathers" visits

subsequent generations in the form of physical vulnerabilities (Exodus 20:5), not as divine punishment for the children's sins, but as a consequence of a corrupted created order.

- **Chronic Illness and Nutritional Deficiencies:** A body wracked with unrelenting pain, a system starved of essential vitamins like B12 or Vitamin D, a gut microbiome thrown into dysbiosis—these somatic realities can be the direct and sole cause of profound anxiety and depressive symptoms. The spirit is willing, but the flesh is not only weak; it is sick, and its sickness cries out through the faculties of the mind.

A pastoral response to potential somatic causes must be one of practical wisdom. It begins with a simple, compassionate question: "Have you seen a medical doctor? Have you had a physical recently?" This is not a lack of faith; it is an act of stewardship over the temple of the Holy Spirit. It honors God's common grace revealed through the medical sciences.

The second domain in our taxonomy is that of **Spiritual and Relational Causes**. Here, we move into the realm of the heart, the will, and our relationship with God and others. This is the domain most familiar to the church, but it must be handled with extreme care, lest we revert to the simplistic spiritualization we have already condemned.

- **Unrepentant Sin and Guilt:** While not the cause of all affliction, the weight of unconfessed sin is a real and powerful burden on the soul. The Psalmist David, after his sin with Bathsheba, lamented, "For when I kept silent, my bones wasted away through my groaning all day long. For day and night your hand was heavy upon me; my strength was dried up as by the heat of summer" (Psalm

32:3-4). This is a classic description of psychosomatic distress rooted in a troubled conscience. True, divinely-sourced conviction leads to repentance and life (2 Corinthians 7:10), while false, accusatory guilt or shame can lead to a destructive spiral.

- **Bitterness and Unforgiveness:** To harbor resentment is to drink poison and expect the other person to die. It is a spiritual and psychological cancer. The writer of Hebrews issues a grave warning: "See to it that no one fails to obtain the grace of God; that no 'root of bitterness' springs up and causes trouble, and by it many become defiled" (Hebrews 12:15). This root can choke the life out of a soul, leading to anger, cynicism, and a depression born of a hardened heart.
- **Demonic Oppression:** We must tread here with biblical sobriety, avoiding both sensationalism and denial. The New Testament clearly depicts instances where spiritual forces directly impact a person's mental and physical state (e.g., the Gerasene demoniac in Mark 5, the boy with a spirit in Matthew 17). Demonic activity often exploits pre-existing vulnerabilities—whether somatic, psychological, or spiritual—and can manifest in sudden, severe shifts in personality, intense and irrational aversions to spiritual things, or voices of accusation and self-harm. However, the key pastoral principle is this: *not all mental affliction is demonic, but some may have a demonic component.* Discerning this requires deep prayer, wisdom, and often the involvement of mature, seasoned ministry leaders.
- **Crisis of Faith and Meaning:** This is an affliction of the *pneuma*, the human spirit. When foundational beliefs about God, the world, and one's purpose are shattered by tragedy, intellectual doubt, or the slow

erosion of disappointment, a profound existential despair can set in. It is the "dark night of the soul" described by St. John of the Cross, where the sensory comforts of faith vanish, and the soul feels abandoned by God. This is not necessarily a sign of failure, but can be a painful stage of purgative growth.

The third domain is the **Psychological Causes**, the realm of the *psyche* itself—the mind, emotions, and memories as shaped by our personal history and learned patterns.

- **Unhealed Trauma:** The human person is designed for attachment and safety. When these are violently ruptured through abuse, neglect, combat, or catastrophic loss, the psyche can fracture. Post-Traumatic Stress Disorder (PTSD) is a complex psychological and physiological injury. The traumatic memory becomes a "splinter in the mind," causing hypervigilance (anxiety), emotional numbness (depression), and intrusive flashbacks. This is not a sin; it is a wound. The sufferer needs the safety and skilled care of trauma-informed therapy to facilitate integration and healing.
- **Maladaptive Cognitive Patterns:** Our minds develop "schemas" or core beliefs about ourselves, others, and the world, often formed in childhood. A person raised by a critical parent may develop a core belief of "I am defective." Someone who experienced abandonment may believe "I am unlovable." These deeply ingrained patterns, what Paul might call "strongholds," automatically filter experiences, leading to predictable cycles of negative thinking, self-sabotage, and emotional distress. This is the territory of Cognitive Behavioral Therapy, which can be seen as a form of

common grace to help fulfill the biblical mandate to be transformed by the renewing of the mind (Romans 12:2).

- **Overwhelming Life Stressors:** The human nervous system has a finite capacity for stress. Chronic financial pressure, caring for a loved one with a debilitating illness, or a season of relentless professional demands can deplete the psychological resources of even the most resilient individual, leading to burnout, anxiety, and depression. This is the soul's cry of "Enough! I have no more to give," echoing Elijah's exhaustion under the broom tree (1 Kings 19:4).

Finally, we have the **Situational Causes**, the external circumstances that press upon the soul.

- **Grief and Loss:** The deep sorrow following the death of a loved one, the end of a marriage, or the loss of a career is a normal, human response to having a part of one's world torn away. The book of Lamentations and the Psalms of lament give divine sanction to this grief. To pathologize normal grief is to fail to understand the cost of love in a fallen world.
- **Poverty and Persecution:** The relentless grind of material deprivation, the constant fear of violence, or the social isolation of being a persecuted minority are external realities that create internal anguish. This is the suffering of the oppressed, and the Bible is replete with God's specific concern for such individuals. Their despair is not a medical condition to be medicated away, but a social evil to be confronted with justice and compassionate action.

Beloved, the reason for this detailed taxonomy is to drive us to a place of profound humility. The human heart, in its complexity, is as the prophet Jeremiah declared: "The heart is deceitful above all things, and desperately sick; who can understand it?" (Jeremiah 17:9). We cannot. Therefore, our pastoral response must always begin not with assumption, but with compassionate, patient inquiry. We must become gentle detectives of the soul, asking questions, listening deeply, and holding space for the complex, messy, and often contradictory story of the sufferer. We must be willing to say, "I don't know the primary cause, but I am here with you, and we will seek the Healer together, using every good gift He has provided—whether through prayer, community, therapy, or medicine." A complex condition requires a nuanced diagnosis, and only the Great Physician, who searches mind and heart (Revelation 2:23), can ultimately untangle the threads. Our role is to be His humble, attentive, and well-equipped assistants.

12.3 The Sin of Simplification: Errors to Avoid in Pastoral Care

Beloved, as we continue to navigate the complex and sacred terrain of ministering to the mentally anguished, we must now, with pastoral courage and theological precision, confront the most common and destructive pitfalls that litter this landscape. These are the errors of simplification—the well-intentioned but deeply harmful attempts to reduce the profound, multi-dimensional agony of a suffering soul to a single, manageable cause, for which we then presume to have a single, straightforward solution. This "sin of simplification," as we shall term it, is a failure of love, a failure of wisdom, and ultimately, a failure to grasp the comprehensive nature of the Fall and the correspondingly comprehensive scope of the gospel's healing power. It is a pastoral strategy born not out of malicious intent, but out of our own deep-seated anxiety in the face of another's pain, our own helplessness, and our fallen desire for clean, controllable answers. Let us examine these errors with the sober clarity they demand, for to be forewarned is to be forearmed for the sake of those we are called to shepherd.

First, and perhaps most pernicious, is **The Error of Moralization**. This is the reflexive, almost instinctual response within certain strands of Christian culture that automatically attributes profound depression or debilitating anxiety to a specific, unconfessed sin in the sufferer's life. This is the error of Job's comforters, who, in their rigid theological framework, could only interpret his catastrophic suffering as evidence of hidden iniquity. Eliphaz the Temanite articulates this position with chilling certainty: "Remember: who that was innocent ever perished? Or where were the upright cut off? As I have seen, those who plow iniquity and sow trouble reap the same" (Job 4:7-8). Their entire ministry to Job was an extended, painful exercise in moral detective work, seeking to uncover the sin that must be at the root of his affliction.

The pastoral damage wrought by this error is catastrophic. It compounds the existing, often unbearable, burden of mental anguish with the crushing weight of spiritual condemnation and guilt. The sufferer, who may already be wrestling with feelings of worthlessness and despair, is now presented with a theological rationale for their self-loathing: "My suffering is proof of my failure. God is punishing me. I am being judged." This drives the individual deeper into isolation, as shame convinces them they are unworthy of community, and fear tells them they will be further judged if they reveal the true depth of their struggle. It creates a vicious cycle where the mental affliction itself generates feelings of guilt and spiritual inadequacy, which are then confirmed and amplified by the misguided counsel of the community, thereby deepening the depression and anxiety. It is a pastoral strategy that, in its attempt to cure, actively poisons the well. It ignores the clear teaching of Jesus in John 9 and the testimony of Paul's thorn in 2 Corinthians 12, which shatter any simplistic, one-to-one correlation between personal sin and personal suffering. To commit this error is to stand in the place of God, claiming a knowledge of His secret counsels that we do not possess, and in doing so, we become not comforters, but accusers of the brethren, echoing the very voice of the Satan whose name means "adversary."

The second grave error is **The Error of Exorcism**. This is the assumption, often fueled by a sensationalist and unbalanced reading of the Gospels, that all severe mental illness is primarily or solely the result of demonic oppression or possession. While we must hold, with biblical fidelity, to the reality of the demonic and the necessity of spiritual warfare, to universalize this principle is to venture into dangerous and unbiblical territory. The New Testament is remarkably discerning in its descriptions of demonic activity; it is never presented as the default explanation for epilepsy, muteness, or physical deformity, even though first-century culture may have interpreted them as such. Jesus and the apostles consistently differentiate between healing sickness and casting out demons (e.g., Matthew 4:24).

When this error is applied in pastoral practice, the consequences can be traumatic. It can lead to intense, confrontational, and fear-based "deliverance ministries" that seek to cast out a "spirit of depression" or a "spirit of anxiety" from a person whose brain chemistry is dysregulated or whose psyche has been shattered by trauma. This approach fails to address the underlying biological or psychological needs, leaving the root cause untreated. Furthermore, it can be spiritually violent. To tell a traumatized individual that their symptoms are the manifestation of a demonic entity can reinforce their feelings of being invaded, contaminated, and unsafe in their own body and mind. It can create a profound spiritual terror, where every negative thought or emotion is interpreted as a demonic attack, leading to a life of paralyzing fear and hyper-vigilance. This error represents a failure of discernment and a neglect of the other channels of affliction. It ignores the reality that the demonic, while real, often works most effectively not through dramatic possession, but through the more subtle avenues of accusation, deception, and the exploitation of our God-given physical and psychological vulnerabilities. To see a demon behind every manifestation of mental distress is not a mark of spiritual power, but of a theological imagination that has been flattened and impoverished.

Third, we encounter **The Error of Trivialization**. This error manifests in the offering of well-meaning but utterly inadequate spiritual platitudes. It is the response that says, "Just pray more," "You just need to have more faith," "Read your Bible more," or "Choose joy." These statements, while containing a kernel of truth about the importance of spiritual disciplines, become profoundly harmful when offered as the *exclusive* solution to a clinical-level mental health crisis. They minimize the person's suffering. They reduce a complex, multi-faceted affliction of the entire person to a simple matter of willpower or spiritual effort.

This error fails to acknowledge the real, often physical and involuntary, nature of the battle. Telling a person in the grips of a major depressive episode to "choose joy" is like telling a person with a broken leg to "choose to walk." It reveals a fundamental misunderstanding of the condition. The very faculties required to "pray more" or "have more faith"—the ability to concentrate, to feel God's presence, to muster hope—are often the very faculties that the affliction has compromised. The sufferer hears these platitudes as an indictment of their inadequate spiritual performance, and when they find themselves unable to comply, they sink deeper into the conviction that they are a failed Christian. This error represents a denial of the psychosomatic unity. It functionally operates as a form of Gnosticism, treating depression and anxiety as purely "spiritual" problems that can be solved with "spiritual" formulas, while ignoring the groaning of the body and the mind (Romans 8:23). It is a refusal to get our hands dirty with the messy, embodied reality of another's pain, preferring instead the clean, abstract world of spiritual clichés.

Finally, there is **The Error of Secularization**. This is the ditch on the opposite side of the road. In a well-intentioned effort to avoid the first three errors, the church or the pastor may capitulate entirely to a secular, medicalized model. The suffering individual is swiftly and solely referred to a therapist or a psychiatrist, and the community of faith, feeling relieved of a burden it does not understand, abdicates its role. The person is handed over to the "experts," and the spiritual companionship, the ministry of prayer, the reading of Scripture, and the tangible love of the body of Christ are withdrawn or offered only as a superficial afterthought.

This error is a failure of the church's God-given identity and mission. It is a practical denial of the reality that the human person is a *nephesh*, a spiritual being, and that their affliction has a spiritual dimension that cannot be fully addressed by psychotherapy or pharmacology alone. While these are essential tools of common grace, they are not substitutes for the ministry of the Spirit. To refer someone only to a therapist is to imply that the gospel has no unique word of comfort, no power for healing, and no community of support for the despairing soul. It fails to provide the one thing the secular world cannot: the hope of the resurrection, the comfort of the Holy Spirit, the assurance of sins forgiven, and the eschatological promise that every tear will be wiped away. It leaves the sufferer to navigate their deepest existential questions—"Where is God in this?" "What is the meaning of my suffering?" "Is there any hope beyond the grave?"—in a therapeutic context that is often methodologically committed to agnosticism on these very questions. This error creates a fragmented care model, where the soul is treated in one office and the psyche in another, with no integration between the two, thus reinforcing the very disintegration the sufferer is experiencing.

Beloved, each of these errors is a form of the sin of simplification. Each one takes the complex, mysterious, and deeply personal reality of human suffering and forces it into a pre-fabricated, one-size-fits-all box. Our calling is to reject these simplistic paradigms and to embrace the more difficult, more costly, but ultimately more faithful path of holistic, patient, and humble companionship. We are called to be a community that can hold the tension—that can pray for healing while supporting someone in therapy, that can renounce the demonic while ensuring a person takes their prescribed medication, that can proclaim the hope of the gospel while sitting in respectful silence with the one who, for now, can see no light at all.

12.4 A Multi-Disciplinary Ministry Model: The Church as Coordinating Center

Beloved, having diagnosed the errors of simplification, we now turn to the constructive task of building a robust, wise, and truly holistic model of care. If the previous section was a warning against building on sand, this section is a blueprint for building upon the rock of a comprehensive biblical anthropology. The local church, as the embodied presence of Christ in the world, must reclaim its God-given vocation as the primary community of care for the broken and afflicted. However, this does not mean the church must possess all expertise within its own institutional walls. Such a view leads to arrogance and incompetence. Rather, the church must function as the **coordinating center**, the integrative hub that lovingly and humbly brings together the diverse resources God has provided for human healing. This requires a posture of holy humility—the humility to acknowledge the limits of our own expertise, and the wisdom to recognize that all truth, whether revealed in Scripture or discovered in His creation, is ultimately God's truth, and therefore, all legitimate healing arts can be received as gifts of common grace to be stewarded for His glory and the good of His people.

This multi-disciplinary model is not a pragmatic compromise but a theological necessity. It flows directly from our understanding of the human person as a complex, multi-dimensional unity—spirit, soul, and body. A problem that exists across multiple dimensions requires a response that engages all those dimensions. To address only the spiritual while ignoring the psychological and biological is a form of Gnosticism. To address only the psychological and biological while ignoring the spiritual is a form of secular materialism. The church, as the guardian of a holistic gospel, is uniquely positioned to hold these dimensions together, ensuring that the suffering person is loved and treated as a whole *nephesh*. Let us then delineate the distinct but complementary roles within this collaborative model of care.

First and foremost, we have **The Role of the Pastor and Elders**. These are the shepherds of the flock, the primary spiritual physicians charged with the care of souls. Their ministry is irreplaceable and foundational, providing the ultimate framework of meaning within which all other forms of care take place. Their specific responsibilities include:

- **Spiritual Direction and Discernment:** The pastor and elders are tasked with walking alongside the sufferer, helping them to discern the movements of their own heart and the voice of God in the midst of their darkness. They help the individual interpret their suffering through the lens of the biblical narrative—the drama of Creation, Fall, Redemption, and Consummation. They ask not just "What is wrong?" but "Where is God in this? What might He be forming in you through this fire?"
- **Prayer and the Ministry of the Word:** This is their primary weapon and comfort. They pray *for* the sufferer, invoking the healing power of the Holy Spirit. They also pray *with* the sufferer, teaching them to cling to God when their own words fail them. They administer the ministry of the Word, not as a blunt instrument of exhortation, but as a balm. They read the Psalms of lament, giving voice to the sufferer's unspoken agony. They proclaim the promises of God's presence ("I will never leave you nor forsake you," Hebrews 13:5), His sovereignty ("And we know that for those who love God all things work together for good," Romans 8:28), and His all-sufficient grace ("My grace is sufficient for you," 2 Corinthians 12:9).
- **The Administration of the Sacraments:** In Baptism, they remind the sufferer of their secure identity in Christ—that they are not defined by their affliction but

by their union with Him in His death and resurrection. In the Eucharist, they offer the tangible presence of Christ, the medicine of immortality, a physical sign of a spiritual reality that nourishes the soul in its deepest poverty. The sacraments anchor the sufferer in objective reality of grace, outside the shifting sands of their subjective feelings.

The pastor and elders provide the theological and spiritual foundation. They are the keepers of the story that assures the sufferer they are not alone, their pain is not meaningless, and their final hope is secure.

Second, we have **The Role of the Christian Counselor/Therapist.** This individual operates as a crucial ally, a specialist in the terrain of the *psyche*—the mind, will, and emotions. Their work is not in competition with the pastor's; it is a complementary discipline that addresses the "how" of change in the intricate patterns of the human mind. A well-trained Christian counselor brings:

- **Professional Psychological Expertise:** They are skilled in evidence-based therapeutic modalities that can be harmonized with a biblical worldview. For example, Cognitive Behavioral Therapy (CBT) is a powerful tool for identifying and challenging the "strongholds" and "arguments" that Paul commands us to tear down in 2 Corinthians 10:4-5. It helps a person retrain the maladaptive cognitive patterns that fuel depression and anxiety, teaching them to "take every thought captive." Similarly, therapies like EMDR (Eye Movement Desensitization and Reprocessing) can be profoundly effective in helping the brain to properly process and integrate traumatic memories, releasing the individual from the prison of post-traumatic stress.

- **A Sanctification Ally:** The work of therapy, from a Christian perspective, can be seen as a direct ally in the process of sanctification. If sanctification is the progressive healing and renewal of the whole person into the image of Christ, then therapy addresses the deeply ingrained wounds and sinful patterns that hinder that process. A therapist can help a person understand *how* their childhood experiences shaped their core beliefs about God and themselves, and *how* to develop new, gospel-shaped patterns of relating. They provide the tools for the hard, practical work of putting off the old self and putting on the new (Ephesians 4:22-24).

The Christian counselor works in the space between the theological foundation laid by the pastor and the biological realities addressed by the physician, helping to repair the fractured connections between thought, emotion, and behavior.

Third, we must affirm **The Role of the Medical Doctor/Psychiatrist**. This is a ministry to the *soma*, the physical body, including the brain. To engage medical help is not a lack of faith; it is an act of stewardship and wisdom, a humble acknowledgment that we live in fallen bodies within a fallen creation.

- **Diagnosis and Biological Treatment:** A psychiatrist is trained to diagnose the complex interplay of neurochemistry, genetics, and physiology that undergirds many mental disorders. The prescription of an SSRI for major depression, for instance, is not a "crutch" but a legitimate attempt to correct a physiological malfunction, much like insulin for a diabetic. It is an application of common grace, utilizing the knowledge God has allowed humanity to discover about His creation.

- **Stewarding the Temple:** To seek medical and psychiatric care is to take seriously the biblical mandate to care for our bodies as temples of the Holy Spirit (1 Corinthians 6:19-20). If the temple's wiring (the nervous system) is malfunctioning, causing fires of anxiety, or if its foundation (the endocrine system) is cracked, leading to the collapse of depression, it is an act of faithfulness to call in the experts God has provided to help with the repairs. Medication can often provide the necessary biochemical stability that allows a person to then engage effectively in the spiritual and psychological work of healing.

Finally, and fundamentally, is **The Role of the Small Group/Community**. While the professionals provide targeted expertise, the community provides the ecosystem of love in which healing can take root and flourish. The small group, the family of God, is the frontline of incarnational ministry.

- **Practical Help:** The community embodies the love of Christ through tangible acts of service: providing meals, helping with childcare, assisting with household chores. This lifts practical burdens from the sufferer and their family, freeing up emotional and physical energy for the hard work of recovery. It is the outworking of Galatians 6:2: "Bear one another's burdens, and so fulfill the law of Christ."
- **Consistent Presence and Faithful Listening:** The community provides the antidote to the toxic isolation of mental illness. They are called to be "quick to hear, slow to speak, slow to anger" (James 1:19). This means

showing up, not with answers, but with ears to listen and hearts to empathize. It means being a non-anxious presence, a safe harbor where the sufferer can be honest about their despair without fear of judgment or trivialization.

- **A Non-Shaming Environment:** The community's unconditional acceptance communicates the unconditional love of God. When a person struggling with mental illness is embraced, included, and loved within the body of Christ, even in their brokenness, it powerfully refutes the lies of shame that tell them they are unacceptable, too damaged, or a burden. This communal love is a tangible foretaste of the grace that justifies the ungodly.

In this multi-disciplinary model, the church acts as the coordinating center. The pastor ensures all efforts are oriented toward the ultimate goal of Christlikeness and are grounded in the gospel. The church community creates the context of love and practical support. And the church, in its humility, joyfully partners with the Christian counselor and the medical doctor, recognizing them as fellow laborers in God's world, agents of His common grace, working together for the healing of the whole person. This is the church at its best: not a fortress against the world, but a healing center for the world, wisely and lovingly integrating every resource God provides to bring His shalom to a fractured soul.

12.5 The Ministry of Presence and Lament

Beloved, we have spoken of models, of roles, of disciplines and diagnoses. We have constructed a framework for a multi-faceted, integrative approach to mental affliction. Yet, there is a dimension of care that undergirds and transcends all these structures, a ministry so fundamental, so primal, that without it, even the most sophisticated care model rings hollow. It is the ministry that requires no advanced degree, no specialized training, but demands the entirety of a compassionate heart. It is the **Ministry of Presence**. And its most sacred language is the grammar of **Lament**.

In an age addicted to answers and obsessed with efficiency, the call to simply *be with* the suffering feels counter-intuitive, even wasteful. Our pastoral impulse, often fueled by our own anxiety in the face of another's pain, is to *do* something, to *say* something, to fix, to explain, to resolve. We reach for Scripture promises like bandages, we offer prayers like prescriptions, we proffer advice like a surgeon's scalpel, all in a frantic effort to close the wound we see before us. But what if the wound is too deep for a quick closure? What if the soul's fracture requires not a suture, but a steady, patient hand to simply hold the broken pieces together until the Great Physician arrives to perform His deeper work?

The ministry of presence is the discipline of doing nothing but being there. It is the intentional, prayerful decision to "sit shiva" with those who mourn, to descend into the ashes of their despair and take up residence there with them, as Job's friends did in their one moment of true wisdom: "And they sat with him on the ground seven days and seven nights, and no one spoke a word to him, for they saw that his suffering was very great" (Job 2:13). For seven days, their silent presence was their ministry. It communicated a truth more profound than any theological discourse: "You are not alone. Your suffering is seen. I will not abandon you in this place."

This silent, steadfast presence is profoundly Christlike. It is an incarnational ministry. The Gospel of John tells us the most theologically dense statement ever uttered: "The Word became flesh and dwelt among us" (John 1:14). Before Jesus preached the Sermon on the Mount, before He performed a single miracle, He *dwelt*. He pitched His tent in the midst of our brokenness. His very presence was the initial and fundamental act of redemption. So too, our physical, emotional, and spiritual presence with the suffering is a tangible sacrament of God's "with-ness." It is a living parable of Immanuel, God with us. When we sit in silence with the depressed, when we walk slowly beside the anxious, we are making visible the invisible reality of the God who promises, "I will never leave you nor forsake you" (Hebrews 13:5). Our non-anxious presence in the room with their turmoil becomes a sanctuary, a small, holy space where the demon of isolation is cast out by the ministry of shared humanity.

But this presence cannot remain entirely silent forever. The pain within the sufferer demands an outlet, a voice. And when that voice emerges, it is rarely a voice of praise or theological clarity. It is often a cry of anguish, a scream of "Why?", a guttural groan of despair. This is where the church must recover the lost language of Lament. Lament is not the absence of faith; it is the cry of faith in a context of pain. It is the stubborn refusal to let go of God even when He seems to have let go of you. It is the raw, unfiltered, and God-directed expression of grief, anger, confusion, and protest.

The Psalter, the prayer book of God's people, is saturated with lament. Nearly forty percent of the Psalms are laments. This is not an accident; it is divine revelation. God, in His wisdom, has given us a vocabulary for our suffering. He has authorized our complaints. He has invited our questions. Consider the brutal honesty of the sacred text:

- "How long, O LORD? Will you forget me forever? How long will you hide your face from me?" (Psalm 13:1)
- "My God, my God, why have you forsaken me? Why are you so far from saving me, from the words of my groaning?" (Psalm 22:1)
- "You have put me in the depths of the pit, in the regions dark and deep. Your wrath lies heavy upon me, and you overwhelm me with all your waves." (Psalm 88:6-7)

Psalm 88 is particularly stunning, for it ends without resolution, without a happy ending. The final verse is, "You have caused my beloved and my friend to shun me; my companions have become darkness." The darkness remains. The lament is unanswered. And yet, it is included in the canon of Scripture. This tells us that God is big enough to handle our despair. He is not threatened by our anger or our grief. He would rather we scream at Him in faith than politely ignore Him in despair.

Therefore, a crucial part of our pastoral ministry is to **create spaces for corporate lament**. Our worship services and small groups are often dominated by the language of victory, praise, and thanksgiving. These are essential, for they point to the ultimate reality of God's kingdom. But when they become the *only* permitted language, we inadvertently exile the suffering. We force them to wear a mask of okay-ness, to sing songs of victory they cannot feel, while their inner world is a funeral dirge. We must intentionally create liturgies of lament—times of worship where songs in a minor key are sung, where prayers of anguish are prayed aloud, where silence is held for the groans that have no words.

In such a space, the person battling clinical depression can finally breathe. They can say, "I feel like God is far from me," without being met with a corrective Bible verse. They can weep without being told to "rejoice in the Lord always." This validation is a radical act of grace. It says, "Your pain is real. Your experience is valid. You are not crazy, and you are not a second-class Christian for feeling this way." By giving them permission to voice their "How long, O Lord?", we are doing two things simultaneously: we are validating the reality of their pain in a fallen world, and we are directing that pain toward the only One who can ultimately bear it and answer it. Lament is faith in a storm. It is the act of turning your face toward God, even if only to ask, "Why have you turned your face from me?"

This ministry of presence and lament is spiritually and psychologically transformative. Psychologically, it facilitates the integration of traumatic and painful emotions. Unexpressed grief and anger become toxic, festering in the unconscious and manifesting as depression, anxiety, or physical illness. Lament provides a safe, held container for this emotional material to be expressed and processed, preventing it from being turned inward as self-hatred or outward as rage. It is a form of psycho-spiritual hygiene.

Spiritually, lament keeps the lines of communication with God open. The greatest danger in suffering is not the pain itself, but the silent turning away from God, the internal withdrawal born of the belief that He does not care or cannot be spoken to honestly. Lament is the antithesis of this. It is a violent, passionate engagement with the Divine. It is the prayer of the Israelite slaves in Egypt, whose "cry for rescue from slavery came up to God" (Exodus 2:23). God did not rebuke their cry; He descended in power to deliver them. Our lament, offered in the presence of a compassionate community, becomes a participation in the sufferings of Christ, who Himself lamented on the cross with the words of Psalm 22. It is in this sacred space of shared presence and honest lament that the soul, though still in darkness, finds it is not alone, and in that realization, finds the first, fragile thread of hope.

12.6 The Sufficiency of Grace in the "Thorn"

Beloved, we now arrive at the most profound and existentially demanding frontier of pastoral theology concerning mental affliction. We have discussed the multi-faceted model of care, the ministry of presence, and the language of lament. But what of those for whom the multi-faceted model yields only marginal improvement? What of those for whom the darkness does not lift, the anxiety does not abate, the biochemical and psychological interventions only manage the symptoms but do not provide a cure? What of the soul for whom the lament seems to echo back from a brass heaven, year after year, decade after decade? To minister here, at the very limits of human endurance and therapeutic skill, we require a theological framework that transcends the paradigm of healing and enters the mystery of sustained suffering. For this, we must turn, as the church has for two millennia, to the Apostle Paul and his divinely appointed "thorn in the flesh."

The passage in 2 Corinthians 12:7-10 is the non-negotiable foundation for a theology of chronic, treatment-resistant affliction. Paul writes: "So to keep me from becoming conceited because of the surpassing greatness of the revelations, a thorn was given me in the flesh, a messenger of Satan, to harass me, to keep me from becoming conceited. Three times I pleaded with the Lord about this, that it should leave me. But he said to me, 'My grace is sufficient for you, for my power is made perfect in weakness.' Therefore I will boast all the more gladly of my weaknesses, so that the power of Christ may rest upon me. For the sake of Christ, then, I am content with weaknesses, insults, hardships, persecutions, and calamities. For when I am weak, then I am strong."

Let us unpack this dense, glorious, and challenging text, for it contains a complete reorientation of how we understand the purpose and potential of unrelenting pain. First, we must consider the **nature of the thorn**. The Greek word *skolops* can mean a stake or a splinter—something sharp, piercing, and chronically irritating. While its exact nature is unknown (theories range from a debilitating eye disease to chronic malaria, to a relentless spiritual opponent), its characteristics are clear: it was *persistent*, *painful*, and *humiliating*. It was a "messenger of Satan," a phrase that acknowledges the malevolent, destructive intent of the enemy, yet it was simultaneously "given" to Paul, a passive verb implying God's ultimate, permissive sovereignty. This is the great mystery: the affliction was demonic in its agency, yet divine in its ultimate permission and purpose. It existed within the permissive will of a good God for a specific, holy end: "to keep me from becoming conceited." The thorn was a divinely sanctioned antidote to the poison of pride that could have arisen from Paul's unparalleled spiritual experiences.

Herein lies the first radical shift in perspective for chronic mental suffering. We are often desperate to assign a single, clean cause—it is either *all* biological or *all* spiritual. Paul's thorn resists this categorization. It was both/and. It was a "fleshly" affliction with a "spiritual" purpose. For the person with treatment-resistant depression or a severe anxiety disorder, this means their affliction, while possessing undeniable biological and psychological components—a "messenger of Satan" that harasses the physical and mental faculties—can simultaneously be a context, a classroom, in which God is performing a deep, hidden work of grace that could not be accomplished in a life of ease and perfect mental health. The affliction itself becomes the very condition that prevents a greater spiritual catastrophe, such as pride, self-sufficiency, or a shallow faith.

The core of this passage, and the heart of our pastoral theology for chronic suffering, is Paul's prayer and God's answer. Paul, the great apostle of faith and miracles, the one who had seen visions of paradise, "pleaded with the Lord" for healing. The word "pleaded" (*parakaleō*) is intense; it signifies begging, imploring, calling for help. This was not a lack of faith; it was the raw, human, and utterly faithful response to unremitting pain. He prayed not once, but three times, with persistence and passion. And the answer he received was not what he asked for. The thorn was not removed. The healing did not come.

Instead, he received a revelation: "My grace is sufficient for you, for my power is made perfect in weakness." This is the divine answer to the problem of the unhealed wound. God does not explain *why* the thorn remains. He does not provide a theodicy. He provides Himself. He offers not the removal of the pain, but the provision of His own presence and power *within* the pain. The Greek word for "sufficient" (*arkei*) means "it is enough." It is a present-tense reality. The grace is not a stockpile for the future; it is a daily, moment-by-moment infusion of divine strength that meets the exact measure of the day's weakness. It is the manna of the soul—enough for today, with the promise of more tomorrow.

This is where the pastoral goal must undergo a fundamental shift. For those in the grip of a chronic "thorn," the goal can no longer be a cure as the primary object of hope. To continually hold out the promise of complete healing as the only acceptable outcome is to set the sufferer up for a crisis of faith when that healing does not materialize. It can lead them to believe that God has failed them or that their faith is inadequate. Instead, the pastoral goal must shift to the Pauline paradigm: fostering endurance and revealing the present-tense sufficiency of Christ's grace. The question changes from, "God, why won't You take this away?" to "God, how will Your grace be sufficient for me in this today? How will Your power be made perfect in my present weakness?"

This is not a passive resignation. It is not a grim, stoic acceptance of fate. It is, as Paul demonstrates, an *active, faith-filled clinging*. His response to the divine revelation is one of the most counter-intuitive statements in all of Scripture: "Therefore I will boast all the more gladly of my weaknesses, so that the power of Christ may rest upon me." The word "boast" (*kauchaomai*) means to glory in, to celebrate. Paul moves from pleading for the thorn's removal to celebrating its existence. Why? Because the thorn has become the precise condition that makes room for the "power of Christ" to "rest upon" him. The Greek for "rest upon" (*episkēnoō*) means to pitch a tent upon, to take up residence. The chronic weakness becomes the dwelling place for Christ's power. The very thing that disqualifies him in the eyes of the world (his weakness) becomes the qualification for a manifestation of divine power that the world cannot explain.

For the believer with a chronic mental affliction, this is the path to a hope that cannot be extinguished by the persistence of their illness. Their depression, their anxiety, their bipolar disorder—

their "thorn"—is not a sign of God's abandonment. It can become, through a miracle of grace, the very platform upon which the strength of Christ is most clearly displayed. Their daily battle to get out of bed, to choose life, to trust God when their emotions scream otherwise, to love their family through the fog of medication—this is not a failure of faith. This is the very theater where faith performs its most heroic acts. When they endure, when they cling to a shred of hope, when they demonstrate a love that is not sourced in their fickle emotions but in the steadfast character of God, they are not weak. They are, in fact, showcasing a strength that is not their own—the power of Christ resting upon them.

This understanding transforms the meaning of "strength" and "weakness." The world's definition of strength is autonomy, self-sufficiency, and the absence of need. The gospel's definition of strength is the exact opposite. It is found in acknowledged dependence. "For when I am weak, then I am strong." The chronic affliction systematically dismantles the illusion of self-sufficiency. It forces a daily, hourly dependence upon Christ. It makes the believer a living testament to the truth that we are jars of clay, and the transcendent power belongs to God and not to us (2 Corinthians 4:7). The "thorn" keeps the jar cracked, ensuring that no one mistakes the clay for the treasure inside.

Therefore, our pastoral task with those who bear a lifelong thorn is to help them make this profound paradigm shift. We must help them to see their struggle not as a meaningless curse, but as a context for grace. We must point out the evidence of that sufficient grace in their lives—the moments they didn't give up, the kindness they showed when they were in anguish, the scripture that comforted them for a fleeting moment. We must celebrate their endurance as the victory it is. We must stop trying to cure them into a version of Christianity that doesn't need grace, and instead, help them to discover the depths of a grace that is made perfect not in their health, but in their acknowledged sickness; not in their strength, but in their confessed weakness. In doing so, we participate with the Spirit in the great work of revealing that the power of the crucified and risen Christ is most gloriously manifested not in the absence of suffering, but in its very midst.

12.7 A Harbor in the Storm

Beloved, as we draw this critical chapter to its culmination, we must gather up the threads of our exploration and weave them into a final, clarifying vision of the church's sacred calling in a world fractured by mental and emotional anguish. The journey we have undertaken—through the complexities of taxonomy, the perils of simplistic error, the architecture of a multi-disciplinary model, the profound ministries of presence and lament, and the mysterious sufficiency of grace in the unremitting "thorn"—all converges upon one fundamental, identity-shaping truth. The church of Jesus Christ is not, and was never intended to be, a pristine gallery displaying the finished masterpieces of sanctification. It is not a community of the perfectly healthy, the emotionally stable, and the spiritually triumphant. To project such an image is a lie, a denial of our shared reality as *simul iustus et peccator*—simultaneously righteous and sinner. Rather, the church's true and glorious calling is to be a **hospital for sinners and sufferers**. It is a field hospital, as Pope Francis has aptly noted, stationed on the front lines of a cosmic battle, and its primary mission is triage, healing, and restoration for all who are wounded in the conflict.

This hospital-identity fundamentally reorients our posture. A hospital is not a place of judgment for those who are sick; it is a place of refuge. Its staff are not scandalized by the presence of disease; they are trained to expect it, diagnose it, and treat it with every tool at their disposal. The atmosphere is not one of shame, but of focused compassion. So it must be with the church. We must shed the last vestiges of the illusion that robust mental health is a prerequisite for fellowship, and instead embrace the biblical reality that the fellowship itself *is* the context God has ordained for healing. The question is not, "Are you well enough to belong here?" but rather, "In your brokenness, will you allow this community to belong to you, to bear your burdens with you, and to point you relentlessly to the Chief Physician?"

A theologically robust and pastorally compassionate approach to mental affliction, therefore, is one that first and foremost **embraces complexity**. It willingly enters the messy, non-linear, and often paradoxical reality of human suffering. It rejects the seductive simplicity of the four errors we outlined—moralization, exorcism, trivialization, and secularization—because it understands that the human *nephesh* is a profound mystery, a unity of spirit, soul, and body, and a rupture in one dimension inevitably causes reverberations throughout the entire person. To embrace complexity is to have the humility to admit that we do not always know why a particular soul is afflicted, and that the "why" may be less important than the "how"—how we can love, support, and point to Christ in the midst of the mystery. It is to sit comfortably with the tension of Paul's thorn—a "messenger of Satan" yet given by God for a holy purpose. It is to acknowledge that a person can be both spiritually mature and clinically depressed, that they can be filled with the Holy Spirit and also require medication to regulate their brain chemistry. This embrace of complexity is not a descent into relativistic confusion; it is an ascent into a higher wisdom that recognizes the limits of human understanding and rests in the boundless, often inscrutable, sovereignty of God.

This robust approach then **leverages all of God's provisions** with gratitude and wisdom. It operates from a theology of common grace that joyfully recognizes that all truth is God's truth, whether it is revealed in the special revelation of Scripture or discovered in the general revelation of His creation. The insights of neuroscience, the techniques of trauma-informed therapy, the stabilizing power of psychopharmacology—these are not threats to a spiritual worldview, but gifts from a benevolent Creator to a fallen world. They are tools in the divine toolkit, and it is the height of folly and ingratitude to refuse to use them. The church, as the coordinating center of care, must become fluent in the language of these disciplines, not to be mastered by them, but to master them for the sake of the gospel, to harness them for the holistic healing of the person.

Simultaneously, this approach never relinquishes the unique, irreplaceable resources of the Spirit. It wields the ministry of the Word not as a blunt instrument, but as a precise scalpel and a healing balm—speaking the Psalms of lament to the despairing, the promises of God's presence to the abandoned, and the sufficient grace of Christ to those with a chronic thorn. It practices the ministry of prayer, invoking the power of the Holy Spirit to heal, to comfort, and to sustain where human effort reaches its limit. It administers the sacraments, those tangible means of grace that anchor the sufferer in the objective reality of Christ's finished work, outside the shifting sands of their subjective emotional state. And it mobilizes the community, the *koinonia*, to be the hands and feet of Jesus, providing the practical help, the faithful listening, and the non-shaming presence that combat the isolation which is the native habitat of despair.

Ultimately, a truly compassionate pastoral approach **points unwaveringly to the hope that our present sufferings are producing an eternal weight of glory** (2 Corinthians 4:17). This is the North Star that guides the entire enterprise. Without this eschatological hope, our care, no matter how compassionate or multi-faceted, is ultimately palliative. It can only offer better management of a terminal condition. But the gospel announces that the terminal condition of a fallen creation has been dealt a deathblow in the cross and resurrection of Jesus Christ. Our present sufferings, therefore, are not the final word. They are, in the mysterious economy of God, actually *productive*. Paul uses the language of weight: a "light momentary affliction" is, paradoxically, "preparing for us an eternal weight of glory beyond all comparison." The agony of depression, the relentless grip of anxiety, the exhausting battle with a disordered mind—these are the "light and momentary" afflictions? This is only comprehensible from the vantage point of eternity, when the scales of God's justice will be balanced and the true, staggering mass of the glory that awaits us will be revealed. This hope does not remove the pain in the present, but it re-contextualizes it. It assures the sufferer that their pain is not wasted, that it is being mysteriously, sovereignly woven into the grand tapestry of redemption, and that it is, even now, producing a glory so heavy, so substantial, and so eternal that the memory of this suffering will be utterly eclipsed by its radiance.

Therefore, the church, as a harbor in the storm, offers not easy answers, but a faithful companionship. It cannot always still the waves or silence the wind, but it can provide a safe anchorage, a place where the ship of the soul can ride out the tempest without being dashed upon the rocks. This faithful companionship is our highest calling. It is the practical outworking of the love of Christ, the Man of Sorrows who is intimately acquainted with grief (Isaiah 53:3). He did not stand at a distance and shout instructions to us in our pain. He entered into it. He became the ultimate Sufferer. And now, as our Great High Priest, He is able to sympathize with our weaknesses (Hebrews 4:15). Our ministry to the mentally afflicted is, at its core, a participation in His ministry. We are called to embody His sympathetic presence, to be a living sacrament of His "with-ness." We are to be a community that can look into the abyss of another's despair and not look away, a people who can bear the weight of another's grief without buckling, a family that can hope fiercely for another when they have no hope left for themselves. This is the church at its most authentic and most beautiful: a harbor of hope in the storm of affliction, a living testament to the One who walks with us through the valley of the shadow of death, and who will, one glorious day, wipe away every tear from every eye.

PART IV

PHYSICAL DISCIPLINE: THE FAITHFUL BODY IN ACTION

CHAPTER 13

The Theology of Physical Labor and Exercise: "Train Yourself for Godliness" (1 Timothy 4:7)

Beloved, we now pivot our theological exploration from the inner landscape of the mind and emotions to the tangible, visible, and often contentious domain of the physical body in motion. We have established that the body is a temple of the Holy Spirit, a sacred vessel. But a temple is not a static museum piece; it is a living, functioning center of worship and service. How, then, are we to understand the deliberate, disciplined use of this physical vessel? How do we reconcile the call to bodily stewardship with the stark warnings against the "works of the flesh"? We stand at a cultural crossroads, where the human body is simultaneously worshipped and despised, curated as an object of desire and dismissed as a biological machine. In this cacophony of conflicting messages, the church has often remained silent, or worse, has implicitly endorsed a new form of Gnosticism that views physical exertion as, at best, irrelevant to spiritual life and, at worst, a dangerous distraction from "more important" spiritual pursuits.

This chapter represents a deliberate and forceful argument against such a disembodied spirituality. We will contend that physical discipline—a category encompassing both the sanctification of our daily, God-given labor and the intentional practice of physical exercise—is a vital, non-optional component of holistic Christian discipleship. It is a form of *askēsis*—a spiritual training—that finds its ultimate justification not in the mirror of self-admiration, nor in the metrics of performance, but in the sanctuary of divine purpose. The sweat of our brow, the strain of our muscles, the rhythm of our breath—all of this can be, and indeed *must* be, taken up into the economy of grace and offered as a living sacrifice. We will explore how the disciplined body becomes a more effective instrument for the Great Commandment, a more resilient vessel for the trials of mission, and a more vivid proclamation of the goodness of the Creator who formed us from the dust. Our guiding star will be the Apostle Paul's provocative and often misunderstood command to his young protégé Timothy: "Rather, train yourself for godliness; for while bodily training is of some value, godliness is of value in every way, as it holds promise for the present life and also for the life to come" (1 Timothy 4:7-8). This text does not dismiss the physical; it properly orders it, subordinating it to its ultimate end: a life wholly oriented toward God.

13.1 From the Gym to the Sanctuary

We begin our exploration by confronting the dominant cultural narrative that surrounds the human body, a narrative that has seeped, often undetected, into the consciousness of the modern church. We live in an age of what can only be described as a **therapeutic-aesthetic complex**. This is a powerful cultural force that reduces the body to one of two primary categories: either a **project for self-optimization** or a **canvas for self-expression**.

On one hand, the body is treated as a machine to be fine-tuned, a system to be hacked. We are bombarded with messages about "bio-hacking," "peak performance," and "optimized wellness." The gym becomes a secular cathedral of self-worship, where the rituals of the lift, the run, and the diet are performed with a religious fervor, all in pursuit of longevity, vitality, and a physique that meets the ever-shifting standards of cultural approval. The goal is autonomy—the creation of a self-sufficient, high-performing individual who is the master of their own biological destiny. This is the religion of the self, dressed in the language of health, and its telos, its ultimate end, is the self.

On the other hand, the body is treated as a canvas upon which to paint one's identity. Tattoos, piercings, surgical alterations, and curated fashion styles are used to signal tribe, to express internal feelings, or to rebel against societal norms. Here, the body's value is found in its utility as a medium for communicating a personal narrative. The goal is authenticity, defined as the external manifestation of the internal, subjective self. Its telos is self-expression.

Both of these paradigms, while containing elements of truth about the importance of health and the legitimacy of artistic expression, are fundamentally anthropocentric. They begin and end with the self. The body exists for my performance, my longevity, my expression, my identity. This stands in stark, radical opposition to the biblical vision. The Apostle Paul issues a thunderous corrective to this entire way of thinking in his first letter to the Corinthians: "You are not your own, for you were bought with a price. So glorify God in your body" (1 Corinthians 6:19-20).

This declaration shatters the foundations of the therapeutic-aesthetic complex. My body is not my own project. It is not my own canvas. It is **Christ's purchased possession**. I am a steward, a caretaker, a tenant in a property that belongs to Another. The fundamental question of my physical existence, therefore, shifts from "What do I want to do with my body?" to "How does the Owner want me to use His body?" The purpose of my physical being is not self-glorification, but the glorification of God. This is the great theological pivot that must inform every rep, every step, every hour of labor.

When we view physical discipline through this lens, it is transformed from a project of self-improvement into a **form of asceticism aimed at cultivating godliness**. The word "asceticism" comes from the Greek *askēsis*, which simply means "training" or "exercise." It was the word used for an athlete's rigorous preparation for the games. In the Christian tradition, asceticism has never been about punishing the body because it is evil—that is the heresy of Gnosticism. True Christian asceticism is about *training* the body, and the appetites associated with it, so that it becomes a willing, responsive, and effective instrument of the will, which is itself being progressively aligned with the will of God.

Physical discipline, therefore, is a school of virtue. It is a tangible, lived-out arena where we practice the fruit of the Spirit. When we discipline ourselves to get out of bed for a morning run when every fiber of our flesh screams to stay under the covers, we are practicing **self-control**. When we push through the burning fatigue of the last few reps, not for the sake of vanity but as an act of stewardship, we are cultivating **perseverance**. When we choose a nourishing meal over a degrading one because we honor the body as a temple, we are exercising **faithfulness** to our divine Tenant. When we accept the limitations of our aging frame or our genetic makeup without despair or rage, we are learning **gentleness** and **peace**. The gym, the garden, the workshop—these become laboratories for sanctification, places where the abstract commands of Scripture become concrete, physical realities.

This training, in turn, **enhances our capacity for service**. A body that is weak, lethargic, and perpetually unwell is a limited instrument for the kingdom of God. The Great Commandment to love God with all our strength and to love our neighbor as ourselves is irreducibly physical. It requires energy, vitality, and resilience. To lift a heavy burden for a neighbor, to play actively with our children, to endure long hours of ministry without collapsing into exhaustion, to have the physical and mental clarity that comes from cardiovascular health for prayer and study—all of this is facilitated by a body that has been diligently and wisely trained. Physical discipline is, in this sense, a profound act of love. We steward our strength not for ourselves, but for the sake of others, that we might have more to give, for longer, and with greater joy.

Thus, the journey from the gym to the sanctuary is not a long one. It is, in fact, the same path. The sweat of our brow, offered to God, becomes a liquid prayer. The disciplined body becomes a living doxology. We are called to move beyond a culture that worships the body for its own sake, and to recover a theology that worships God *with* the body, presenting it as a living sacrifice, holy and acceptable to Him, which is our spiritual worship (Romans 12:1).

13.2 Creational Foundations: Work as a Pre-Fall Vocation

Beloved, to construct a truly robust theology of physical labor and exercise, we must journey back before the curse, before the thorn and the thistle, before the sweat of the brow became a symbol of futility. We must return to the pristine goodness of the Garden, to the original design, where the relationship between the human body and its purpose was untainted by sin and unclouded by toil. It is here, in the second chapter of Genesis, that we find the non-negotiable foundation for all our subsequent thinking: **Physicality is not a curse.** The body and its labor are not part of the problem introduced by the Fall; they are an essential, glorious component of the original, "very good" creation. To view physical exertion as inherently base, burdensome, or spiritually inferior is to succumb to a heresy that denies the goodness of God's material world and the dignity of His embodied image-bearers.

Our foundational text is Genesis 2:15, a verse of monumental significance that is often read but whose theological weight is rarely felt: "The LORD God took the man and put him in the garden of Eden **to work it and keep it**." Let us pause and feel the tectonic implications of this statement. This divine assignment was given *before* the serpent, *before* the forbidden fruit, *before* the rupture of relationships. Work was not a punishment; it was a **pre-fall vocation**. It was the first thing God gave Adam to do. His identity as God's image-bearer was to be expressed, in part, through the purposeful engagement of his physical body with the physical world.

To understand the profound nature of this vocation, we must delve into the rich Hebrew words used here. The English translation "to work it and keep it" is accurate, but it fails to capture the dense theological and cultural freight these terms carried.

The first word is ***avad*** (עָבַד). While it is correctly translated "to work," its semantic range is far broader and more profound. *Avad* fundamentally means to serve, to labor, to worship. It is the word used for the service of a slave to a master, for the Levitical priesthood in the tabernacle, and for the worship of Yahweh. This is staggering. Adam's work in the Garden was not merely horticultural maintenance; it was an act of *service* to God and *worship* of God. By tending the Garden, he was fulfilling his role as a vice-regent, serving the Creator by lovingly cultivating His creation. His physical labor—the tilling, the planting, the pruning—was a form of liturgy. It was an extension of the divine creativity, a co-operative act with God in bringing the potential of the earth to its fullest, most beautiful fruition. The dirt under his fingernails was a badge of his priestly office. The sweat on his brow (which at this point would have been the pleasant perspiration of engaged effort, not the anguished sweat of cursed toil) was an anointing oil, consecrating him to his task. To *avad* the garden was to image forth the God who Himself worked for six days and rested on the seventh. It was to participate in the ongoing, sustaining work of the Creator.

The second word is ***shamar*** (שָׁמַר). Translated "to keep," it carries the strong connotations of guarding, protecting, watching over, and preserving. It is the word used for the cherubim who *guard* the way to the Tree of Life after the Fall (Genesis 3:24). It is used of God, who *guards* His people (Psalm 121). Adam was placed in the Garden not just as a worker, but as a guardian. His vocation was one of protection and preservation. He was to exercise a priestly dominion that "kept" the harmony and integrity of the created order. This implies a world that, while "very good," was not static or risk-free. It was a dynamic ecosystem that required wise, attentive stewardship to maintain its *shalom*. Adam's physical presence, his watchful eye, his protective intervention—all were part of this *shamar* responsibility. He was the earth's first custodian, its divinely appointed steward, charged with ensuring that the goodness of God's creation was nurtured and protected from any potential disorder.

Therefore, the original human vocation, as encapsulated in *avad* and *shamar*, was a holistic, integrated calling. It was:

1. **Physically Engaged:** It required a body. It demanded the expenditure of caloric energy, the use of muscular strength, the coordination of hand and eye. The body was the essential instrument for fulfilling the cultural mandate.
2. **Intellectually Stimulating:** To work and keep the garden required observation, learning, problem-solving, and creativity. Adam had to learn the properties of plants, the patterns of growth, the interplay of soil and water. He was, in a sense, the first scientist and artist.
3. **Spiritually Significant:** This labor was not secular. It was inherently sacred, a primary means of worshipping and serving God. His daily work was his worship. There was no sacred-secular divide.

This creational foundation radically reframes our understanding of all physical labor and discipline today. When we engage in physical work—whether it is tilling a field, building a cabinet, writing code, or cleaning a home—we are, at their most fundamental level, participating in this original, pre-fall vocation of *avad* and *shamar*. We are serving God by cultivating and bringing order to His world. We are acting as His image-bearers. The curse in Genesis 3:17-19 did not introduce work; it introduced *frustration*, *pain*, and *futility* into work. "Cursed is the ground because of you; in pain you shall eat of it all the days of your life; thorns and thistles it shall bring forth for you... By the sweat of your face you shall eat bread." The work itself remains part of our God-given design, but it is now stained with the reality of the Fall. It is often frustrating, exhausting, and seemingly futile.

This understanding also sanctifies intentional physical exercise. If our bodies were designed for the active, purposeful labor of *avad* and *shamar*, then exercise can be seen as a form of "creational practice." In a modern, sedentary world where our daily work often does not require full physical engagement, disciplined exercise becomes a way of maintaining the instrument for its original purpose. It is a way of honoring the creational design of our musculoskeletal, cardiovascular, and nervous systems. When we lift weights, we are stewarding the strength that would have been used to *shamar*—to build, to protect, to guard. When we run or engage in cardio, we are maintaining the endurance that would have been required to *avad*—to cultivate, to explore, to serve across vast territories. Exercise, from this perspective, is not about creating a body that is useful; it is about maintaining a body that is *faithful* to its original, creational calling. It is an act of remembering what we were made for and a hopeful anticipation of the day when the curse of futility will be lifted, and our labor—physical, intellectual, and spiritual—will once again be purely and perfectly an act of *avad* and *shamar* in the New Heavens and New Earth.

13.3 The Curse and the Redemption of Toil

Beloved, having gazed upon the pristine beauty of humanity's original vocation in the Garden, we must now, with sober realism, confront the catastrophic fracture that rent this divine harmony asunder. The pre-fall symphony of *avad* and *shamar*—of worshipful work and priestly keeping—was violently disrupted by the dissonant chord of human rebellion. The creational goodness of physical labor was not erased by the Fall, but it was profoundly and painfully corrupted. It was subjected to a curse, a divine judgment that introduced a new and agonizing quality to the human experience of work. To understand the full scope of Christ's redemptive work, we must first comprehend the depth of this curse, for we cannot appreciate the glory of the redemption until we have felt the weight of the bondage.

The pronouncement of judgment in Genesis 3:17-19 is unequivocal and devastating: "And to Adam he said, 'Because you have listened to the voice of your wife and have eaten of the tree of which I commanded you, "You shall not eat of it," **cursed is the ground because of you; in pain you shall eat of it all the days of your life; thorns and thistles it shall bring forth for you; and you shall eat the plants of the field. By the sweat of your face you shall eat bread, till you return to the ground**, for out of it you were taken; for you are dust, and to dust you shall return.'"

Let us parse the anatomy of this curse upon work. First, God pronounces a curse upon the **ground** itself (*ha'adamah*). This is profoundly significant. The very material from which Adam (*ha'adam*) was formed and over which he was to exercise his priestly dominion now becomes his adversary. The creation, which was designed to respond willingly and fruitfully to his touch, now becomes resistant. It will now produce "thorns and thistles"—useless, painful, obstructive growth that competes with and chokes out the life-giving plants. This is the origin of what we might call systemic frustration. Work is no longer a seamless flow of co-creative effort with a responsive creation; it becomes a struggle, a wrestling match with a recalcitrant earth. The ground, which was meant to be a partner in bringing forth abundance, is now an opponent that must be wrestled into submission.

Second, the nature of the labor itself is transformed. The joyful, fulfilling work of *avad* is now described as "painful toil." The Hebrew word here, *itsabon*, conveys grievous labor, sorrow, and pain. It is the same word used to describe the pain of childbirth for Eve in the preceding verse. Work becomes agonizing. It is now characterized by "the sweat of your face." Sweat, in this context, is not the healthy perspiration of vigorous effort; it is the sign of anguished struggle, of a body straining against a creation that is pushing back. Work becomes exhausting, depleting, and often demeaning. The creational purpose of work remains, but the experience of it is now shot through with the reality of struggle, fatigue, and frustration.

Finally, the curse introduces the specter of **futility** and **death**. The entire endeavor is now framed by the ultimate return to the dust. "Till you return to the ground..." All of Adam's labor, all his sweat and struggle, is now shadowed by the grim reality that he himself will ultimately be reabsorbed by the very ground he struggles to cultivate. His work will not last. He will die, and his accomplishments will, in the grand scheme, turn to dust. This is the existential weight of the curse: the haunting sense that our labor is, in the final analysis, meaningless, a "striving after wind" as the Preacher in Ecclesiastes so poignantly laments.

The Apostle Paul, centuries later, would describe this cosmic condition with theological precision in Romans 8:20: "For the creation was subjected to **futility**, not willingly, but because of him who subjected it, in hope." The Greek word for futility, *mataiotēs*, means emptiness, vanity, transitoriness. It is the same concept Ecclesiastes explores. The entire created order, including our work within it, has been subjected to this frustrating cycle of decay and death. A field carefully cultivated will eventually be overrun by weeds. A building meticulously constructed will eventually crumble. A report brilliantly written will eventually be filed away and forgotten. This is the "groaning" of creation, and it is the groaning that echoes in the heart of every worker who has ever asked, "What is the point of all this effort?"

Yet—and this is the glorious, gospel-saturated "yet"—the story does not end with the curse. The redemptive work of Jesus Christ extends its sovereign reach into the very realm of our toil. In Christ, work is **redeemed**. This does not mean the curse is magically lifted and our work becomes effortless and perpetually fulfilling in this age. The thorns and thistles remain. The sweat still pours from our brow. The specter of futility still looms. But what changes, radically and fundamentally, is the *meaning*, the *context*, and the *purpose* of our labor.

The Apostle Paul, in his letter to the Colossians, unveils the transformative key: "**Whatever you do, work heartily, as for the Lord and not for men**, knowing that from the Lord you will receive the inheritance as your reward. You are serving the Lord Christ" (Colossians 3:23-24).

This single verse performs a cosmic shift in the orientation of all human labor. Work is no longer merely a cursed activity to be endured, a necessary evil for survival. It is now a **domain for worship**. The primary audience for our work is no longer our human boss, our client, or even ourselves. The primary audience is the Lord Christ. When we dig a ditch, we are digging it for Jesus. When we type a report, we are typing it for Jesus. When we change a diaper, we are changing it for Jesus. When we write code, we are writing it for Jesus. The nature of the task is secondary; the primary reality is the One for whom it is done.

This sanctifies *all* faithful labor. There is no longer a hierarchy of "spiritual" work (preaching, missionary service) and "secular" work (farming, accounting). All work, when done "heartily, as for the Lord," becomes a sacred offering. The motivation shifts from self-glorification, mere financial gain, or social approval to the pleasing of our divine Master. The quality of our work is transformed, for we are no longer working for a fallible human supervisor but for the perfect, all-seeing Christ. We become concerned with integrity, excellence, and diligence not because it earns a promotion, but because it reflects the character of the God we serve.

This redemptive perspective also reframes the **frustration and futility** of work. The sweat, the thorns, the resistance—these are no longer meaningless punishments. They become our participation in the sufferings of Christ, who Himself entered into a cursed creation and labored unto death, sweating great drops of blood in the Garden of Gethsemane. Our daily struggles with a frustrating project, a difficult colleague, or a resistant material can be offered up to God as a share in the "fellowship of his sufferings" (Philippians 3:10). Furthermore, the futility is now held within the context of hope. We know that the creation itself will be set free from its bondage to decay (Romans 8:21). Our work, though it may turn to dust in this age, is not lost. It is, in ways we cannot fully see, being taken up into God's redemptive economy. A faithfully built cabinet that lasts a hundred years speaks of a God of order and beauty. A diligently managed business that provides for families reflects God's providential care. Our labor, offered to Christ, becomes a seed that will bear fruit in the New Creation, in ways that transcend our present understanding.

Therefore, the redemption of toil in Christ transforms it from a curse to be endured into a **vocation to be fulfilled**. It is an act of obedience. It is a spiritual discipline. It is a tangible way to love our neighbor by providing good and useful goods and services. And it is a profound act of worship, a daily, physical offering of our whole selves—our minds, our hands, our strength—to the Lord who bought us. The curse introduced the sweat, but redemption sanctifies it, turning it into a liquid prayer, a sacrifice of praise offered upon the altar of our daily labors.

13.4 Exegesis of 1 Timothy 4:7-8: The Athletic Metaphor

Beloved, we now arrive at the exegetical heart of our theology of physical discipline, the very words of the Apostle Paul that have been both a source of guidance and, tragically, a source of profound misunderstanding for centuries. In his first letter to his young protégé Timothy, Paul writes: "Have nothing to do with irreverent, silly myths. Rather, **train yourself for godliness; for while bodily training is of some value, godliness is of value in every way, as it holds promise for the present life and also for the life to come**" (1 Timothy 4:7-8). This passage is the linchpin, the divine commentary that connects the creational goodness of the body with the ultimate purpose of all discipline. To misread it is to risk either an idolatry of the physical or a Gnostic dismissal of it. Therefore, we must approach this text with the utmost care, allowing the richness of the Greek language and the cultural context to illuminate its true, balanced, and empowering meaning.

The first and most critical word to grasp is the imperative verb at the beginning of Paul's positive command: **"Train yourself..."** The Greek word is *gymnaze* (γύμναζε). This is not a generic word for "try hard" or "be disciplined." It is a highly specific, culturally loaded term drawn directly from the world of Greek athletics. It means to exercise naked, to train in the gymnasium. In the first-century Greco-Roman world, the gymnasium was the center of civic and cultural life, where young men trained their bodies for the athletic games, which were religious festivals dedicated to the pagan gods. The training was rigorous, systematic, and all-consuming. It involved strict dietary regimens, repetitive drills, and painful conditioning—all aimed at winning a perishable wreath, a crown of leaves that would soon wither.

By choosing this word, Paul is performing a brilliant act of cultural appropriation. He is taking a concept familiar to every person in the Hellenistic world—the concept of intense, focused, bodily discipline for a temporal prize—and he is baptizing it. He is redirecting it. He is saying, "You understand what it means to train your body for a race that lasts a few minutes, for a prize that will rot. Now, I command you to apply that same mentality, that same intensity, that same commitment to repetition and pain, to the development of your inner being, to the cultivation of godliness." The command *gymnaze* implies that the pursuit of godliness is not a passive, effortless process of spiritual osmosis. It is *askēsis*. It requires a plan. It requires sweat. It requires saying "no" to certain things and "yes" to others, even when it is painful. It requires getting up early for prayer when you want to sleep. It requires meditating on Scripture when you would rather be entertained. It requires forgiving when you want to retaliate. This is the *gymnaze* of the soul.

Having established this powerful metaphor, Paul then makes his famous comparative statement: **"for while bodily training is of some value, godliness is of value in every way..."** It is here that a superficial reading has led many in the church to a tragic error. The common interpretation has been to hear this as a dismissal: "Bodily training? Oh, that's of *some* value, I suppose, but it's really not very important. The real thing is godliness." This reading has provided a theological excuse for generations of Christians to neglect the physical temple of the Holy Spirit, leading to poor health, a lack of energy for service, and a functional Gnosticism that denies the goodness of God's creation.

But this is a profound misreading, born of a failure to engage the Greek text with precision. The phrase translated "of some value" is the Greek *pros oligos* (πρὸς ὀλίγον). The key to understanding this phrase lies in the preposition *pros*, which primarily means "for" or "toward," often with a sense of limitation or purpose. A more accurate and nuanced translation would be **"for a little,"** or **"for a short time."** The contrast Paul is making is not between "a little value" and "a lot of value." The contrast is between **temporal value** and **eternal value**. Between **limited scope** and **comprehensive scope**.

Let us be unequivocally clear: Paul is *not* saying bodily training is of negligible value. He is affirming its genuine, real, and God-given value, while properly contextualizing its *duration* and *scope*. Bodily training has value *for a little*—for the few decades of this present life. The benefits are real: strength, health, vitality, endurance, mental clarity. These are good gifts from a good Creator. A strong, healthy body is a better instrument for loving one's neighbor, for working diligently, and for enduring hardship than a weak and sickly one. Paul, who himself used the metaphor of an athlete running to win a prize (1 Corinthians 9:24-27), would not deny this.

However, its value is circumscribed. It is for *this* life. When this body returns to dust, the benefits of its physical training cease. The muscular strength, the cardiovascular endurance—these are for the *pros oligos*, for the short span of our earthly pilgrimage.

Godliness, on the other hand, is of value *pros panta*—"for all things" or "in every way." Its value is not limited to the present life. It holds promise "for the present life *and also for the life to come*." The character formed through the *gymnaze* of godliness—the love, joy, peace, patience, kindness, goodness, faithfulness, gentleness, and self-control—this is not a perishable wreath. This is an imperishable character that transcends the grave. The soul that has been trained in godliness enters eternity with the fruits of that training intact. The value of godliness is comprehensive and eternal.

Therefore, the relationship between bodily training and godliness, as Paul presents it, is not one of opposition but of **ordered priority and integrated purpose**. The error is to pursue bodily training as an end in itself, for its value is temporary. The wisdom is to pursue bodily training *in service of* godliness, for when the body is well-stewarded, it becomes a more effective vessel for the eternal work of the Spirit.

We can think of it this way: Bodily training is like maintaining the tools in a workshop. Keeping the tools sharp, clean, and in good repair is of genuine value. It is "for a little"—for the duration of the projects in that workshop. But no one confuses maintaining the tools with the purpose of the workshop, which is to create beautiful and useful objects. The ultimate value is in the craftsmanship, the creation, the art that is produced. Similarly, bodily training maintains the tool—the body—for the ultimate purpose of godliness: loving God and loving neighbor. A well-maintained tool allows for more skillful, enduring, and effective craftsmanship in the art of godly living.

Thus, Paul's metaphor is not a denigration of the physical but a proper ordering of it. He is calling us to be spiritual athletes, to bring the same discipline and intentionality we might apply to our physical bodies to the far more important training of our hearts and minds. And in doing so, he implicitly sanctifies physical discipline itself, when it is taken up as part of this larger, integrated project of holistic stewardship. We are to *gymnaze* our bodies not for the applause of the crowd or the crown of leaves, but so that this jar of clay can be a more resilient, capable, and enduring vessel for the transcendent treasure of the gospel, both for this life and for the life to come.

13.5 The Patristic and Monastic Witness: Ora et Labora

Beloved, as we continue to trace the golden thread of a theology of physical labor through the tapestry of church history, we now come to a pivotal moment—the rise of monasticism. In the centuries following the apostolic era, as the church moved from the catacombs to the halls of imperial power, a profound counter-cultural movement emerged. Men and women, sensing the spiritual complacency and worldliness seeping into the church, fled to the deserts of Egypt, the caves of Syria, and the forests of Europe to wage a new kind of warfare: the warfare of the heart. These Desert Fathers and Mothers, and later the great monastic founders like St. Benedict, did not see the body as an enemy to be conquered in a Gnostic sense, but as a stubborn, recalcitrant mule that must be trained to carry the soul to God. In their wisdom, they developed a holistic spirituality that seamlessly wove together the life of prayer and the life of physical labor. Their legacy, crystallized in the Benedictine motto **Ora et Labora** (Pray and Work), provides a profound historical and theological witness to the integration we have been advocating.

To understand the monastic view of labor, we must first appreciate the specific spiritual malady it was designed to combat: the sin of *acedia*. Often translated as sloth, *acedia* was far more than mere laziness. The desert monastics called it the "noonday demon," a state of spiritual apathy, listlessness, and restlessness that would descend upon a monk in the heat of the day. It was a deep-seated sorrow about the spiritual life itself, a loathing of one's cell, a paralyzing boredom that made prayer feel futile and the scriptures seem dry. It was a temptation to abandon one's vocation, to seek distraction in gossip, sleep, or pointless wandering. *Acedia* was understood as a fundamental dis-integration of the person, where the will became detached from its ultimate Good, which is God.

In this spiritual diagnosis, manual labor was prescribed as a powerful **antidote to *acedia***. The physical exertion of tilling a garden, weaving a basket, or chopping wood was seen as a divine medicine for the soul. Why? Because *acedia* is a sickness of disordered desire and dissipated attention. It pulls the soul inward upon itself in a spiral of melancholic self-preoccupation. Physical labor, by its very nature, forces the person outward. It requires engagement with the real, material world. The feel of the soil, the rhythm of the breath, the strain of the muscle—these tangible sensations ground the soul in the present moment and disrupt the toxic, inward-focused cycle of *acedia*. The fatigue that comes from honest labor is a healthy, ordered fatigue that leads to restorative sleep, unlike the exhausting restlessness of the slothful soul. By engaging the body in purposeful work, the monk was quite literally working his way out of a spiritual stupor, re-integrating his will with the physical reality of God's creation and breaking the demonic spell of listlessness.

Furthermore, within the cenobitic (communal) monastic tradition established by St. Benedict, manual labor served the crucial practical purpose of **self-support**. The Benedictine Rule is explicit on this point. Chapter 48, "On the Daily Manual Labor," begins: "Idleness is the enemy of the soul. Therefore, the brothers should have specified periods for manual labor as well as for prayerful reading." The community was to be self-sustaining. The monks were to be "of the same mind as the Apostle," who commanded, "Anyone unwilling to work should not eat" (2 Thessalonians 3:10). This was not a harsh economic principle but a spiritual one. It fostered humility, destroying any sense of aristocratic entitlement. It ensured the monastery did not become a burden on the surrounding community, but rather a source of blessing and economic stability. The work of their hands—in the fields, the bakery, the brewery, the scriptorium—was an act of love for their brothers and a testimony to the dignity of all labor before God. It sanctified the mundane, transforming the baking of bread and the copying of manuscripts into acts of worship that sustained the body and the soul of the community.

Perhaps the most profound spiritual insight of the monastic tradition regarding labor was its role in **humbling the body and focusing the mind**. The fallen human condition is one of pride. We are naturally inclined to vanity, to a preoccupation with our own comfort, appearance, and importance. The disciplined, often repetitive and menial, labor of the monastic life was a direct assault on this pride. Scrubbing floors, weeding gardens, and mending fences were not glamorous tasks. They forced the monk to engage in work that held no worldly prestige. This was a school of humility. It was a tangible way of "dying to self," of conforming to the image of Christ, who took the form of a servant and humbled himself (Philippians 2:7). The blisters on the hands, the ache in the back, the dirt on the robe—these were the sacramental signs of a prideful will being broken and reshaped into the gentle and lowly heart of Jesus.

Simultaneously, this humble labor was understood to **focus the mind on God**. The repetitive nature of many manual tasks—the steady rhythm of scything a field, the back-and-forth motion of a plane on wood—could create a space for prayer. The body, engaged in a familiar, almost automatic activity, could free the mind and the heart for uninterrupted communion with God. This was not an emptying of the mind as in some Eastern meditative traditions, but a filling of it with the presence of Christ. The work itself became a kind of moving meditation, a prayer without ceasing. The monk learned to pray not only in the choir during the Divine Office but also in the field, the workshop, and the kitchen. The distinction between sacred and secular time and space collapsed. All of life, including physical labor, became a continuous liturgy offered to God.

Through this integrated life of *Ora et Labora*, the monastic tradition cultivated a suite of Christlike virtues. The daily grind of labor taught **perseverance**—the ability to continue in a task when it became difficult or monotonous, a direct parallel to the perseverance required in the long journey of sanctification. It instilled **diligence**—a commitment to doing a task well, not for human praise but as an offering to God, reflecting His own character as a God of excellence and order. And as we have seen, it rooted out the deep taproot of pride, nurturing the fundamental virtue of **humility**.

The Patristic and Monastic witness, therefore, stands as a powerful corrective to both the modern idolatry of the body and the ancient heresy of its denigration. It presents a vision where the sweat of the brow is not a curse to be avoided, but a means of grace to be embraced. It shows us that the path to God is not an escape from the physical world, but a journey through it, where the disciplined use of our bodies in faithful labor becomes one of the primary ways we cooperate with the Holy Spirit in the transformation of our souls. In the rhythmic harmony of prayer and work, we find a holistic spirituality that honors the Creator by fully engaging with the good creation He has given us, and in which He is to be found.

13.6 A Reformed Theology of the Body in Action: For Glory and for Neighbor

Beloved, as we bring our theological exploration of physical labor and exercise to its culmination, we must now ground it within a distinctly Reformed framework—a worldview that sees all of life as a sacred theater for the glory of God. The central pillar of this perspective is the Latin phrase *coram Deo*: "before the face of God." This is not a mere theological abstraction; it is the orienting reality for every thought, word, and deed, including every rep completed, every mile run, and every hour of faithful labor. In the Reformed vision, there is no sacred-secular divide. There is no realm of "spiritual" activity that is inherently more pleasing to God than the realm of the "physical." All of life, from the most exalted moment of Eucharistic adoration to the most mundane task of washing dishes, is to be lived as an act of worship before the sovereign, all-seeing God. It is from this foundational principle that we derive a powerful, twofold purpose for the disciplined stewardship of our bodies: it is an act undertaken **for the glory of God** and **for the service of our neighbor**.

First and foremost, a Reformed theology frames physical discipline as an act lived **For the Glory of God**. This immediately purges the endeavor of the self-referential narcissism that characterizes the world's approach to fitness. Our culture screams that the body is for self-expression, self-gratification, and self-optimization. The gospel whispers, and then thunders, a different truth: "You are not your own, for you were bought with a price. So glorify God in your body" (1 Corinthians 6:19-20). The ultimate purpose of bodily training, therefore, is doxological. It is about rendering the physical vessel that houses the Holy Spirit a fit instrument for the manifestation of divine excellence.

This transforms physical fitness from a pursuit of vanity into a discipline of **stewardship**. To be a steward is to manage a possession that belongs to another. Our bodies are Christ's purchased property. How then, shall we manage them? Would a faithful steward allow a magnificent, intricate, God-designed instrument to rust from disuse, to seize up from neglect, or to become clogged and dysfunctional through willful abuse? Of course not. Faithful stewardship implies active, intentional, and wise maintenance. It means providing the body with the movement, rest, and nourishment it requires to function at its God-given capacity. A body that is strong, healthy, and resilient is a well-maintained tool. It is a temple where the lights are on, the floors are clean, and the systems are in good working order, ready for the Owner's use.

And what is that use? The Apostle Paul provides the answer in Ephesians 2:10: "For we are his workmanship, created in Christ Jesus for good works, which God prepared beforehand, that we should walk in them." A healthy, capable body is simply better able to perform these God-prepared good works. It has the energy to engage in prolonged prayer and study. It has the vitality to serve in ministry without being constantly sidelined by fatigue and illness. It possesses the resilience to endure hardship, persecution, and the general "light and momentary afflictions" that are part of the Christian walk (2 Corinthians 4:17). When the body is weak and perpetually unwell, our capacity to "walk in" these good works is severely diminished. We become like a skilled craftsman with broken tools; the will is present, but the means are compromised. Therefore, the disciplined care of our physical frame is an act of faith and obedience. It is our active preparation, our "getting the tools ready," for the good works God has already sovereignly ordained for us. We glorify Him not only by doing the works, but by being diligent stewards of the instrument through which those works are accomplished.

This Godward orientation naturally and inevitably flows outward into a second purpose: physical discipline for **the Service of Neighbor**. The Reformed faith holds in beautiful tension the vertical dimension of life (coram Deo) with the horizontal dimension (coram mundo, before the world). The great commandment to love God with all our heart, soul, mind, and *strength* is inextricably linked to the second: to love our neighbor as ourselves (Mark 12:30-31). And we must be utterly clear about this: love is not merely a sentiment; it is an action. It is *agape* made tangible. And tangible love is physically demanding.

Consider the concrete realities of loving our neighbor:

- It requires the **energy** to care for young children through sleepless nights, to sit with a grieving friend for hours, or to mentor a young person.
- It requires the **strength** to help a family move into a new home, to build a ramp for a disabled neighbor, or to assist in disaster relief efforts.
- It requires the **stamina** to serve meals at a homeless shelter, to participate in a short-term mission trip, or to maintain a consistent, presence-based ministry in a challenging context.
- It requires the **mental and emotional resilience** that is so often tied to physical health—the clarity of mind to offer wise counsel, the emotional

stability to de-escalate a conflict, the patience that is frayed by poor sleep and poor nutrition.

When we are physically depleted, our capacity for this kind of costly, tangible love shrinks. We become inwardly focused, conserving our dwindling energy for ourselves. We are more likely to be irritable, impatient, and quick to withdraw from the demands of others. Conversely, a body that has been trained and disciplined has a greater reservoir from which to draw. Bodily training is, in this profound sense, an act of love. It is the sharpening of the axe before attempting to fell the tree for the community. It is the conditioning of the rescuer before diving into the turbulent waters to save a drowning soul. By increasing our physical capacity—our strength, our endurance, our energy—we are directly increasing our capacity to incarnate the love of Christ to a world in need.

This Reformed synthesis provides a powerful and motivating framework. It saves us from the idolatry of self-worship by directing our physical efforts toward the glory of God. And it saves us from a pietistic withdrawal from the world by channeling our physical strength into the self-giving service of our neighbor. The gym, the running path, the workspace—these are not escapes from the spiritual life. They are training grounds for it. Every disciplined choice is a small death to self-interest and a small resurrection of the body as a tool for divine glory and human flourishing. We are called to be whole-person disciples, and this means offering our bodies, in their strength and vitality, as living sacrifices, ready and able to do whatever good works, in whatever sphere, our sovereign God has prepared for us to walk in.

13.7 The Sin of Asceticism and the Sin of Indulgence

Beloved, as we seek to faithfully navigate the path of embodied stewardship, we find ourselves walking a narrow ridge with two treacherous and alluring chasms on either side. These are not mere errors of emphasis; they are theological heresies with profound practical consequences for how we view and use our bodies. They represent two demonic perversions of the good gift of physicality, and the church has, at various times in her history, fallen prey to both. To faithfully glorify God in our bodies, we must be able to clearly identify these opposing errors, understand their theological roots, and consciously reject them in favor of the biblical *via media*—the path of grateful stewardship and sanctified use.

On one side of the ridge lies the chasm of **Gnostic Asceticism**. This ancient error, which plagued the early church and continues to manifest in subtle forms today, is fundamentally a denial of the goodness of the material world. Gnosticism, in its various forms, posits a radical dualism between spirit and matter. Spirit is seen as inherently good, divine, and eternal, while matter—including the human body—is viewed as inherently evil, corrupt, or at best, a temporary and worthless prison for the immortal soul. From this foundational error flows a particular disdain for the body and its needs, including physical exercise and strength.

When this Gnostic impulse infiltrates Christian thought, it produces a spirituality that is suspicious of the physical. It disparages physical exercise as "unspiritual," a waste of time that could be better spent in prayer or Bible study. It views the body as a problem to be managed, a source of temptation to be suppressed, rather than as a good creation to be stewarded. This perspective often leads to a neglect of physical health, justified by a misguided piety that believes such neglect is a form of spiritual discipline. The body is treated as an enemy to be conquered, rather than as a partner to be trained.

This Gnostic Asceticism constitutes a direct assault on core Christian doctrines. First, it is a **denial of the goodness of creation**. The opening chapter of Genesis, with its repeated refrain "And God saw that it was good," culminates in the creation of humanity as the pinnacle of this good material order. The body is not an afterthought or a tragic compromise; it is the skillful handiwork of a benevolent Creator. To despise the body is to insult the divine Artisan. Second, and even more catastrophically, it is a **denial of the doctrine of the resurrection**. The Christian hope is not the escape of a disembodied soul from its physical shell. Our hope is the resurrection of the body—the redemption, transformation, and glorification of this very physical frame. As the Apostle Paul argues so forcefully in 1 Corinthians 15, if there is no resurrection of the body, then our faith is futile and we are still in our sins. The Gnostics, by treating the body as a disposable container, undermine the very heart of the gospel, which is the redemption of the entire created order, including our physical selves. A spirituality that degrades the body is, therefore, not a "higher" spirituality; it is an anti-incarnational heresy.

On the opposite side of the ridge lies the equally perilous chasm of **Narcissistic Indulgence**. If the first error hates the body, this error worships it. This is the dominant religion of our secular age, and it has powerfully infiltrated the church, often masquerading as "stewardship." Narcissistic Indulgence makes the body an idol. It pursues fitness, not for God's glory or for the service of neighbor, but for the purposes of pride, sensuality, and self-worship. The body becomes a project for self-glorification, a canvas for self-expression, and a source of personal identity and worth.

This idolatry manifests in the gym as a pursuit of physical perfection defined by cultural standards of beauty and performance. The mirror becomes the altar, and the reflection the object of devotion. It is driven by vanity, by the desire to be admired, desired, and envied. It is the "works-righteousness" of the body, where one's value is earned through the sweat of one's brow and displayed in the sculpting of one's physique. This is the very vanity condemned so powerfully by the Preacher in Ecclesiastes: "Then I considered all that my hands had done and the toil I had expended in doing it, and behold, all was vanity and a striving after wind, and there was nothing to be gained under the sun" (Ecclesiastes 2:11). The pursuit of a perfect body, severed from its transcendent purpose, is ultimately as meaningless as any other endeavor "under the sun."

Furthermore, this indulgence can manifest as a slavery to sensuality and comfort. Here, the body is not trained but pacified. Its every appetite for pleasure, ease, and comfort is indulged. This is the sin of gluttony, of sloth, of a life organized around the avoidance of discomfort and the pursuit of sensory gratification. The body is not an idol to be sculpted, but a master to be obeyed. Its demands for rich food, for endless entertainment, for prolonged sleep, and for the avoidance of strenuous effort dictate the course of life. This, too, is a form of idolatry, for it places the creature's comfort above the Creator's command.

Both of these errors—the hatred of the body and the worship of the body—are, at their core, failures to understand the body's true purpose. Gnostic Asceticism fails to see the body as a *temple of the Holy Spirit*, a sacred vessel designed for divine indwelling and holy use. Narcissistic Indulgence fails to see the body as *not its own*, a purchased possession that belongs to Christ and is to be used for His purposes.

The biblical path, the narrow ridge we are called to walk, steers clear of both chasms. It affirms the goodness of the body without making it a god. It acknowledges the reality of bodily brokenness and the presence of sinful desires without treating the body itself as the enemy. It calls us to a disciplined stewardship that is motivated by worship and directed toward love. We are to care for the body diligently, not because we worship it, but because we worship the God who made it and indwells it. We are to train it and discipline it, not to attract the admiration of the world, but to increase our capacity to serve the world in the name of Christ. We are to present our bodies as a living sacrifice, which is our spiritual worship (Romans 12:1)—a sacrifice that is holy precisely because it is a *living*, breathing, physical offering, set apart for the Master's use.

13.8 Discipline for a Purpose

Beloved, as we draw this foundational chapter to its culmination, we are now positioned to synthesize its myriad threads into a single, cohesive, and transformative vision. The journey we have undertaken—from the creational mandate of *avad* and *shamar*, through the curse and its redemption in Christ, past the wisdom of the monastic *ora et labora*, and navigating the twin perils of Gnostic asceticism and narcissistic indulgence—all converges upon one powerful, practical, and doxological conclusion. A robust Christian theology of physical discipline performs a radical act of **reframing**. It takes the secular, culturally-conditioned pursuit of exercise and bodily training and relocates it from the realm of vanity and self-optimization to the sacred realm of **stewardship and worship**. It is the decisive act of tearing down the "stronghold" of the world's arguments about the body and taking every thought about our physical existence "captive to obey Christ" (2 Corinthians 10:5).

This reframing is not a minor adjustment; it is a Copernican revolution in our understanding of physical exertion. The world orbits around the self. Its gravitational center is the individual's desire for aesthetic perfection, performance metrics, longevity, and social validation. In this paradigm, the body exists for the self. The Christian paradigm, revealed in Scripture, places God at the center. The body, as a creation of God and a possession of Christ, exists for His glory. Therefore, the entire enterprise of physical discipline undergoes a fundamental reorientation. It is no longer "bodily training" for its own sake, a closed loop of self-referential effort. It is "bodily training" with a *telos*—an ultimate end, a purpose that transcends the self. This *telos* is nothing less than **to cultivate a body that is a fit instrument for God's use**.

Consider the profound implications of this shift. When you engage in strength training, you are not merely building muscle for the mirror; you are forging the physical capacity that may be called upon to bear a brother's burden, to build a house for the homeless, or to endure persecution with resilience. When you engage in cardiovascular exercise, you are not merely improving your VO2 max for personal pride; you are building the endurance that will allow you to serve your family after a long day, to persist in prayer through the night, or to walk alongside a suffering friend without succumbing to compassionate fatigue. When you discipline your eating, you are not merely following a diet for weight loss; you are practicing the self-control that is a fruit of the Spirit, honoring the temple of the Holy Spirit by refusing to defile it with gluttony, and maintaining the mental clarity necessary for discerning the will of God. Every drop of sweat, every aching muscle, every resisted craving, when offered to God, becomes a physical prayer, a tangible act of saying, "This body is Yours. Prepare it. Strengthen it. Use it."

This purpose-driven discipline cultivates a body characterized by three essential qualities for kingdom service:

First, a body capable of **diligent work**. We recall that work is our original, pre-fall vocation. A body weakened by chronic neglect is a poor instrument for the *avad* and *shamar* to which we are called, even in a fallen world. Physical discipline restores the body's functional capacity for the daily labor that provides for our needs, serves our community, and reflects the creative, industrious nature of our God. It is the difference between the sharp axe and the dull one; both can swing, but one accomplishes its purpose with far greater efficiency and joy.

Second, a body capable of **enduring service**. The way of the cross is a way of costly love, and love is often exhausting. It demands that we have something left to give when our natural reserves are depleted. The disciplined body possesses a deeper well from which to draw. It has the resilience to serve when it is inconvenient, to love when it is costly, and to persevere when the mission is long and the results are slow to appear. This endurance is not merely a matter of willpower; it is a physiological reality. A body trained in perseverance has a greater capacity for it, just as a soul trained in the spiritual disciplines has a greater capacity for faith, hope, and love.

Third, a body capable of **resilient witness**. Our physical presence in the world is a testament to what we believe about

God and His creation. A body that is either ascetically despised or narcissistically worshipped preaches a false gospel. But a body that is strong, healthy, and joyfully disciplined—a body that is clearly *cared for* but not *worshipped*—becomes a silent but powerful apologetic. It testifies to a God who made the material world good, who redeems it in Christ, and whose Spirit empowers us for faithful stewardship. It demonstrates that the gospel is not a disembodied spirituality but a reality that encompasses and transforms our entire existence, from the inner man to the outermost physical cell.

Ultimately, this holistic vision of physical discipline is the most practical, tangible expression of the imperative in Romans 12:1: "I appeal to you therefore, brothers, by the mercies of God, to present your bodies as a living sacrifice, holy and acceptable to God, which is your spiritual worship." The language of "presenting your bodies" is irreducibly physical. It is not merely our souls or our intentions that we are to offer, but our very bodies. A "living sacrifice" is one that is active, breathing, and engaged in the world. The discipline of physical training is the daily, ongoing process of placing this living, breathing, working, resting body upon the altar of God's service. It is the act of making it "holy"—set apart for His exclusive use. And Paul stunningly labels this physical offering our "spiritual worship" (*logiken latreian*). The worship God desires is not confined to a church building or a quiet time; it is the rational, logical, and fitting offering of our entire embodied existence back to the God of all mercy. Therefore, the repetition in the weight room, the rhythm of the run, the choice of a nourishing meal—these are not secular interruptions in a spiritual life. They are the very stuff of which a spiritually worshipful life is made. They are the physical grammar of our doxology, the embodied Amen to the goodness of God's creation and the redemption that is in Christ Jesus, our Lord.

CHAPTER 14

Designing a Life-Stage Appropriate Regimen: Stewardship from Youth to Old Age

Beloved, we have now laid a comprehensive theological foundation for the stewardship of the physical body. We have established its sacred status as a temple, its creational purpose for labor and service, and the redemptive framing of its discipline as an act of worship. Yet, a critical pastoral and practical question remains: What does this stewardship look like when lived out across the full span of a human life? The body of a sprightly child, the burgeoning frame of an adolescent, the capable strength of a young adult, the seasoned resilience of midlife, and the fragile dignity of advanced age—are these all stewarded in the same way? The clear and biblical answer is a resounding no. To impose a single, rigid template of physical discipline upon every stage of life is to ignore the wisdom of the Creator, who Himself has woven a dynamic and purposeful progression into the very fabric of our biological existence.

This chapter, therefore, moves from the universal principles of embodied stewardship to their particular and prudent application across the lifespan. We will argue that faithful stewardship is not a static state to be achieved, but a dynamic, unfolding process of attentive and wise adaptation. It requires listening to the body as it journeys through the seasons God has ordained, and responding with regimens of care that honor the unique capacities, vulnerabilities, and divine purposes inherent to each stage. From the boundless energy of youth, which must be channeled and formed, to the declining strength of age, which must be conserved and honored, our calling is to cooperate with God's design, not to fight against its inherent chronology. We will explore how the core principles of stewardship—that the body is for God's glory and the service of neighbor—remain constant, while their practical outworking must be as fluid and responsive as the life God has given us to live.

14.1 The Unfolding Stewardship of the Lifespan

The foundational truth upon which this entire chapter rests is a theological reading of our biology: **The human body is not a static entity.** It is a divinely orchestrated narrative, a living story of growth, maturation, and eventual decline. To treat it as a machine that should perform at a constant level from puberty until death is to embrace a modern, mechanistic myth that is foreign to the biblical witness. The Preacher in Ecclesiastes grounds this reality in the sovereign wisdom of God: "For everything there is a season, and a time for every matter under heaven: a time to be born, and a time to die... a time to break down, and a time to build up" (Ecclesiastes 3:1-3). This is not merely poetry about the social rhythms of life; it is a profound theological statement about the ontology of the created order, including our own physical being. There is a God-appointed time for the building up of the body—the seasons of childhood, adolescence, and young adulthood. And there is a God-appointed time for the "breaking down"—the gradual, inevitable kenosis, or self-emptying, of strength and vitality that characterizes middle and old age.

This divinely ordained process is not a flaw in the design, nor is it solely the result of the Fall. While the Fall introduced the *sting* of death and the *frustration* of decay, the underlying rhythm of life—the movement from potential to actuality to legacy—is part of the creational pattern. We see this even in the unfallen narrative of Genesis, where Adam is formed from dust, filled with the divine breath, and given a vocation that implies a future. The trajectory of life is built into the original good design, albeit now experienced through the painful lens of sin and mortality. Therefore, to resent the aging process, to wage a frantic war against every wrinkle and every waning capacity, is ultimately a form of rebellion against the Creator's wise and sovereign ordering of our days. It is to reject the "time to break down" as somehow less sacred or less filled with purpose than the "time to build up."

Faithful stewardship, therefore, must be **dynamic, not static**. It is the opposite of a one-size-fits-all prescription. It is the spiritual discipline of *attentive discernment*. It requires that we learn to listen to the narrative our body is telling in each season. The stewardship of a child involves protecting a delicate, rapidly developing system and channeling its explosive energy toward healthy formation. The stewardship of a young adult involves building a foundation of strength and endurance for a lifetime of service and responsibility. The stewardship of midlife involves a strategic shift from building peak capacity to maintaining functional resilience and managing the slow creep of metabolic decline. The stewardship of old age involves a holy acceptance of increasing limitation, a focus on conserving dignity and function for as long as possible, and a redefinition of "strength" from physical power to spiritual fortitude and wisdom.

This dynamic approach is an act of cooperation with the Holy Spirit, who is at work in us throughout our entire lifespan. It is to ask, in each new season: "Lord, what is the particular purpose for this body at this time? What capacities have You given that I am to maximize for Your glory? What limitations have You permitted that I am to accept with grace, offering them back to You as a part of my 'living sacrifice'?" The goal is not to cling to the physical prowess of twenty-five when one is sixty-five. The goal is to be a faithful, five-talent steward at twenty-five, and an equally faithful, one-talent steward at eighty-five, investing whatever capacity one has—whether great or small—with the same wholehearted devotion to the Master.

Thus, the unfolding stewardship of the lifespan is a profound exercise in practical theology. It is where the doctrines of Creation, Fall, and Redemption meet the daily reality of our aching joints, our changing metabolism, and our shifting energy levels. It is a call to worship God not only with the vibrant strength of youth but also with the grateful, dependent fragility of age, recognizing that in our weakness, His power is made perfect, and in every season, our bodies can be a testimony to the faithfulness of the God who sustains us from our first breath to our last.

14.2 Childhood and Adolescence: Cultivating Joyful Embodiment

Beloved, as we begin our journey through the lifespan, we start at its dawn: the seasons of childhood and adolescence. This is a period of breathtaking dynamism, where the body is not merely growing but *unfolding* according to a divine blueprint of astonishing complexity. The theological task during this formative stage is not to impose a rigid, adult-style regimen of discipline, but to lay a foundation that will support a lifetime of faithful stewardship. The primary goal for these years is not the cultivation of peak performance or aesthetic perfection, but something far more profound and enduring: **to instill a positive, joyful understanding of the body as God's good gift and to develop the foundational motor skills and coordination that form the basis for a lifetime of physical activity.** This is the season for sowing the seeds of what we might call *joyful embodiment*.

Theologically, this stage is about rooting a child's identity in the creation narrative of "very good," before the complications of the Fall and the cultural pressures of performance-based identity take hold. A child should learn that their ability to run, leap, shout, and tumble is a reflection of the God who is Himself dynamic, creative, and overflowing with life. The Psalms are filled with this language of creation's joyful movement—the mountains skipping like rams, the hills girding themselves with joy (Psalm 114:4,6). A child's uninhibited play is a participation in this creational chorus. It is a pre-theological doxology, a worship enacted through the body itself. The goal is for the child to internalize a fundamental truth: *My body is not a problem to be solved or a project to be perfected. It is a gift to be explored, a instrument of discovery, and a vehicle for joy.* This positive foundation is the single greatest bulkhead against the Gnostic disdain for the physical and the narcissistic obsession with it that will assault them in later years.

Practically, this theological goal is achieved through several key applications, each designed to align with the developmental needs and natural inclinations of the young.

First and foremost is the primacy of **Play-Based Activity**. In our hyper-structured, achievement-oriented age, we must recover the sacred wisdom of unstructured play. For a child, play is not a frivolous distraction from "real" activity; it *is* their primary physical and spiritual "work." When a child chases a butterfly, scrambles up a tree, or invents a game with friends, they are not just passing time. They are engaging in a divinely appointed process of neuromuscular development, spatial awareness, risk assessment, and creative problem-solving. They are developing what physical educators call "physical literacy"—the innate, confident ability to move their bodies through space with competence and joy. This is the natural, God-given means by which a child learns to steward the physical capacity they have been given. The prophet Zechariah, in his vision of the restored Jerusalem, paints a picture of this very scene: "And the streets of the city shall be full of boys and girls playing in its streets" (Zechariah 8:5). This is not a minor detail; it is a sign of shalom, of a community where children are safe, free, and joyful in their embodied existence. To rush a child out of this stage with premature formal training is to rob them of this sacred, formative ground.

Second, we move to the gentle and broad **Introduction of Skills**. As a child grows, particularly into later childhood and early adolescence, there is a place for introducing structured activities. However, the emphasis must be on *variety* and *exposure*, not on specialization or intense competition. The goal is to build a broad movement vocabulary. Swimming teaches breath control and a unique relationship with a different element. Basic gymnastics develops body awareness, flexibility, and kinesthetic sense. Throwing and catching a ball develops hand-eye coordination. The objective is not to produce a star athlete by age twelve, but to equip the young person with a diverse toolkit of physical competencies. This approach prevents the "all your eggs in one basket" peril of early specialization, which often leads to overuse injuries and psychological burnout. It allows the adolescent to discover what activities they genuinely enjoy, fostering an intrinsic motivation to be active that will far outlast the extrinsic motivation of parental pressure or the pursuit of trophies.

Third, and of paramount importance, is **Family Integration**. The most powerful curriculum for physical stewardship is not written in a book; it is modeled in the home. When a family goes for a hike together, they are doing more than getting exercise. They are communing with God's creation, building shared memories, and silently communicating that movement is a normal, enjoyable part of life. When parents bike with their children, play catch in the backyard, or simply dance in the living room, they are building positive neural and emotional associations with physical activity. This models stewardship in its most winsome form. It demonstrates that caring for the body is not a solitary, grim duty, but a shared family value, a source of connection and fun. It answers the "why" of physical activity with the powerful testimony of relationship and joy, long before the child is capable of understanding the theological "why" of 1 Corinthians 6:19-20.

This holistic approach requires a conscious and counter-cultural commitment to avoiding specific pitfalls. The most dangerous of these is the trap of **Early Specialization and Intense Competition**. The modern youth sports industrial complex often pushes children into a single sport with year-round training at a very young age. This is profoundly at odds with a theology of joyful embodiment. It replaces the delight of play with the pressure of performance. It exchanges a broad-based physical literacy for a narrow, repetitive skill set that maximizes the risk of physical injury. Most damningly, it forges a performance-based identity. The child learns that their value is tied to their wins, their stats, and their standing on the team. This lays a foundation for either pride or shame, both of which are alien to the gospel identity of being a beloved child of God, accepted in Christ irrespective of athletic achievement. When the body becomes primarily a tool for winning, it is a short step to viewing it as a tool for attracting admiration, leading directly to the narcissistic indulgence we must reject. The burnout, anxiety, and broken relationships that often result from this pressure are a testament to its anti-human design.

Therefore, the stewardship of childhood and adolescence is a ministry of protection and cultivation. It is about protecting the sacred space of play, protecting the child from premature pressure, and protecting their identity from being fused with their performance. And it is about cultivating joy, cultivating a wide range of physical competencies, and cultivating a deep-seated, unshakeable belief that their body—in all its clumsy, energetic, growing glory—is a very good gift from a very good God, made for His pleasure and their joyful exploration.

14.3 Young Adulthood: Building a Foundation for Service

Beloved, we now enter the season of young adulthood—a time of immense energy, burgeoning responsibility, and the forging of a life's trajectory. This is the stage where the physical potential cultivated in youth is called upon to bear the weight of real-world vocation and service. The body, having passed through the developmental unfolding of adolescence, now stands at its peak capacity for strength, endurance, and resilience. The theological goal for this season, therefore, shifts from the joyful exploration of childhood to a more focused and intentional purpose: **To build peak physical capacity for maximum effectiveness in the demanding seasons of career-building, family-raising, and ministry service.** This is the time to forge the body into a robust, reliable, and highly capable instrument, ready for a lifetime of demanding use in the Kingdom of God.

Theologically, this stage is an active outworking of the cultural mandate and the Great Commandment. The body is the primary tool through which we "work and keep" our various domains—our careers, our homes, our churches. It is the vessel through which we love our neighbor with tangible, often physically demanding, acts of service. The young adult years are a unique window of biological opportunity to build a deep reservoir of physical capital. This is not for self-glorification, but for stewardship of the high calling God places upon this season. It is about being like the faithful servant in the Parable of the Talents, who took the five talents given to him and traded with them, generating more for his master (Matthew 25:16-21). The "five talents" of young adulthood are these very capacities—the energy to work long hours building a career or a business, the strength to lift a child or move a neighbor's furniture, the stamina to serve in ministry after a full day's work, and the resilience to endure the intense pressures that often characterize this life stage without collapsing into burnout or illness. To neglect the body during this season is to bury this talent in the ground. It is a failure to invest the physical resources

God has provided for the work He has prepared in advance (Ephesians 2:10).

Practically, this theological goal is achieved through a regimen that is more structured, intense, and purposeful than in previous stages, always with the end of service in view.

First, there must be a focus on **Structured Strength and Conditioning**. This is the time to build a foundation of functional strength that will support a lifetime of labor and protect the body from injury. The emphasis should be on compound, multi-joint movements that mirror the demands of real life: the squat (for lifting), the deadlift (for picking objects up from the ground), and the various presses (for pushing and carrying). These movements do not merely build muscle for appearance; they build a body that is truly useful. They forge a strong musculoskeletal system that can handle the physical strain of demanding work, whether that is construction, nursing, or simply the cumulative load of parenting young children. This functional strength is a direct expression of the creation mandate to *avad*—to work and serve. A strong back and capable legs are tools for co-laboring with God in the cultivation and keeping of His world.

Second, a commitment to **Cardiovascular Health** is paramount. The demands of young adulthood are not just bursts of strength, but often long, sustained efforts. Building stamina through regular aerobic training (like running, cycling, or swimming) and anaerobic conditioning (like high-intensity interval training) equips the body to endure. This cardiovascular resilience has profound spiritual and practical parallels. It builds the physical capacity for longsuffering and endurance. It provides the energy to be present and engaged with family after a draining workday, to pursue a graduate degree while working, or to lead a small group without being perpetually exhausted. A healthy cardiovascular system supports cognitive function and emotional regulation, which are essential for making wise decisions in a high-pressure season of life. This is the stewardship of one's inner resources, ensuring that the "outer self" has the energy required to fuel the work of the "inner self" (2 Corinthians 4:16).

Third, the young adult stage presents a unique opportunity to leverage **Community and Discipline**. This is a naturally social period of life. Harnessing this social drive for physical stewardship can be a powerful means of grace. Engaging in group sports, joining a fitness class, or committing to a regular workout with a partner or "accountability brother or sister" provides motivation, camaraderie, and a structure that reinforces discipline. This communal aspect transforms a solitary chore into a shared pursuit. It provides a context for mutual encouragement, where believers can "stir up one another to love and good works" (Hebrews 10:24), and in this case, the "good work" is the faithful stewardship of the physical temple. This community provides accountability, helping the individual to remain consistent when motivation wanes, which is a crucial spiritual discipline in itself.

However, this season of building capacity is fraught with two particularly potent pitfalls that must be navigated with gospel wisdom.

The first pitfall is **Neglect Due to Busyness**. The young adult years are often a whirlwind of career advancement, relational development, and possibly starting a family. It is dangerously easy to view physical stewardship as a dispensable luxury, the first thing to be sacrificed on the altar of a crowded schedule. This is a short-sighted and ultimately destructive choice. To neglect the body during this high-demand season is to burn the candle at both ends without ever replacing the wax. It leads to premature burnout, chronic fatigue, and a weakened constitution that will have negative repercussions for decades to come. It is a failure to see that the time invested in exercise is not lost, but redeemed, as it creates a more energetic, resilient, and productive individual for all other spheres of life.

The second, and more subtle, pitfall is the **Idolatry of Fitness**. In a reaction against neglect, it is easy to swing to the opposite extreme and make physical training a central idol. When the gym becomes the primary community, when workout schedules become inflexible and consume excessive time and financial resources, when self-worth becomes tied to physical appearance or performance metrics, then stewardship has curdled into self-worship. This is the vanity of Ecclesiastes, a "striving after wind." It represents a failure to remember that bodily training is "for a little" (1 Timothy 4:8)—for the temporary season of this life—and that its ultimate purpose is service, not self. When fitness compromises one's ability to be present for family, to serve the local church, or to fulfill vocational duties, it has ceased to be a tool for the Kingdom and has become a rival kingdom itself.

Therefore, the stewardship of young adulthood is a delicate and crucial balance. It is a call to vigorous, intentional investment in the body's capacity, viewing this investment as a sacred trust for the work of the Kingdom. But it is simultaneously a call to constant heart-checking, ensuring that this powerful tool remains a servant to the greater goals of glorifying God and loving one's neighbor, and never becomes a master that demands its own worship.

14.4 Middle Adulthood: Preserving Function and Managing Stress

Beloved, we now arrive at the pivotal season of middle adulthood, a time often marked by the peak of one's influence and responsibility, yet accompanied by the first undeniable whispers of the body's mortality. This is the stage where the relentless forward momentum of youth begins to encounter the sobering reality of entropy. The metabolic furnace that once burned so brightly now cools a degree; the joints that were once supple now speak with the creaking grammar of wear and tear; the recovery that was once overnight now requires days. The theological goal for this season, therefore, undergoes a strategic and crucial shift. It is no longer primarily about *building* peak capacity, but about **actively combating the natural decline of muscle mass and bone density, managing stress, and preventing the onset of chronic lifestyle diseases, thus preserving the body's ability to serve and lead.** This is the season of wise, defensive stewardship—a long, obedient campaign to hold the line against decay, ensuring that the vessel remains seaworthy for the continued journey of discipleship and service.

Theologically, this stage is a profound lived-out lesson in the "already but not yet" of redemption. We feel the "not yet" in our very bones—the groaning of a creation still subject to futility (Romans 8:20-23). The slow decline is a tangible, daily reminder that our hope is not in the preservation of this earthly tent, but in the building of our eternal, heavenly dwelling (2 Corinthians

5:1-2). Yet, in the "already," we are called to a holy defiance. We are called to steward this aging temple with the same diligence as we did in our youth, not because we can stop the clock, but because we honor the God who created time itself. The fight against sarcopenia and osteoporosis is not a vain attempt to achieve immortality; it is an act of faithfulness, a way of ensuring that this instrument can continue to play its part in the symphony of God's kingdom for as long as the Conductor appoints. It is the practical application of Paul's exhortation that "though our outer self is wasting away, our inner self is being renewed day by day" (2 Corinthians 4:16). We acknowledge the wasting away without surrendering to it, all the while focusing on the renewal of the inner person, which gives purpose to the outer struggle.

Practically, this theological goal demands a regimen that is more strategic, more preventative, and more attuned to the body's changing signals than ever before.

First and foremost is the non-negotiable **Emphasis on Strength Training**. If there is one single most important physical discipline for this season, it is resistance training. The natural physiological process of sarcopenia—the age-related loss of muscle mass and strength—begins in earnest during these years. This is not merely an aesthetic concern; it is a direct assault on functional capacity. Muscle is the body's metabolic engine; losing it slows the metabolism and increases the risk of weight gain and type 2 diabetes. More critically, muscle strength is the foundation of independence—the ability to get out of a chair, to climb stairs, to carry groceries, to lift a grandchild. Strength training is the God-given antidote. By challenging the muscles with resistance, we signal the body to maintain and even rebuild this precious tissue. Similarly, weight-bearing exercise is the primary defense against osteoporosis, the weakening of bones. In a very real sense, lifting weights is an act of spiritual warfare against the physical consequences of the Fall, a way of saying "no" to the slow creep of frailty and "yes" to a life of continued strength and service.

Second, there must be a strategic shift in **Cardiovascular** approach. The high-impact running and intense sports of youth may now begin to exact a heavy toll on the knees, hips, and back. Wisdom dictates a pivot towards **Low-Impact Cardio**. Activities like cycling, swimming, brisk walking, and using the elliptical trainer provide the essential benefits of cardiovascular health—strengthening the heart, improving circulation, and managing weight—without the joint-pounding that can lead to chronic pain and injury. This is not a retreat, but a tactical repositioning. It is the stewardship of longevity, choosing activities that can be sustained for decades to come, rather than those that offer short-term intensity at the cost of long-term function.

Third, this is the season to formally **Incorporate Flexibility and Balance**. These are the unsung heroes of midlife physical stewardship. As connective tissues lose elasticity and the nervous system's reaction time slows, the risk of debilitating injuries from simple falls or strains increases dramatically. Practices like yoga, Tai Chi, or dedicated stretching routines are no longer optional "extras"; they are essential maintenance. They preserve the range of motion necessary for daily life, preventing the body from becoming stiff and rigid. More importantly, they train the body's proprioception—its sense of its own position in space—which is the key to preventing falls. A fall in one's sixties can have life-altering consequences, and the discipline of balance training is a profound act of preventative stewardship and a practical expression of loving one's future self and one's family, who would otherwise bear the burden of care.

Underpinning all of these applications is the governing principle of **Consistency Over Intensity**. The glory days of setting personal records in the weight room or on the race course are often past. The new metric of success is not the weight on the bar, but the number of years one can continue to lift safely and effectively. A sustainable, consistent routine—perhaps four days a week of moderate activity—is infinitely more valuable than sporadic, heroic workouts that leave one injured and sidelined for weeks. This requires a sanctification of the ego. It demands humility, the acceptance of new limits, and the wisdom to listen to the body's warnings. This consistent, plodding faithfulness is a spiritual discipline in itself, mirroring the long obedience in the same direction that characterizes the mature Christian life.

This season, however, presents its own unique set of pitfalls that must be vigilantly avoided.

The first is the temptation to **Use Age as an Excuse for Complete Inactivity**. It is easy to look at the slowing metabolism, the new aches, and the increased effort required and simply give up. This is a surrender to the curse, a passive acceptance of decay. It is a failure to fight the good fight of stewardship. The mantra becomes, "I'm just getting old," and physical discipline is abandoned, leading to an accelerated decline that unnecessarily truncates one's capacity for service and joy.

The second, more subtle pitfall, is **Ignoring New Aches and Pains**. The machismo of youth, which taught us to "push through the pain," becomes a dangerous liability in midlife. A new kind of pain is no longer a signal of growth but a warning of breakdown. To ignore a persistent ache in the shoulder, a twinge in the knee, or a nagging pain in the back is folly. It reflects a refusal to accept the body's new reality and a prideful insistence on training like a twenty-five-year-old. This almost inevitably leads to a significant injury that forces a much longer and more drastic period of inactivity than would have been required by a simple modification of the regimen. It is a failure of the wisdom that should characterize this season (Proverbs 16:31).

Thus, the stewardship of middle adulthood is a call to wisdom, humility, and strategic, persistent faithfulness. It is about trading the explosive power of youth for the enduring strength of the oak. It is about listening to the body with discernment, caring for it with patience, and honoring God by preserving this temple for the continued work of leadership, mentorship, and service to which He has called us in this rich and fruitful season of life.

14.5 The Senior Years: Stewarding Wisdom and Maintaining Independence

Beloved, we now approach the sacred and poignant season of the senior years, a time when the narrative of the body reaches its final, profound chapters. This is a stage that our youth-obsessed culture often fears and marginalizes, viewing it as a period of mere decline and loss. But the biblical vision for this season is radically different, imbued with dignity, purpose, and a unique form of stewardship. The body, now bearing the marks of a long journey, may be frailer, its steps slower, its strength diminished. Yet, its sacred status as a temple of the Holy Spirit remains undiminished. The theological goal for this season is not to recapture the vigor of youth, but to fulfill the Proverbial wisdom: **"Gray hair is a crown of glory; it is gained in a righteous life" (Proverbs 16:31).** Our goal is to honor this "crown of glory" by maintaining functional independence, managing the symptoms of age with grace, and continuing to contribute to the community for as long as possible. This is the stewardship of legacy, where the focus shifts from building capacity to preserving dignity and offering the hard-won wisdom that can only be forged in the crucible of a long life.

Theologically, this stage is a powerful lived-out testimony to the sufficiency of God's grace in weakness. The Apostle Paul's declaration, "My grace is sufficient for you, for my power is made perfect in weakness" (2 Corinthians 12:9), finds its most tangible expression here. The gradual weakening of the physical frame is not a sign of God's abandonment, but can become the very platform upon which the strength of Christ is most clearly displayed. When a believer in their eighties, with aching joints and failing eyesight, continues to pray fervently, to offer gentle counsel, to testify to God's faithfulness over decades, their witness carries a weight and authenticity that the robust energy of youth cannot replicate. The stewardship of the senior years is, therefore, an exercise in dependent strength. It is about drawing deeply from the well of God's sustaining grace and demonstrating that a life's value is not contingent on physical capability, but on faithful relationship with the Eternal God. It is a season to embody the truth that "though our outer self is wasting away, our inner self is being renewed day by day" (2 Corinthians 4:16), and to allow that renewed inner self—character refined by a lifetime of walking with God—to shine through the increasing fragility of the outer self.

Practically, this theological goal demands a regimen that is gentle yet deliberate, focused not on performance but on the profound gift of functional autonomy.

The single most important focus becomes **Priority on Balance and Strength**. In the senior years, a fall is not a simple mishap; it is often a catastrophic event that can lead to a fracture, a loss of independence, and a rapid decline in overall health. Therefore, exercises specifically designed to improve balance and maintain leg strength are paramount. This is a direct, practical outworking of the command to love your neighbor; by preventing a fall, you prevent becoming a burden and you preserve your ability to contribute. Simple, life-saving exercises include:

- **Chair Rises:** Practicing standing up from a seated position without using hands builds the crucial leg strength needed for daily life.
- **Heel-to-Toe Walking:** Walking in a straight line, placing the heel of one foot directly in front of the toes of the other, dramatically improves balance.
- **Light Resistance Training:** Using light weights or resistance bands to maintain muscle mass in the arms, legs, and core. This is not for building bulk, but for preserving the functional strength to carry a bag of groceries, lift a kettle, or get up from the floor.

Alongside this, **Moderate, Consistent Movement** remains a cornerstone. The simple, God-given act of walking is one of the most powerful medicines for the aging body. A daily walk, even if slow and short, maintains cardiovascular health, supports joint mobility, improves mood, and fosters a connection with the outside world. It is a rhythm of grace, a testament to the fact that while the body slows, it does not have to stop. This consistent movement is an act of hope, a declaration that this day, too, is a gift from God to be actively received and inhabited.

Furthermore, the importance of **Social Exercise** cannot be overstated. Loneliness and social isolation are silent epidemics among the elderly, with devastating effects on both mental and physical health. Group exercise classes designed for seniors—such as water aerobics, gentle yoga, or SilverSneakers programs—provide a double benefit. They offer the physical stimulus of movement while simultaneously providing the vital, life-giving nutrient of community. In these settings, exercise becomes a means of *koinonia*, of fellowship. It combats the despair of isolation and reinforces the biblical truth that we are made for relationship. The body of Christ can manifest beautifully in a room of seniors moving together, encouraging one another, and sharing life.

Finally, the entire regimen must have a razor-sharp **Focus on Function**. Every exercise should be chosen for its direct translation to the activities of daily living (ADLs). The question is not, "Will this help me look better?" but "Will this help me live better?" Can I:

- Get in and out of a car easily?
- Reach for a plate on a high shelf without losing my balance?
- Carry my laundry basket without strain?
- Stand up from the toilet without assistance?

This functional focus makes the discipline of exercise profoundly meaningful. It is no longer an abstract pursuit of health, but a concrete investment in continued independence and the ability to serve one's family and community in simple, yet essential, ways.

This season, however, is fraught with particularly insidious pitfalls that require spiritual discernment to overcome.

The first is the temptation toward a **Sedentary Lifestyle Born from Fear of Injury**. After a lifetime of activity, the increased risk of a fall or a strain can breed a debilitating fear. The thought becomes, "It's safer to just stay in my chair." This is a lie from the enemy, a temptation to surrender one's God-given agency. Inactivity is the fastest path to losing the very independence one fears losing. Muscle atrophies, balance worsens, and confidence plummets. The stewardship of this season requires courage—the courage to move, carefully and wisely, in the face of fear, trusting that God has given us a spirit not of fear, but of power and love and self-control (2 Timothy 1:7).

The second pitfall is **Failing to Consult with Healthcare Providers**. The uniform training regimens of younger years are no longer appropriate. The senior body is often managing multiple chronic conditions: arthritis, hypertension, osteoporosis, heart disease. To embark on an exercise program without the guidance of a doctor or physical therapist is foolishness, not faith. It is a refusal to avail oneself of the common grace of medical wisdom. A tailored approach, which respects the unique limitations and needs of one's body, is an act of wise stewardship. It honors God by honoring the complex and fragile temple He has entrusted to us, ensuring that our efforts to preserve it do not inadvertently cause it harm.

Thus, the stewardship of the senior years is a beautiful, slow, and deliberate dance of grace and effort. It is about offering the body, in its fragility, back to God as a living sacrifice. It is about fighting for every step, every ounce of strength, and every moment of balance, not for the sake of vanity, but for the sake of love—love for God, love for family, and love for a community that still needs the priceless gift of a life well-lived and a faith deeply rooted. It is the final, faithful act of tending the temple, until the day it is finally and gloriously replaced by a building from God, a house not made with hands, eternal in the heavens (2 Corinthians 5:1).

14.6 A Theology of Diminishment: Finding Grace in Weakness

Beloved, as we conclude our journey through the lifespan, we must confront a theological reality that underpins every stage but becomes overwhelmingly present in the later years: the reality of bodily diminishment. We have spoken at length of stewardship—of building, preserving, and maintaining the temple of the body. Yet, a faith that speaks only of strength and preservation is a half-truth, a gospel that has not yet fully engaged with the groaning of a fallen creation. No matter how diligent our stewardship, no matter how wise our regimen, the trajectory of this earthly tent is ultimately one of decay. The muscles will atrophy, the senses will dim, the organs will falter. To face this reality without a robust theological framework is to risk despair, to see the body's failure as a personal failure or, worse, as a sign of God's abandonment. Therefore, we must now develop what can only be called a **Theology of Diminishment**, a spiritual lens through which to view the inevitable weakening of the physical frame, not as a defeat for faith, but as a unique and sacred arena for the manifestation of divine grace.

This theology requires us to hold two seemingly contradictory truths in a dynamic, gospel-informed tension. On one hand, we are called to the faithful, active stewardship we have outlined—the *gymnaze* of the body, the fight against decay, the preservation of function. This is our duty, our "working out" of our salvation with fear and trembling. On the other hand, we must simultaneously embrace the sobering reality so eloquently stated by the Apostle Paul: **"So we do not lose heart. Though our outer self is wasting away, our inner self is being renewed day by day" (2 Corinthians 4:16).** The "wasting away" (Greek: *diaphtheirō*—to decay, to corrupt, to destroy) is not a hypothetical. It is the present, active experience of every human being, a direct consequence of the Fall and the curse upon the ground from which we were taken. A theology that only emphasizes stewardship without acknowledging this "wasting away" leads to a theology of glory, a performance-based righteousness where our value is tied to our physical vitality, and where aging becomes a source of shame and frantic denial. But a theology that only acknowledges the "wasting away" without the call to stewardship leads to a passive fatalism, a surrender to decay that fails to honor God with the time and capacity we are given.

The resolution to this tension is found in the purpose of the decay. The body's failure is not a random, meaningless tragedy. It is part of the corporate **groaning of creation** that awaits its final redemption. Paul expands on this in Romans 8:22-23: "For we know that the whole creation has been groaning together in the pains of childbirth until now. And not only the creation, but we ourselves, who have the firstfruits of the Spirit, groan inwardly as we wait eagerly for adoption as sons, the redemption of our bodies." Our aching joints, our failing eyesight, our diminishing strength—these are not signs of God's displeasure with us as individuals. They are our personal, embodied participation in the collective sigh of a universe subjected to futility. Our groans are not cries of faithlessness; they are the birth pangs of a new creation, the eager longing for the fulfillment of God's promise. When we groan, we are in good company; we are joining the chorus of the cosmos, and the Spirit Himself intercedes for us with groanings too deep for words (Romans 8:26).

This divine perspective transforms the experience of weakness from a curse to be resented into a classroom of grace. It is in the very experience of our physical limits that we are taught the most profound spiritual lessons. When we are strong and capable, it is easy to rely on our own energy, our own plans, our own prowess. But when the body weakens, when the capacities we once took for granted are stripped away, we are confronted with our fundamental creatureliness and dependence. It is here, in this place of acknowledged weakness, that the gospel shines with its brightest hope. This is the ultimate fulfillment of Christ's word to Paul: **"My grace is sufficient for you, for my power is made perfect in weakness" (2 Corinthians 12:9).** The Greek word for "perfect" here is *teleitai*, meaning "brought to its end, completed, fulfilled." God's power finds its ultimate purpose, its perfect fulfillment, not when it is added to our human strength, but when it becomes the sole source of strength in the vacuum of our own inability.

Therefore, the slow diminishment of the body is not God's failure to keep us healthy; it is often His chosen instrument to wean us from self-reliance and to school us in the radical dependence that is the essence of faith. The steward who has diligently cared for their body their entire life must, in the end, learn the hardest lesson of all: to be a good steward of their own weakness. This means offering our fatigue, our pain, our frustration, and our dependence to God as part of our spiritual worship. It means allowing others to serve us, thus giving them the opportunity to fulfill the law of Christ. It means redefining "productivity" not in terms of physical output, but in terms of love, prayer, patience, and the quiet testimony of a heart that trusts God when the body can no longer perform.

A Theology of Diminishment, therefore, does not negate the call to physical stewardship; it envelops it in a larger, more hopeful story. We steward the body diligently for as long as we are able, as an act of worship and love. But when stewardship can no longer prevent the decline, we do not despair. We see the weakening of the "outer self" as the very condition that makes space for the renewal of the "inner self." We understand that our groans are not the end of the story, but a faithful longing for the final chapter: the redemption of our bodies, the resurrection, when this perishable body will put on the imperishable, and this mortal body will put on immortality (1 Corinthians 15:53-54). Until that day, we live in the tension, stewarding the strength we have, and finding, in the midst of the strength we have lost, the surprising, sufficient, and perfected power of Christ.

14.7 Faithfulness Across the Generations

Beloved, as we bring our exploration of life-stage stewardship to a close, we are left not with a rigid, one-size-fits-all prescription, but with a profound and flexible principle: **faithful stewardship is a dynamic conversation of wisdom with the body God has given us, across the entire span of our earthly pilgrimage.** This life-stage approach is far more than a pragmatic health strategy; it is a deep and practical act of theological wisdom. It is the lived-out expression of the fear of the Lord, which is the beginning of wisdom (Proverbs 9:10), applied to the flesh and bone of our daily existence. It requires that we listen to the narrative God has written into our biology—the explosive growth of youth, the resilient strength of young adulthood, the strategic preservation of midlife, and the dignified conservation of the senior years—and that we respond with regimens of care that honor the unique purpose and capacity of each season.

This approach stands as a bulwark against the two great errors of our age: the modernist lie that the body is a machine to be optimized according to our own will and for our own glory, and the ancient Gnostic temptation to despise the body as a prison for the soul. Instead, we affirm that the body is a sacred trust, a divine design, and its changing nature is not a flaw but a feature of God's creational and providential order. To impose the high-intensity training of a twenty-five-year-old upon a sixty-five-year-old frame is not faithfulness; it is folly, a refusal to accept the God-ordained "time to break down" (Ecclesiastes 3:3). Conversely, to allow a child to forsake the holy, kinetic joy of play for sedentary entertainment is to stifle the divine impulse for movement and discovery woven into their very being. Wisdom, therefore, is the key that unlocks appropriate stewardship at every age. It is the capacity to ask and answer the question, "Heavenly Father, what is the particular calling for this body, in this season, and how can I care for it in a way that maximizes its capacity to bring You glory and love my neighbor?"

When we embrace this wisdom, we see that the form of our physical offering changes, but its fundamental nature as worship remains constant. It is a **tangible offering of worship across the entire lifespan.** For the child, worship is the unrestrained, joyful play that explores the goodness of a created world, a kinetic doxology of running, jumping, and shouting. For the adolescent, worship is the disciplined channeling of newfound strength and energy into skill-building and cooperative sports, learning to offer their burgeoning capabilities to God and others. For the young adult, worship is the intense, focused building of a resilient and capable instrument, forging a body ready for a lifetime of demanding service in career, family, and ministry. For the middle-aged, worship is the wise, often humbling, work of preservation—the lifting of weights to combat decay, the choosing of low-impact cardio to protect joints, the patient stretching to maintain mobility—all as an act of defiance against the futility of the Fall and a commitment to remain useful in God's kingdom. For the senior, worship is the courageous, daily movement that fights for independence, the acceptance of help with grace, and the powerful testimony of a spirit that is being renewed even as the outer body wastes away, demonstrating that the source of true life has never been the flesh, but the Spirit.

This generational vision of stewardship weaves a beautiful tapestry of faithfulness. It presents a picture of the people of God, from the youngest to the oldest, collectively embodying the full spectrum of physical life as an offering to their Creator. The church should be a community where the joyful noise of children at play is recognized as liturgy, where the sweat of a young adult serving on a mission trip is seen as a sacrifice of praise, where the consistent, plodding walk of an elder is honored as a faithful pilgrimage. This holistic view destroys the sacred-secular divide entirely, demonstrating that there is no realm of physical life—from the playground to the deathbed—that cannot be sanctified and offered back to God.

Therefore, the goal is not to arrive at a final, static state of perfect health. The goal is **faithfulness across the generations.** It is to be a five-talent steward in the season of five talents, investing that abundant physical capital vigorously for the Kingdom. It is to be a two-talent steward in the season of two talents, investing that more modest capacity with no less diligence. And it is to be a one-talent steward in the season of one talent, offering even the last remnants of physical strength back to the Master with the same trust and devotion, knowing that His assessment of our stewardship will be based not on the absolute magnitude of our capacity, but on the faithfulness with which we invested whatever we were given. From the first unsteady steps of a toddler to the last measured steps of a nonagenarian, the disciplined, loving, and wise care of the body remains our spiritual worship, a lifelong hymn of gratitude to the God who formed us from dust, redeemed us by blood, and will one day raise us in glory.

CHAPTER 15

Sabbath Rest and Sleep: Divine Rhythms for Human Restoration

Beloved, we now turn our attention from the active disciplines of labor and exercise to a dimension of stewardship that is, in our modern context, perhaps even more radical and counter-cultural: the sacred disciplines of rest. In a world that worships at the altar of relentless productivity, that equates busyness with importance, and that offers the seductive glow of the screen as a substitute for the deep, healing darkness of sleep, the biblical call to Sabbath and restorative slumber is a prophetic word. It is a word that cuts against the grain of our deepest anxieties and our most ingrained habits. This chapter will argue a truth that we have largely forgotten: that rest is not a passive void, a mere cessation of activity born of exhaustion. It is, rather, an active, trust-filled, and deliberate cessation from labor that is woven into the very fabric of God's created order. Both the weekly Sabbath and the daily gift of sleep are not spiritual luxuries or signs of laziness; they are non-negotiable components of holistic stewardship, designed by God to physically restore the body He has given us and to spiritually reorient the soul He has redeemed.

15.1 The Sanctification of Rest

We begin by confronting the dominant spiritual pathology of our age: the idolatry of productivity. This is a spirit that measures human worth by output, that views time as a commodity to be maximized, and that sees rest as wasted time. It is a worldview that is fundamentally at odds with the gospel of grace, which declares that our value is not in what we produce, but in whose we are—the beloved children of a sovereign God. This idolatry has seeped into the church, creating a culture of burnout where pastors and laypeople alike wear their fatigue as a badge of honor, mistakenly believing that their ceaseless activity is a testament to their devotion.

In stark opposition to this stands the divine pattern established at the dawn of creation. The Genesis narrative culminates not with the creation of humanity, but with God's own rest. "And on the seventh day God finished his work that he had done, and he rested on the seventh day from all his work that he had done. So, God blessed the seventh day and made it holy, because on it God rested from all his work that he had done in creation" (Genesis 2:2-3). This is one of the most theologically significant acts in all of Scripture. The omnipotent God, who does not faint or grow weary (Isaiah 40:28), chooses to rest. His rest is not due to fatigue; it is an act of contemplation, enjoyment, and declaration. He rests to behold the goodness of what He has made and to establish a rhythm that is now inherent to the structure of reality itself. The Sabbath is not an afterthought; it is the crown of creation. By blessing and hallowing the seventh day, God sanctified rest itself. He set it apart as a sacred space in time, a weekly testimony that our world is, and always will be, fundamentally dependent on His creative and sustaining power, not our frantic efforts.

Therefore, to rest is an act of *imitatio Dei*—the imitation of God. It is a conscious, willful alignment with the grain of the universe. When we Sabbath, we are not merely taking a break; we are participating in a divine rhythm. We are declaring with our bodies and our schedules that we are not the ultimate masters of our world. We are ceasing from our work to remember that God is the one who ultimately builds the house and keeps the city (Psalm 127:1). This is why Sabbath-keeping and trust are inextricably linked. To stop working requires a profound trust that God will provide for our needs in six days what we fear we cannot accomplish in seven. It is a tangible repudiation of the anxiety that drives our culture of overwork.

Similarly, the daily rhythm of sleep is a miniature, enacted Sabbath. Every night, we are compelled to surrender our consciousness, our control, and our productivity. We lie down in a state of profound vulnerability, entrusting our safety, our very lives, and the ongoing care of the world to God. Sleep is a forced confession of our creatureliness. We are not machines that can run perpetually; we are dependent beings who must regularly acknowledge our limits and our need for sustenance from a source outside ourselves. The Psalmist captures this beautifully: "It is in vain that you rise up early and go late to rest, eating the bread of anxious toil; for he gives to his beloved sleep" (Psalm 127:2). Sleep is here portrayed as a gift from a loving Father to His beloved children, a gift that the striving, anxious heart refuses.

Thus, proper sleep and Sabbath observance are foundational to holistic stewardship. Physically, sleep is the non-negotiable mechanism God has built into our biology for cellular repair, memory consolidation, metabolic regulation, and cognitive restoration. To chronically deprive ourselves of sleep is not a mark of dedication; it is an act of violence against the temple of the Holy Spirit, willfully disregarding the most basic maintenance protocol hardwired into its design. Spiritually, Sabbath and sleep reorient the soul. They break the addictive cycle of work and achievement. They create a space for gratitude, for worship that is not task-oriented, for relationship that is not utilitarian, and for the quiet reception of grace. They are the great equalizers, reminding the CEO and the janitor alike that they are dust, utterly dependent on the God who neither slumbers nor sleeps (Psalm 121:4), so that they, His beloved, can. In a culture of relentless doing, the sanctification of rest is the necessary corrective that teaches us the blessedness of simply *being*—being His children, held and sustained by His unwavering grace.

15.2 The Theology of Sabbath: Ceasing, Resting, Feasting, Embracing

Beloved, having established the sanctity of rest as a divine principle, we must now delve into its most profound and structured expression: the Sabbath. The fourth commandment, given at Sinai, is not an arbitrary restriction but a gracious invitation into a rhythm that is both therapeutic and theological. "Remember the Sabbath day, to keep it holy. Six days you shall labor, and do all your work, but the seventh day is a Sabbath to the LORD your God. On it you shall not do any work... For in six days the LORD made heaven and earth, the sea, and all that is in them, and rested on the seventh day. Therefore the LORD blessed the Sabbath day and made it holy" (Exodus 20:8-11). This command is rooted not in the soil of the Mosaic covenant alone, but in the bedrock of creation itself, in the very pattern of God's own work (Genesis 2:2-3). To understand the Sabbath is to understand the heart of God for His people—a heart that desires not slaves for endless production, but children who can enter into His rest. The practice of Sabbath, therefore, is not a mere day off, but a rich, four-part liturgy of time, involving the sacred movements of Ceasing, Resting, Feasting, and Embracing.

First, and most fundamentally, the Sabbath begins with **Ceasing**. This is the most difficult and counter-cultural act. It is a deliberate, willful stop. It is the laying down of tools, the closing of laptops, the silencing of the internal to-do list. But it is far more than a cessation of productive labor. It is a cessation of anxiety, of the need to be in control, of the relentless drive to define ourselves by our accomplishments. To cease is to enact a powerful, non-verbal declaration of faith. It is to proclaim to the world, to our own anxious hearts, and to the principalities and powers that the universe does not ultimately depend on our labor for its continued existence. It is a tangible confession that God is sovereign, that He holds all things together by the word of His power (Colossians 1:17), and that His kingdom will advance not by our frantic striving, but by His sovereign grace. Every unpaid bill, every unfinished project, every unresolved conflict is, for this twenty-four-hour period, placed squarely in the hands of our capable Father. This ceasing is an act of war against the idolatry of self-sufficiency. It is the practical outworking of Jesus' invitation: "Come to me, all who labor and are heavy laden, and I will give you rest" (Matthew 11:28). We lay down our heavy burdens of productivity and control, and in doing so, we find that the world continues to spin on its axis, held firmly in the grip of the One who never slumbers.

From this foundational act of ceasing flows the second movement: **Resting**. This is the positive reception of the gift that ceasing makes space for. It is physical, mental, and emotional recuperation. This is not the same as collapse from exhaustion, which is a symptom of a disordered life. Sabbath rest is a purposeful, joyful reception of peace. It may involve a nap without guilt, a leisurely walk in nature without a step-counting goal, reading a book for pleasure, or engaging in a hobby that truly restores the soul. It is crucial to distinguish this from mere entertainment or distraction. The modern "day off" is often filled with noise, screens, and activities that, while perhaps enjoyable, do not necessarily restore the deep wells of the spirit. Sabbath rest is qualitatively different. It is characterized by peace, quietness, and activities that replenish rather than deplete. It is the restoration of the *nephesh*, the whole person. It is the practice of *being* rather than *doing*, allowing the nervous system to descend from a state of constant sympathetic arousal (fight-or-flight) into the parasympathetic state of rest-and-digest. This is how we "recharge our batteries," not as a grim necessity for another week of productivity, but as a joyful participation in the peace of God which surpasses all understanding (Philippians 4:7).

The third movement of the Sabbath liturgy is **Feasting**. If ceasing is the negative space and resting is the receptive space, then feasting is the celebratory filling of that space. The Sabbath is not a fast; it is a feast. It is a day to joyfully celebrate with family and community, to enjoy the good gifts of God's creation with intentional delight. This means preparing a special meal, setting a beautiful table, opening a good bottle of wine, and sharing it with loved ones. It is a time for laughter, for storytelling, for unhurried conversation. This feasting is a profound theological act. It is a declaration that God is not an ascetic tyrant, but a generous Father who gives us all things richly to enjoy (1 Timothy 6:17). It is a defiant act of joy in a world marred by sorrow. And most significantly, it is a **foretaste of the eschatological marriage supper of the Lamb** (Revelation 19:9). Every Sabbath feast is a rehearsal for the great, eternal banquet in the New Jerusalem. It points our hearts forward, stoking our hope and reminding us that the ultimate goal of redemption is not a disembodied eternity, but a glorious celebration in resurrected bodies, in perfect community, in the direct presence of God. The Sabbath feast is a weekly anchor of hope, pulling the future joy of heaven into the present reality of our lives.

Finally, the Sabbath finds its ultimate fulfillment in **Embracing**. This is the intentional, focused turning of the entire person toward God. It is the heart of the command to "keep it holy"—to set it apart. This involves the corporate embrace of God's presence in worship with the people of God. It involves the personal embrace of His Word through unhurried reading and meditation. It involves the intimate embrace of His person through extended, conversational prayer. This is the time for re-centering. Throughout the week, our identity is constantly under assault. We are defined by our jobs, our roles, our successes, and our failures. The Sabbath, through the movement of embracing, forcibly reorients us. We are reminded that our primary identity is not that of a worker, a parent, or a consumer, but that of a **beloved creature** and a redeemed child of God. We are human *beings*, not human *doings*. In His presence, we remember that we are loved not for what we produce, but because we are His. This embrace repairs the soul, healing the fractures of a week's worth of performance-based living and grounding us anew in the solid rock of grace.

Thus, the theology of the Sabbath presents it not as a legalistic burden, but as a liberating rhythm. It is a weekly pilgrimage through the movements of faith (Ceasing), restoration (Resting), joy (Feasting), and love (Embracing). It is a divine prescription for the healing of our souls and the reordering of our lives around the reality of God's sovereignty and goodness. It is a twenty-four-hour sanctuary in time, a gift from a loving Father who knows that we, His fragile children, need regular, structured reminders to stop, to rest, to celebrate, and to remember who we truly are in Him.

15.3 The Neurobiology of Sabbath: General Revelation Confirms Special Revelation

Beloved, the wisdom of God, revealed in the sacred text of Scripture, is not confined to the spiritual realm alone. It is woven into the very fabric of the physical universe He created. The principle of General Revelation—that God makes Himself known through His creation—assures us that when we examine the natural world with the tools of science, we should find echoes and confirmations of the truths declared in Special Revelation. The Sabbath command is a stunning example of this divine harmony. What God ordained for our spiritual and communal health millennia ago, modern neurobiology now confirms as essential for our physical and psychological well-being. The Sabbath is not an arbitrary religious rule; it is a divinely engineered safety protocol for the human organism, and the data from our own bodies bears witness to this profound truth.

To understand this, we must first grasp the physiology of the stress that the Sabbath is designed to interrupt. Our bodies are equipped with a magnificent, God-given system for handling acute danger: the hypothalamic-pituitary-adrenal (HPA) axis. When faced with a threat, this system triggers the release of cortisol, the primary stress hormone. Cortisol is a lifesaver in the short term. It sharpens focus, mobilizes energy stores, and modulates the immune system for a rapid response. This is the "fight-or-flight" mechanism, and it is a testament to the Creator's foresight.

However, this system was designed for acute, short-lived crises—escaping a predator, facing a sudden conflict. It was not designed for the chronic, low-grade, psychological stress that characterizes modern life: the relentless inbox, the financial pressures, the constant connectivity, the traffic jams, the performance anxiety. When the HPA axis is perpetually activated, we exist in a state of **chronic stress**, and the lifesaving cortisol becomes a slow-acting poison. The very hormone that once saved us begins to dismantle us from the inside out.

The devastating effects of elevated cortisol without rest are now well-documented. It **impairs cognitive function**, particularly in the prefrontal cortex—the seat of executive functions like decision-making, emotional regulation, and focused attention. This is why we feel mentally foggy, irritable, and unable to concentrate when we are chronically stressed. Cortisol also **weakens the immune system**. It suppresses the production of lymphocytes and directs immune resources away from long-term defense, making us more susceptible to infections and, over time, increasing the risk of autoimmune disorders. Furthermore, sustained high cortisol **increases the risk of heart disease** by raising blood pressure, promoting the buildup of arterial plaque, and contributing to weight gain, particularly dangerous visceral fat. And perhaps most insidiously, it is a direct contributor to **depression and anxiety**, as it can disrupt the delicate balance of neurotransmitters like serotonin and dopamine, which are essential for mood stability.

This is the physiological reality of a life without Sabbath. It is a life of constant, low-grade alarm, a state of being where the body is perpetually preparing for a battle that never culminates, slowly eroding its own foundations.

Into this reality, the Sabbath rhythm speaks with the authority of divine medicine. A weekly day of deliberate rest—a true cessation from productive labor, anxiety, and the performance-driven mindset—acts as a powerful circuit breaker for the HPA axis. The practices of Sabbath—the ceasing, the resting, the feasting, the embracing—directly counteract the physiological ravages of chronic stress.

When we truly cease, we signal to the deepest parts of our brain that the "threat" is over. The nervous system, no longer perceiving demands and deadlines, can descend from a state of sympathetic overdrive (fight-or-flight) into the parasympathetic state (rest-and-digest). This shift is measurable. **Cortisol levels drop significantly.** Heart rate variability, a key marker of resilience and healthy autonomic function, improves. The body begins the essential work of repair that is impossible when it is constantly on alert. The immune system is given a reprieve, allowing it to re-calibrate and strengthen. The prefrontal cortex, freed from the cortisol bath, can restore its cognitive capacities. This is not merely "feeling relaxed"; it is a fundamental biological reset.

This weekly reset is not a luxury; it is a necessity for sustainable human function. The science of ultradian rhythms—the 90-120 minute cycles of alertness and fatigue our bodies move through each day—suggests that we are designed for regular breaks. The Sabbath is the macro-level application of this principle. Just as the body requires sleep each night to repair itself, it requires a longer, deeper weekly rhythm to recover from the cumulative stress of six days of labor. Without it, we are like a machine run continuously without maintenance, destined for a premature breakdown.

Therefore, the findings of modern neurobiology do not explain away the Sabbath; they illuminate its profound wisdom. They demonstrate in the language of hormones and neural pathways what God declared in the language of covenant: "And now, Israel, what does the LORD your God require of you, but to fear the LORD your God, to walk in all his ways, to love him, to serve the LORD your God with all your heart and with all your soul, and to keep the commandments and statutes of the LORD, which I am commanding you today **for your good**?" (Deuteronomy 10:12-13, emphasis added).

The Sabbath is "for your good." The lowered cortisol, the reset nervous system, the improved well-being—these are not accidental benefits. They are the gracious design of a loving Father who knows the frame of His children (Psalm 103:14). He knows that we are dust, and He has given us a rhythm to prevent us from returning to dust prematurely. The General Revelation of neurobiology stands as a powerful witness, confirming the life-giving truth of the Special Revelation of Scripture. In a world pushing us toward burnout, the ancient command to remember the Sabbath day and keep it holy is revealed to be not a relic of a bygone era, but a prophetic, essential, and scientifically-validated prescription for human flourishing in the twenty-first century.

15.4 The Theology of Sleep: The Vulnerability of Faith

Beloved, if the Sabbath is the weekly sanctuary of rest, then sleep is its daily, non-negotiable counterpart. We have explored the sacred rhythm of ceasing from labor for one day in seven, but each night, God in His wisdom compels us to a far more profound and intimate cessation. Sleep is not merely a biological necessity; it is a theological reality, a daily, physical parable of the gospel itself. In the vulnerable, unconscious state of slumber, we enact the deepest truths of our faith—our dependence, our mortality, and our hope for redemption. To understand sleep theologically is to transform it from a passive state of recharge into an active discipline of faith, a nightly ritual of surrender that lies at the very heart of what it means to be a creature before the Creator.

First and foremost, sleep is a profound **Act of Humility**. In a culture that worships productivity, control, and self-sufficiency, sleep is a scandal. It is a state of utter unproductivity. For six to nine hours each day, we contribute nothing to the economy, achieve no goals, and advance no projects. We are, by the world's standards, completely useless. Furthermore, we are in a state of profound vulnerability. We are unaware of our surroundings, defenseless against potential dangers, and entirely dependent on our environment for safety. This forced relinquishment of control is a divine rebuke to our pride. We cannot will ourselves to stay awake indefinitely. The body, in its God-given wisdom, eventually shuts down, overriding our arrogant attempts to master time and circumvent our own limits.

In this, sleep is a tangible enactment of the truth proclaimed in Psalm 127:2: "It is in vain that you rise up early and go late to rest, eating the bread of anxious toil; for he gives to his beloved sleep." The "bread of anxious toil" is the fruit of a life lived in the delusion of self-sufficiency. It is the belief that our security and provision depend on our frantic, ceaseless effort. But the Psalmist declares this vain, futile. True provision and security come from the Lord, who *gives* to His beloved the gift of sleep. To receive this gift is an act of faith. It is to say, "I am not the master of my destiny. I am a dependent being. I entrust my life, my family, my work, and my world to the care of my faithful God while I am incapable of managing them." Each night, as we close our eyes, we confess our creatureliness and affirm God's sovereign lordship over all that we cannot control. It is the ultimate act of letting go, a daily practice in the humility that is the foundation of all wisdom.

Secondly, sleep serves as a powerful **Picture of Death and Resurrection**. The parallels are inescapable and deeply woven into the biblical narrative. Each night, we "die" to the world. Our consciousness ceases. Our engagement with loved ones is severed. Our plans and activities come to a complete halt. Our body lies in a state that, to any observer, is a mere semblance of life. This is a daily memento mori, a reminder that "you are dust, and to dust you shall return" (Genesis 3:19). Sleep is a gentle, gracious rehearsal for the final sleep of death, a way to become familiar with the relinquishment that will one day be required of us.

But the parable does not end in the darkness. Each morning, by God's grace, we are "raised" to new life. The return of consciousness is a miracle we take for granted. We open our eyes to a new day, a new beginning, with the past day's failures and successes behind us. The fatigue of the previous evening is often washed away, and we are given a fresh start. This daily resurrection is a tangible foretaste of our ultimate hope. Just as we trust that the sun will rise and that we will awaken, we trust by faith in the promise of the bodily resurrection. Paul makes this connection explicit in his teaching on the final resurrection, using the language of sleep for those who have died in Christ (1 Thessalonians 4:13-14). The hope of the gospel is that the night of death is not the end; the morning of resurrection is coming. Therefore, every sunrise is a divine object lesson, a physical confirmation of God's faithfulness and His power to bring life from death. Our nightly journey into unconsciousness and our daily return to wakefulness is a God-ordained rhythm that preaches the gospel to our bodies and souls every single day of our lives.

Finally, we must recognize sleep as a **Divine Provision for Processing and Healing**. God, in His intricate design of the human person, did not create us as simple machines that can run perpetually. He built into us a complex, essential maintenance cycle that occurs almost exclusively during sleep. Modern science has illuminated the wonders of this design, revealing that sleep, and particularly the Rapid Eye Movement (REM) stage, is not a passive state but a period of intense activity crucial for our wholeness.

During sleep, our brain engages in critical **memory consolidation**, sorting through the experiences of the day, solidifying important learning, and discarding irrelevant information. It is the time when the raw data of our experiences is integrated into the narrative of our lives. Furthermore, sleep is fundamental for **emotional regulation**. The amygdala, the brain's fear center, is recalibrated during sleep, allowing us to process the emotional charge of the day's events. This is why a problem so often seems more manageable after a night's sleep; the brain has literally detoxified the emotional intensity attached to it. And on a purely physical level, sleep is when the body performs the majority of its **cellular repair and restoration**. Growth hormone is released, tissues are rebuilt, and the immune system is strengthened.

To willfully and chronically deprive oneself of sleep, then, is not merely a bad health habit; it is an act of profound folly and a rejection of a fundamental mechanism of God's grace. It is to say, "I know better than my Creator how to manage my mind and body." It is to refuse the gift of emotional healing, cognitive integration, and physical repair that God has so lovingly provided. The anxiety, irritability, poor judgment, and weakened health that result from sleep deprivation are the natural consequences of living out of sync with our divine design. They are the fruit of the pride that insists we can thrive while ignoring the very rhythm God established for our restoration.

Therefore, the pursuit of good sleep is a spiritual discipline. It is an act of obedience that requires us to surrender our illusion of control, to trust in God's sustaining grace through the night, and to receive the gift of daily resurrection and healing that He so freely offers. In a world that prizes the 24/7 hustle, choosing to prioritize sleep is a counter-cultural declaration of faith—a confession that we are not God, that we are dust, and that our true rest, our true security, and our true hope for renewal are found not in our own striving, but in the hands of the One who gives His beloved sleep.

15.5 The Spirituality of Sleep Disorders: When Rest Eludes

Beloved, having established the profound theology of sleep as a gift, a parable, and a divine provision, we must now, with great pastoral sensitivity, turn to the agonizing reality that for many, this gift feels cruelly withheld. The prevalence of chronic insomnia, sleep anxiety, and restless nights is a modern epidemic, and the church must be a place of understanding and wisdom, not simplistic judgment. To tell a suffering insomniac to simply "trust God and go to sleep" is as helpful as telling a drowning man to simply swim. The inability to rest is a complex affliction that often exists at the intersection of body, mind, and spirit. While poor sleep hygiene—the overuse of screens, the consumption of caffeine and alcohol, and erratic schedules—is a common and often addressable cause, we must look deeper. The state of our soul has a direct and powerful bearing on the state of our sleep. The night watches can become a stark mirror, reflecting back to us the true condition of our inner world. When rest eludes us, it can be a manifestation of a profound spiritual state, a divine alarm calling us to attend to the deeper disquiet within.

First, sleeplessness can be the symptom of **A Conscience Troubled by Sin**. The human conscience, that God-given internal witness, is not easily silenced. When we harbor unconfessed sin, nurture bitterness, or refuse to walk in the light of repentance, a spiritual dissonance is created. This dissonance does not remain confined to the "spiritual" realm; it reverberates through our entire psychosomatic unity. The Psalmist Asaph gives voice to this experience in Psalm 77:4: "You hold my eyelids open; I am so troubled that I cannot speak." His wakefulness is directly linked to his inner turmoil. The guilt, shame, and fear associated with sin activate the very same physiological stress response—the hyper-arousal of the sympathetic nervous system—that is the antithesis of the peaceful state required for sleep. The mind races with thoughts of exposure, consequences, and self-condemnation. The body is flooded with cortisol and adrenaline, making the vulnerable surrender of sleep feel impossible. In such cases, the insomnia is not the problem; it is a merciful symptom. It is the flashing red light on the soul's dashboard, warning of a deeper malfunction. The path to rest in this context is not a sleeping pill, but the gospel. It is the difficult, humble work of self-examination, confession, and receiving the cleansing forgiveness that is ours in Christ (1 John 1:9). The peace that comes from a conscience cleansed by the blood of Jesus is the most powerful sedative known to the human soul. To lie down after genuine confession is to enact the faith that we are, in that moment, fully accepted and reconciled, and that we can therefore safely entrust ourselves—and our reputations—to God while we sleep.

Second, chronic insomnia can be a manifestation of **An Anxious Lack of Trust**. We return to the wisdom of Psalm 127:2, but now from the perspective of its violation: "It is in vain that you rise up early and go late to rest, eating the bread of anxious toil." The insomniac who lies in bed mentally rehearsing tomorrow's meeting, worrying over a child's well-being, or fretting about a financial burden is, in essence, eating the "bread of anxious toil" in the middle of the night. Their mind is a factory of "what if" scenarios, a control center desperately trying to solve problems that are, for the moment, entirely outside of its control. This is a functional atheism. It is a life lived as if God were not sovereign, as if His promises to provide and sustain were not true. The inability to sleep is the body's testimony to a heart that refuses to relinquish the helm. It is a stubborn, fearful clutching of control, a refusal to practice the vulnerability that sleep requires. In this case, the spiritual discipline is one of active, volitional surrender. It is the practice of what St. John of the Cross called "the dark night of the senses," where we must learn to trust God not by feeling His presence, but by faith in His character, even in the midst of our anxiety. It is to take each worrying thought captive to the obedience of Christ (2 Corinthians 10:5), to replace the litany of fears with the recitation of Scripture—"You will keep him in perfect peace whose mind is stayed on you, because he trusts in you" (Isaiah 26:3). It is to pray, not with a demand for immediate sleep, but with a relinquishment of our burdens: "Father, into your hands I commit my spirit, my family, my work, and this night" (cf. Luke 23:46).

Finally, we must acknowledge that for some, sleeplessness is **A Season of Affliction** that is not directly tied to personal sin or a failure of trust. The Psalms are filled with the raw cries of the righteous who are simply overwhelmed by the pain of existence. Psalm 6:6 declares, "I am weary with my moaning; every night I flood my bed with tears; I drench my couch with my weeping." Here, the insomnia is born of sheer grief, loss, or depression. It is the groan of a soul under a weight too heavy to bear. In such seasons, the well-meaning advice to "just relax" or "confess your worry" is not only unhelpful, it is pastorally cruel. It adds the burden of spiritual failure to the already crushing weight of sorrow. For the one in this dark night, the spiritual discipline is not to *achieve* sleep, but to *sanctify* the wakefulness. The long, lonely hours of the night can be transformed from a torture of anxiety into a watch of lament. This is the practice of bringing our raw, unfiltered anguish to God, following the pattern of the Psalmist. It is to cry out, "How long, O LORD?" (Psalm 13:1). It is to use the time for extended, honest prayer, not to demand a change in circumstances, but to pour out the heart before the Lord who sees our tears (Psalm 56:8). In this context, the insomnia becomes a paradoxical place of intimacy, a shared vigil with the Man of Sorrows who Himself knew what it was to sweat great drops of blood in the darkness of Gethsemane. The goal shifts from seeking the gift of sleep to seeking the Giver in the midst of the sorrow, trusting that His grace is sufficient even for the exhaustion of the next day (2 Corinthians 12:9).

Therefore, a compassionate and theologically robust response to sleep disorders requires discernment. It calls for practical wisdom in addressing habits, for the courage to engage in spiritual self-examination, for the faith to practice active surrender, and for the grace to sit in compassionate silence with those whose nights are flooded with tears. In all cases, the answer is not to condemn the sleepless, but to point them to the One who neither slumbers nor sleeps (Psalm 121:4), who keeps watch over them in the darkest of nights, and who invites them to find their ultimate rest, not in a perfect night of sleep, but in His own wounded side.

15.6 Practical Disciplines for Sanctified Rest

Beloved, we have now arrived at one of the most pastorally urgent and practically demanding applications of our entire theology of Embodied Stewardship: the sanctification of our rest. We have spoken at length about the body as a temple, about the integration of body, soul, and spirit, and about the rupture of *Shalom* and its restoration in Christ. Yet, I tell you, all of this lofty theology crumbles into pious dust if it does not descend into the daily, nightly, and weekly rhythms of our exhausted lives. The great heresy of our age is not merely a theoretical Gnosticism, but a *practical* one—a lived frenzy that functionally denies the goodness of limits, the holiness of cessation, and the divinity of the pause. We are a people perpetually over-caffeinated, digitally over-stimulated, and vocationally over-committed. We worship at the altar of productivity, and our burnt offering is our own nervous system. We are tired, not merely physically, but to the very core of our souls. And in our exhaustion, we become poor stewards of the temple, irritable neighbors, inattentive spouses, and dull listeners to the still, small voice of God.

Therefore, we must now move from doctrine to discipline, from theology to practice. We must forge, with intentionality and grace, practical disciplines for sanctified rest. This is not a call to self-help relaxation techniques, though some of their insights may be co-opted. This is a call to spiritual warfare against the principalities and powers of hurry, anxiety, and the idolatry of the self. We are to reclaim rest as a sacred trust, a divine ordinance, a non-negotiable pillar of the life that is truly life. We will focus on three foundational disciplines: the holy architecture of Sabbath preparation, the restorative liturgy of sleep, and the redemptive prayer of the night watch.

Sabbath Preparation: Structuring the Week for Holy Ceasing

Beloved, the Sabbath is not merely a day off. It is not a twenty-four-hour period for catching up on errands, binging entertainment, or frantically preparing for the week ahead. To treat it as such is to profane it. The Sabbath is a divine institution, a weekly monument to God's creative power and redemptive grace. It is a foretaste of the eternal rest that awaits the people of God (Hebrews 4:9-11). It is a twenty-four-hour sanctuary in time, a divine "temple of hours" into which we are invited to enter. But you cannot stumble into the sanctuary breathless and frantic. You must prepare to enter. The sanctity of the seventh day is established by the purposeful labor of the six that precede it. Therefore, the first and most critical discipline for sanctified rest is the spiritual and practical architecture of **Sabbath Preparation**.

The pattern is set for us at the very dawn of creation. For six days, God worked. He spoke, He formed, He filled, He ordered. And on the seventh day, He ceased. He did not cease because He was exhausted; He ceased because the work was *finished*, and it was *very good* (Genesis 2:1-3). The cessation was the capstone, the final act that declared the perfection and completeness of His work. Our weekly rhythm is to mirror this divine pattern. Our six days of labor are to be purposeful, directed, and trust-filled, aimed at bringing a measure of order and fruitfulness to our little plot of creation. And then, we are to stop. We cease not because all our work is done—it never will be—but because we trust that the world is upheld by God's sovereign hand, not by our frantic effort.

So, how do we structure our week to ensure the Sabbath can be truly kept? This requires intentionality, what the ancients might have called *ascetical forethought*.

1. **The Culinary Consecration:** A significant part of Sabbath preparation, deeply rooted in the Hebraic tradition, involves the preparation of food *before* the Sabbath begins. The manna in the wilderness provides the paradigm: a double portion was provided on the sixth day, and it did not spoil, so that the people would not have to gather on the seventh (Exodus 16:22-26). This

was a tangible lesson in trust and preparation. Practically, this means that the cooking, the cleaning, the shopping—all the labors of the kitchen—should be largely completed by sundown on the sixth day. The goal is to free the Sabbath from the tyranny of domestic chores. The meals on the Sabbath should be simple, perhaps pre-prepared, or celebratory feasts that require minimal last-minute effort. This is not a legalistic burden; it is a liberating discipline. It transforms the kitchen from a place of work into a place of shared enjoyment and gratitude. When the family gathers around a table that required no one to slave over a hot stove, you are enacting a small but profound parable of grace—enjoying a meal you did not earn by your sweat.

2. **The Digital Detox and the Cleansing of the Temple of Time:** If our bodies are temples, then our time is the sacred space in which that temple exists. To prepare for the Sabbath, we must deliberately wall off this sanctuary from the invasive forces of the digital age. This begins with a conscious, deliberate disconnection. I urge you, establish a "technology Sabbath." Let the screens go dark. Power down the computers, silence the smartphones, and turn off the televisions. The constant ping of notifications, the endless scroll of newsfeeds, the pressure to be perpetually available and informed—this is the very antithesis of rest. It is the "noise" that drowns out the "sound of a low whisper" (1 Kings 19:12). By severing this connection, we declare that our worth is not defined by our productivity or our social currency. We affirm that the world will continue to spin without our constant input. We create a space of silence, a vacuum that God can fill with His presence. This detox should begin, if possible, on Friday evening and extend until

Sunday morning. It is a radical act of faith in a world that equates being online with being alive.

3. **The Completion of Secular Labor:** Make it a spiritual discipline to bring your work to a point of closure by Friday evening. This does not mean that every project is finished, but that you have intentionally tidied your workspace, made a list for Monday, and mentally and emotionally released the burdens of your vocation. This is an act of offering your work to God and trusting Him with the results. It is the practical outworking of Psalm 127:1-2: "Unless the LORD builds the house, those who build it labor in vain. Unless the LORD watches over the city, the watchman stays awake in vain. It is in vain that you rise up early and go late to rest, eating the bread of anxious toil; for he gives to his beloved sleep." The "bread of anxious toil" is the very substance we renounce on the Sabbath. We cease our labor because we believe that the ultimate building and watching is done by the Lord, not by us.

4. **The Intentional Pivot of the Heart:** Finally, Sabbath preparation is an inward reorientation. As the sun sets, light a candle. Offer a specific prayer of transition. Read a Psalm, such as Psalm 92, which is titled "A Song for the Sabbath." Gather the family and speak a blessing over one another. This ritual, however simple, serves as a liturgical threshold. It marks the passage from the realm of doing into the realm of being; from the kingdom of getting and spending into the Kingdom of God where we receive all things as gift. It is a way of telling your soul, "Be still, and know that I am God" (Psalm 46:10).

A Sleep Liturgy: The Sanctification of the Night

Beloved, if the Sabbath is the weekly sanctuary of rest, then sleep is its daily sacrament. Yet, how many of us treat sleep as an inconvenient interruption, a necessary evil, or a state of unconsciousness to be manipulated with pharmaceuticals and stimulants? This, too, is a form of Gnosticism—a disdain for the profound vulnerability and creatureliness that sleep requires. Sleep is a divine ordinance. It is God's daily reminder that we are not God. We are finite, dependent creatures who must, for a third of our lives, relinquish control, consciousness, and the illusion of self-sufficiency. In sleep, we are utterly passive. We do not achieve rest; we receive it. It is a pure gift. Therefore, we must not crash into sleep like a collapsed building. We must prepare for it as we would prepare for a holy encounter—because it is. We need a **Sleep Liturgy**.

A liturgy is a patterned, repetitive form of worship that shapes the affections of the heart through the actions of the body. A sleep liturgy is a deliberate, pre-sleep routine that signals to the entire integrated being—body, soul, and spirit—that the time for wakeful striving is over and the time for trusting surrender has come.

1. **The Technology Curfew: Guarding the Gates of the Mind.** The first and most non-negotiable element of this liturgy is a strict technology curfew, at least one hour, but ideally two hours, before the intended time of sleep. The blue light emitted from screens suppresses melatonin production, the hormone essential for sleep. But the damage is more than physiological. The content we consume—the frantic news cycles, the curated social media feeds, the stimulating entertainment—agitates

the *psyche*. It fills the mind with images, anxieties, and narratives that are antithetical to the peace of Christ. The *nous* (the mind) becomes a crowded, noisy marketplace right at the time it should be becoming a quiet, still sanctuary. You cannot offer a peaceful spirit to God in sleep if you have just fed it a diet of chaos and conflict. Therefore, let the screens go dark. Power them down. Do not merely put them on silent; remove them from the bedroom entirely. This is an act of exorcism against the spirit of the age.

2. **The Calming of the Soma: A Ritual of Embodied Stillness.** The body must be led gently toward rest. This can involve a series of small, physical acts that become sacramental signs of letting go. A warm bath or shower can lower the body's core temperature and trigger the sleep-ready response. Gentle, slow stretching can release the physical tension held in the muscles from the day's stresses. A cup of caffeine-free herbal tea, like chamomile, can be a physical sign of comfort and warmth. The key is consistency. These acts, repeated night after night, become powerful neurological cues that tell the nervous system, "The fight is over. It is safe to stand down."

3. **The Nourishment of the Psyche: Scripture and Examen.** With the body calming and the screens dark, we now turn to the soul. This is not the time for intense theological study or wrestling with complex spiritual problems. That is daytime work. This is the time for the simple, deep nourishment of the soul. Read a portion of Scripture that is comforting, affirming, and peaceful. The Psalms are the perfect companion for this hour. Psalm 4, for example, is a bedtime prayer: "In peace I will both lie down and sleep; for you alone, O LORD, make me dwell

in safety" (Psalm 4:8). Psalm 23: "He makes me lie down in green pastures. He leads me beside still waters. He restores my soul." Read slowly. Meditatively. Let the words wash over you.

Following this, practice a brief Prayer of Examen. This ancient Ignatian discipline is not a morbid introspection but a prayerful review of the day in God's loving presence. Ask the Holy Spirit to bring to light two things: First, a moment from the day for which you are particularly grateful. Savor it. Thank God for it. Second, a moment where you fell short, where you were anxious, angry, or unloving. Confess it briefly, receive God's forgiveness, and release it. The goal is to lay down the emotional and spiritual baggage of the day before you lay down your body.

4. **The Surrender of the Spirit: A Prayer of Trust.** Finally, as you lie down in bed, in the darkness and quiet, offer a simple prayer of total surrender. This is the climax of the liturgy. It is the active handing over of your life, your loved ones, your work, and your very consciousness to God. You might use the words of Christ from the cross: "Father, into your hands I commit my spirit" (Luke 23:46). You are not merely committing your disembodied soul; you are committing your entire, integrated self—your tired body, your overactive mind, your anxious heart—into the faithful hands of your Father. You are acting out the belief that He who watches over Israel, and you, neither slumbers nor sleeps (Psalm 121:4). You can sleep because He is awake. This prayer is the final, decisive act of faith that breaks the power of

insomnia, which is often, at its root, a failure to trust—a desire to remain in control.

The Prayer of the Night Watch: Redeeming Sleeplessness

And yet, beloved, despite our best preparations and most faithful liturgies, there will be nights when sleep does not come. The mind races. The body is restless. Anxiety grips the heart. What then? Are we failures? Has God abandoned us? Absolutely not. The faithful steward must also have a discipline for the sanctification of *sleeplessness*. We must learn the practice of **The Prayer of the Night Watch.**

The "night watches" are a biblical concept (Psalm 63:6, Psalm 119:148, Lamentations 2:19). They refer to the periods of the night when guards would be posted, alert and vigilant. When you find yourself awake in the middle of the night, do not fight it with frustration. Do not immediately reach for a sleeping pill or your phone. Instead, reframe it. See it as a divine appointment. You have been assigned to the night watch. Your post is your bed. Your task is prayer.

1. **From Frustration to Intercession:** Instead of agonizing over your own need for sleep, turn your attention outward. Bring your wakefulness to God as an offering. Use the quiet, uninterrupted time to pray for others. Bring before the Lord your family, your friends, your pastors, your nation, the persecuted church, the lost. Often, our sleeplessness is caused by a subconscious burden for these very things. By giving voice to that burden in prayer, we are cooperating with the Holy Spirit who "intercedes for us with groanings too deep for words" (Romans 8:26). Your insomnia becomes a sanctuary of intercession.

2. **The Prayer of Recollection and Contemplation:** Another path is to move into a more contemplative, receptive prayer. In the darkness, practice the presence of God. Simply rest in the awareness that He is with you. Breathe slowly and prayerfully. You might use a single, short phrase from Scripture as a "prayer word" to anchor your wandering mind. "Jesus." "My Lord and my God." "Your grace is sufficient." When anxious thoughts arise, do not engage them. Gently return to your prayer word. This is not about achieving a spiritual experience; it is about abiding. It is about being content to keep vigil with your Lord, even in the silence and the dark.
3. **The Prayer of Lament and Trust:** Sometimes, our wakefulness is born of deep pain, grief, or fear. In these moments, the most sanctifying thing you can do is to pray the Psalms of Lament. Psalm 77 is a perfect example: "I cry aloud to God, aloud to God, and he will hear me. I seek the Lord in my day of trouble... Will the Lord reject forever and never again show favor? Has his faithful love ceased forever?" (Psalm 77:1, 7-8). Give voice to your despair. Be brutally honest with God. And then, like the Psalmist, force yourself to remember God's past faithfulness: "I will remember the LORD's works; yes, I will remember your ancient wonders. I will reflect on all you have done and meditate on your actions" (Psalm 77:11-12). This movement from lament to recollection is a powerful act of faith that can transfigure a night of terror into a night of wrestling that ends in blessing, much like Jacob's night at Peniel (Genesis 32:22-32).

Beloved, these disciplines—of Sabbath preparation, a sleep liturgy, and the prayer of the night watch—are not magic formulas. They are the practical, gritty, daily and weekly workouts that strengthen our trust muscles. They are how we live out the belief that our bodies are temples, that our time is sacred, and that our rest is ultimately found not in the absence of work, but in the presence of the One who said, "Come to me, all who labor and are heavy laden, and I will give you rest" (Matthew 11:28). Let us then, with intentionality and hope, become stewards not only of our waking hours but of our rest, for the glory of God and the renewal of our whole being.

The Eternal Significance of Temporal Stewardship

The journey through this treatise has sought to establish a singular, foundational truth: the care of the body, mind, and spirit is not a peripheral concern for the spiritually minded, but a central tenet of Christian discipleship. The doctrine of Embodied Stewardship, rooted in the creation narratives, illuminated by the Incarnation, and oriented toward the hope of the Resurrection, provides a comprehensive theological framework that elevates daily health practices from the realm of the mundane to the sphere of the sacred.

We have seen that the human person is an integrated unity—a *nephesh*—where the physical, psychological, and spiritual are inextricably intertwined. To neglect the body is to neglect the vehicle through which the Spirit works, the instrument through which we love our neighbor, and the very self that God created and will redeem. The metaphor of the body as a temple (1 Corinthians 6:19-20) is not merely illustrative; it is prescriptive, charging us with the solemn and joyful duty of maintaining this holy dwelling place.

This stewardship is not a pursuit of vanity or a capitulation to secular healthism. It is, rather, an active participation in God's mission of *Shalom*—the restoration of holistic harmony. Every nutritious meal is a act of receiving God's provision with gratitude. Every moment of managed stress through prayer and cognitive discipline is a declaration that the peace of Christ reigns. Every step taken in exercise is an investment in the physical capacity for service. And every Sabbath rest and night of sleep is a tangible act of faith, a relinquishing of control, and a trust in the God who sustains us even in our vulnerability.

The temporal nature of our bodies—their susceptibility to decay, disease, and eventual death—does not negate the significance of their care. Rather, it frames our stewardship within the "already but not yet" tension of the Kingdom. We care for these "jars of clay" (2 Corinthians 4:7), knowing they are temporary, precisely because they contain the eternal treasure of the Gospel. We fight the disintegrating effects of the Fall not in the hope of achieving immortality through nutrition or fitness, but as an act of faithful witness to the coming restoration of all things.

Therefore, let the reader understand: to choose a salad over gluttony, to walk in nature over sloth, to meditate on Scripture over anxiety, to seek counsel for a troubled mind, and to honor the rhythm of rest is to engage in a profoundly theological act. It is to live out the reality of the Incarnation, whereby God affirmed the goodness of the physical. It is to enact a foretaste of the Resurrection, where the perishable will put on imperishability.

The ultimate calling of the embodied steward is to offer the whole person—body, soul, and spirit—as a "living sacrifice, holy and acceptable to God," which is our "spiritual worship" (Romans 12:1). This is the eternal significance of our temporal stewardship. For the life of faith is lived not in a disembodied state, but in the flesh-and-blood reality of our daily existence. And it is here, in the garden of our own embodied lives, that we are called to work, to keep, and to offer it all back to the Creator, for His glory, for the service of our neighbor, and for our ultimate good.

CONCLUSION

The Eternal Significance of Temporal Stewardship

Beloved, as we stand at the culmination of this extensive theological expedition, we must now gather together the many threads we have carefully unraveled and woven throughout this treatise and bind them with a final, unbreakable cord of conviction. The journey upon which we have embarked—through the doctrines of creation, the fall, redemption, and eschatology, through the intricate architecture of human anthropology, and through the practical domains of nutrition, mental discipline, and physical stewardship—has sought to establish, defend, and illuminate one singular, foundational, and non-negotiable truth: **the care of the body, the mind, and the spirit is not a peripheral concern for the spiritually elite, nor a secondary matter of Christian liberty, but a central, essential, and indispensable tenet of authentic, holistic Christian discipleship.** To relegate the stewardship of our embodied existence to the realm of optional extras or secular preoccupations is to commit a grave theological error, a practical heresy that has crippled the witness of the Church and impoverished the lives of countless believers.

The doctrine of **Embodied Stewardship** that we have labored to construct is not a novel innovation. It is a recovery project, a return to the rich, holistic soil of the biblical witness that has been obscured by the dust of dualistic philosophies and the debris of modern fragmentation. This framework, firmly rooted in the "very good" declaration of the creation narratives (Genesis 1:31), is irrevocably illuminated by the staggering reality of the Incarnation, and is passionately oriented toward the glorious, bodily hope of the Resurrection. It is this comprehensive theological vision that elevates our daily health practices—what we eat, how we sleep, how we manage our thoughts, how we move our bodies—from the mundane realm of personal hygiene and self-help into the sacred sphere of worship, discipleship, and participation in the divine mission. When we understand that our physicality is the chosen medium of divine indwelling, the very act of caring for it becomes a priestly service, a liturgical act performed in the temple of the self.

We have seen, with exegetical and theological force, that the Hebraic concept of the human person as a *nephesh chayyah*—a living being, an animated body, an ensouled entity—shatters the persistent and pernicious heresy of Gnosticism that would relegate the body to a temporary, and often troublesome, container for the "real" self, the soul. This integrated unity, this psychosomatic whole, means that a disruption in one dimension inevitably sends shockwaves through the entire system. An anxious mind (*psyche*) can trigger a cascade of stress hormones that weaken the immune system (*soma*) and create a sense of spiritual distance (*pneuma*). Conversely, a body malnourished by processed foods can cloud cognitive function, dampen emotional resilience, and hinder the receptivity of the spirit to the things of God. Therefore, to neglect the body is not merely to neglect a machine; it is to neglect the integrated vehicle through which the Holy Spirit works, the essential instrument through which we enact the love of our neighbor, and the very self—the unique, particular, physical self—that God fearfully and wonderfully made (Psalm 139:14) and that He has promised to redeem, not discard, on the last day.

The apostolic metaphor of the body as a **temple** (*naos*) of the Holy Spirit in 1 Corinthians 6:19-20 must, therefore, cease to be for us a mere spiritual illustration, a pleasant but ultimately impractical metaphor. It is, we have discovered, a radical ontological claim and a prescriptive ethical mandate. It charges us with a solemn, joyful, and non-negotiable duty: the maintenance, purity, and vitality of this most holy dwelling place. We are the custodians of the inner sanctuary. The gold, the linen, the sacred vessels of this temple are our organ systems, our neural pathways, our hormonal balances. To willfully introduce defilement through gluttony, to allow the walls to crumble through sloth, to let the altar grow cold through the neglect of rest, is not a lack of discipline; it is an act of desecration. Conversely, to nourish, to strengthen, to cleanse, and to rest this temple is an act of profound worship, a tangible expression of gratitude for the price paid to purchase it, and a cooperative venture with the Divine Resident who is at work within us to will and to work for His good pleasure (Philippians 2:13).

This sacred stewardship, we must insist, is categorically distinct from the modern cult of "wellness" or the secular religion of "healthism." Our goal is not the optimization of the body for its own sake, the pursuit of a sculpted physique as an idol of vanity, or the quest for longevity as the ultimate good. These are simply baptized versions of the same self-worship that characterizes the fallen world. No, the telos of Embodied Stewardship is infinitely grander. It is an active, daily **participation in God's cosmic mission of *Shalom***—the restoration of holistic harmony across the four dimensions of existence: with God, with ourselves, with others, and with creation. Every conscious choice for a nutritious, whole food is not just a smart dietary choice; it is an act of receiving God's creational provision with gratitude, a participation in the original goodness of Eden, and often, a choice for ethical consumption that promotes justice and environmental *Shalom*. Every moment where we arrest an anxious thought and take it captive to the obedience of Christ (2 Corinthians 10:5), through prayer and the renewal of our minds, is not merely a stress-management technique; it is a declaration that the peace of Christ, which surpasses all understanding, is the true ruler of our hearts (Colossians 3:15). Every step taken in purposeful exercise, every weight lifted, every mile run, is not an act of vanity; it is an investment in the physical capacity for long-term, tangible service, a strengthening of the vessel so that it might be poured out more abundantly for the sake of the Gospel and the love of our neighbor.

And what of the undeniable, temporal nature of these very bodies? They are subject to decay, to disease, to the relentless onslaught of entropy, and to the ultimate enemy, death. Does this not render our stewardship futile? Is it not, as the cynic might say, merely rearranging the deck chairs on the Titanic? Absolutely not. The very temporality of our bodies frames our stewardship within the profound and dynamic tension of the "already but not yet" of Christ's Kingdom. We care for these "jars of clay," as the Apostle Paul calls them, knowing they are fragile, temporary, and cracking (2 Corinthians 4:7). But why? Precisely because they contain, here and now, the eternal, all-surpassing treasure of the Gospel of Jesus Christ. We fight the disintegrating effects of the Fall—we resist disease, we slow decay, we manage disorder—not with the foolish and ultimately idolatrous hope of achieving immortality through organic kale and weight training, but as an act of faithful, hopeful witness. Our stewardship is a protest against the tyranny of death. It is a living, breathing signpost that points to the coming day when the perishable *will* put on imperishability, and the mortal *will* put on immortality (1 Corinthians 15:54). We tend to the seed, knowing it will die, but believing with all our hearts in the resurrection of the body that will spring forth from it.

Therefore, let the reader understand with crystal clarity: to choose a plate of vibrant vegetables over a gluttonous feast of processed indulgence, to take a walk in God's creation in preference to the lethargy of sloth, to meditate on a verse of Scripture rather than to spiral into an anxious rehearsal of our fears, to seek wise counsel and medical help for a troubled mind rather than to suffer in silent shame, and to honor the God-ordained rhythms of Sabbath and sleep—these are not minor lifestyle choices. They are, each one, **profoundly theological acts.** They are the lived-out reality of the Incarnation, whereby the eternal Word took on flesh and blood, thereby sanctifying material existence forever and revealing that the spiritual and the physical are united in the person of Christ. They are enacted foretastes of the Resurrection, where the groaning of creation and the wasting away of our outer self will be swallowed up by life and glory (2 Corinthians 4:16-17, 5:4).

The ultimate, high calling of the embodied steward, then, is the offering prescribed in Romans 12:1. It is to present our *bodies*—our physical, breathing, eating, sleeping, working, resting bodies—as a *living sacrifice*. This offering is not the presentation of a disembodied soul, but the consecration of the whole, integrated *nephesh*. This offering is holy—set apart from common use, dedicated entirely to God's purposes. And it is acceptable to God, not because of its inherent perfection, but because it is offered through the mercies of God in Christ Jesus. And this act, this daily, hourly offering of our physical lives in acts of conscious, loving stewardship, is nothing less than our *logiken latreian*—our rational, logical, true, and **spiritual worship.**

For the life of faith, from its inception to its consummation, is not lived in a disembodied state, floating in a ethereal realm of pure spirit. It is lived here, in the grit and grace of our daily, flesh-and-blood existence. It is lived in the garden of our own embodied lives, a garden still bearing the scars of the Fall, yet visited by the Gardener who walks in the cool of the day and who has begun a glorious work of restoration. And it is here, in this garden, with these hands, this stomach, this mind, and this heart, that we are called to work and to keep it (Genesis 2:15), to tend it with diligence and love, and to offer it all back to our Creator and Redeemer, for His eternal glory, for the tangible service of our neighbor, and for our ultimate and everlasting good.

APPENDICES

Beloved, having traversed the vast theological landscape of Embodied Stewardship, we now turn from the grand architecture of doctrine to the practical blueprints for its construction in the daily rhythm of our lives. A vision without a pathway remains a mirage. A theology without a methodology is but an intellectual curiosity. Therefore, we provide these appendices not as an afterthought, but as an essential workshop, a set of tools for the faithful artisan who seeks to build a life of integrated wholeness upon the foundation we have laid. These are not rigid, legalistic codes, but flexible, wisdom-based templates designed to facilitate the graceful application of sacred truth to the messy, beautiful reality of our embodied existence.

Appendix A: A Sample Rule of Life for Holistic Stewardship

My dear brothers and sisters, the ancient Christian tradition has long understood that the spiritual life does not flourish in chaos and spontaneity alone. It requires structure, intention, and a rhythm that aligns our habits with our beliefs. This intentional structure is known as a **Rule of Life**. It is not a law to be slavishly obeyed under threat of condemnation, but a gentle, firm trellis upon which the vine of our life can grow upward toward the Son. It is a means of grace, a way of ordering our days so that we might more freely and fully offer our entire selves to God. This sample Rule integrates the core principles of our treatise—theological anthropology, nutritional stewardship, mental renewal, and physical discipline—into a practical, weekly template. Consider it a starting point for prayerful adaptation, a prototype for your own unique journey of Embodied Stewardship.

The Theological Foundation of a Rule: A Rule of Life is grounded in the recognition that we are creatures of habit, and our loves are shaped by our routines. What we do repeatedly, we become. A Rule seeks to sanctify time itself, recognizing that our minutes and hours are the raw material of our offering to God (Ephesians 5:15-16). It is an answer to the question posed by our stewardship: "How, practically, do I glorify God in my body, in my time, with my energy?"

The Daily Rule: The Sanctification of the Mundane

- **Morning Prayer & Scripture Reading (The Vertical Foundation):** The day must not be seized, but received. Before the cacophony of the world intrudes, we intentionally position ourselves as creatures before our Creator. This is not a time for intense study, but for receptive listening. A pattern of Lectio Divina (detailed in Appendix D) on a short passage of Scripture, perhaps from the Psalms or the Gospels, allows the Word to sink beneath the cognitive level to the level of the *nephesh*.

This practice, as we have discussed, renews the mind (Romans 12:2) and sets a trajectory of God-consciousness for the day. It is the daily realignment of our spirit (*pneuma*) with the Divine Spirit, establishing vertical *Shalom* before the horizontal demands begin.

- **Mindful Eating at One Meal (Nutritional Sacramentalism):** We have argued that eating is a theological act. The Daily Rule makes this concrete by designating at least one meal—perhaps the midday lunch or the evening dinner—as an occasion for mindful eating. This means:
    - **Pausing:** Beginning with a genuine prayer of gratitude, acknowledging God as the ultimate source of this provision.
    - **Paying Attention:** Eating slowly, without the distraction of screens or frantic reading. Noticing the textures, flavors, and aromas. This transforms consumption into communion, fostering gratitude and breaking the cycle of mindless fueling.
    - **Stopping:** Learning to recognize the body's signals of satiety, honoring the temple by not overloading it. This single, daily act of intentionality becomes a school for gratitude and self-control, a small but potent rebellion against the gluttony and hurry of the age.
- **Thirty Minutes of Physical Activity (Temple Maintenance):** The body (*soma*) is for the Lord. The Daily Rule commits to a minimum of thirty minutes of intentional movement. This is not necessarily a grueling gym session. It could be a brisk walk, a bike ride, gardening, or gentle yoga. The form can vary, but the principle is constant: we are maintaining the instrument.

This activity acknowledges that the body is not a passive carriage for the soul but an active participant in our discipleship. It boosts cardiovascular health, manages stress hormones, and clears the mind, directly serving the goals of internal and horizontal *Shalom* by increasing our capacity for patient, loving service.

- **Examen & Gratitude Journal Before Bed (Cognitive and Emotional Integration):** As discussed in our chapter on rest, the day should not be ended abruptly. The Prayer of Examen (see Appendix D) provides a structured way to review the day in God's presence. This is followed by the simple discipline of writing down three specific things for which one is grateful. This powerful combination does two things: The Examen allows for the confession and release of the day's failures and anxieties, preventing them from festering in the subconscious through the night. The Gratitude Journal actively trains the *psyche* to notice and dwell on God's goodness (Philippians 4:8), re-wiring the brain for joy and trust. This practice is a direct implementation of the command to "take every thought captive," and it prepares the whole person for sanctified sleep.

The Weekly Rule: The Rhythm of Grace and Strength

- **One Sabbath Day of Ceasing:** This is the non-negotiable weekly pillar of the Rule. As elaborated in our discipline of rest, this is a 24-hour period from sunset to sunset dedicated to delight, worship, relationship, and rest. It is a complete cessation from *productive* work—paid or unpaid. It is a day for corporate worship, for naps, for long walks, for reading for pleasure, for playing with children, for enjoying good food prepared in advance. It is the weekly, physical enactment of the gospel of grace.

- **Two Strength-Training Sessions:** The weekly rhythm includes two focused sessions of resistance training. Theologically, this honors the body as an essential part of our identity and prepares it for service. Strength is a resource for love. It allows us to lift a child, help a friend move, or endure the physical demands of mission work. It fights the sarcopenia (muscle loss) of aging, stewarding the "seed" of the resurrection body for as long as we have it. It is a discipline that teaches perseverance and the principle of delayed gratification.
- **Three Cardiovascular Sessions:** Complementing strength training, three sessions of sustained cardiovascular activity (e.g., running, swimming, cycling) care for the body's engine—the heart and lungs. This enhances stamina, improves mental clarity, and is a powerful mitigator of anxiety and depression. It is an investment in the endurance required to "run with endurance the race that is set before us" (Hebrews 12:1).
- **One Extended Period of Contemplative Prayer:** Beyond the daily morning prayer, the weekly rule sets aside a longer period (e.g., 45-60 minutes) for contemplative or silent prayer. This is a time to move beyond words and petitions, to simply "be still, and know that I am God" (Psalm 46:10). This practice deepens the vertical *Shalom* that fuels all other activity, allowing the soul to find its rest in God alone.

The Monthly & Seasonal Rule: The Review and The Retreat

- **Monthly Review of Dietary Habits:** Once a month, take a sober look at your eating patterns. Are they aligned with the principles of creational goodness and gratitude? Is there a creeping reliance on processed foods? This is not about obsessive calorie counting, but about faithful, conscious stewardship.

- **Monthly "Digital Sabbath":** Beyond the weekly Sabbath, consider a full 24-hour period completely disconnected from all digital devices. This is a more profound detox, a radical act of reclaiming your attention and your time from the digital principalities and powers.
- **Monthly Communal Activity:** Embodied Stewardship is not a solitary pursuit. Join a hiking group, a sports team, or a service project. This fosters horizontal *Shalom* and makes stewardship a shared joy, not a private burden.
- **Seasonal Health Check-up:** Faithful stewardship involves using the means of General Revelation. A seasonal (i.e., quarterly) check-up with a doctor is an act of wisdom and responsibility, honoring the body by attending to its needs with professional help.
- **Seasonal Half-Day Silent Retreat:** Four times a year, withdraw completely for a half-day of silence, Scripture reading, and prayer. This is a time for deeper listening, for re-calibrating the heart, and for allowing God to speak into the rhythms of your life.
- **Seasonal Review of the Rule:** The Rule is a servant, not a master. Each season, review it. What is life-giving? What has become burdensome? Where is God calling you to grow? Adjust the Rule accordingly, with freedom and wisdom. The goal is not the perfect execution of the Rule, but a heart increasingly oriented toward God in every facet of life.

Beloved, the pastoral and personal challenge of mental affliction is one of the most complex arenas where our holistic anthropology must be applied. The simplistic either/or of "it's a spiritual problem, just pray more" or "it's a chemical problem, just take a pill" is a destructive false dichotomy that has wounded many. This appendix provides a framework, a flowchart of questions, to guide a more nuanced, theologically robust, and compassionate discernment process for pastors, caregivers, and individuals.

Foundational Principle: Mental affliction is a disruption of the psychosomatic unity of the *nephesh*. Therefore, it can, and often does, have simultaneous and interacting spiritual, psychological/emotional, and biological/somatic dimensions. Our goal is not to find the *one* true cause, but to wisely discern the primary contributing factors and address them with the appropriate God-given means.

The Discernment Flowchart & Key Questions:

1. **Begin with Compassionate Presence and Prayer:** Before any diagnosis, embody the love of Christ. Listen without judgment. Pray with and for the person, inviting the Holy Spirit, the Divine Physician, into the process.
2. **Explore the Spiritual Dimension (The State of the *Pneuma* and *Psyche*):**
    - **Relational History with God:** Is there unconfessed sin creating a burden of guilt and shame? Is there a history of trauma associated

with "God" or the church? Is there a sense of God's absence or anger?

- **Engagement with Spiritual Practices:** Has there been a cessation of practices that nurture the spirit (prayer, Scripture, worship)? Or have these practices become compulsive, fear-driven, and devoid of grace?
- **Discernment of Spiritual Forces:** Are there indicators beyond typical temptation that suggest demonic harassment or oppression (e.g., intense, irrational aversion to spiritual things, supernatural knowledge, personality shifts tied to specific locations or objects)? *This requires great wisdom and should not be a first resort.*

3. **Explore the Psychological/Emotional Dimension (The State of the *Psyche*):**
   - **Cognitive Patterns:** What are the recurring, automatic negative thoughts? Are there patterns of catastrophic thinking, self-loathing, or perfectionism? (This aligns with the concept of "strongholds" in 2 Corinthians 10:4-5).
   - **Emotional Regulation:** Is the person able to experience and manage a full range of emotions, or are they numb, volatile, or persistently overwhelmed by one emotion (e.g., fear, sadness, anger)?
   - **Life History and Trauma:** Has there been significant loss, abuse, neglect, or other traumatic events that have not been processed? The soul remembers what the mind sometimes tries to forget.

- **Relational Dynamics:** Are current relationships a source of life or of chronic stress, conflict, or abuse?

4. **Explore the Biological/Somatic Dimension (The State of the *Soma*):**
    - **Physiological Basics:** How is sleep? Nutrition? Physical activity? Caffeine and alcohol intake? These are not minor details; they are the foundational physical pillars of mental health. A mind cannot be well when the brain it inhabits is starved, exhausted, or poisoned.
    - **Genetic and Medical History:** Is there a family history of mental illness? Has a medical doctor ruled out physiological causes (e.g., thyroid dysfunction, vitamin deficiencies, hormonal imbalances) that can manifest as psychiatric symptoms?
    - **Neurochemical Considerations:** While we must avoid reductionism, do the symptoms (e.g., pervasive anhedonia, paralyzing fatigue, psychotic features) suggest a strong biological component that may be helped by medication?

Pathways of Care Based on Discernment:

- **Primary Pathway: Spiritual Direction & Pastoral Care:** This is the primary response when the core issue appears to be a disrupted relationship with God, unconfessed sin, or a need for basic discipleship and prayer support. The focus is on repentance, receiving grace, and re-engaging with the means of grace.
- **Primary Pathway: Christian Psychological Counseling/Therapy:** This is indicated when the primary

issues are maladaptive cognitive patterns, unresolved trauma, or dysfunctional relational dynamics. A competent Christian therapist can help "renew the mind" using tools from Cognitive Behavioral Therapy, EMDR for trauma, and other modalities that are compatible with a biblical worldview. This is a ministry of wisdom.

- **Primary Pathway: Medical Intervention:** This is a necessary and God-honoring pathway when there is a clear biological predisposition, when physiological causes have been identified, or when symptoms are so severe (e.g., psychosis, debilitating depression) that they prevent the person from engaging in spiritual or psychological work. Medication can be a gift of common grace that stabilizes the biological substrate, allowing the other dimensions of the person to begin healing. It can be a tool that "makes straight the paths" for the work of the Spirit.
- **The Integrated Pathway (Most Common):** In the vast majority of cases, care will be integrated. A person may meet with a pastor for spiritual encouragement, a therapist for trauma processing, and a doctor for medication to manage severe anxiety. The key is that all these caregivers communicate, if possible, and recognize that they are all tending to different facets of the same, whole person—the *nephesh* for whom Christ died. The goal is not to ask, "Is this a spiritual or a clinical problem?" but to ask, "How is the *Shalom* of this whole person disrupted, and what are the God-given means for its restoration?"

Beloved, in a world obsessed with body image and saturated with conflicting nutritional advice, the Christian must navigate the landscape of "diet culture" with theological discernment, not cultural captivity. This appendix provides a framework for evaluating popular dietary trends—such as Ketogenic, Paleolithic, and Vegan diets—through the lenses of Scripture and the doctrine of Embodied Stewardship. We ask not merely, "Does it work?" but "What story does it tell? What does it assume about the human person, the body, and the goal of life?"

Evaluative Lenses:

1. **The Lens of Creational Goodness (Genesis 1:29-31):** God created a world abundant with diverse foods and declared it "very good." A theology of food begins with gratitude and reception, not fear and restriction.
    - **Critique of Strict Paleo/Keto:** These diets often implicitly (or explicitly) frame certain creational food groups (e.g., grains, legumes, fruits) as inherently harmful or "toxic." This can foster a mindset of fear towards God's provision and an unwarranted asceticism that denies the goodness of what God has made to be received with thanksgiving (1 Timothy 4:4-5).
    - **Critique of Industrial Veganism**: While often motivated by ethical concerns, a veganism reliant on highly processed meat substitutes and refined carbohydrates can fail to honor the body's creational design for a variety of nutrient-dense foods, including those from the animal kingdom

which God provided for consumption after the Fall (Genesis 9:3).

2. **The Lens of the Fall and Redemption (Genesis 3, Romans 8:20-21):** The Fall introduced thorns, thistles, and a corruption of creation's systems. Our bodies and our food systems are not in their pristine, Edenic state.
    - **Application to Paleo:** The "Paleo" narrative of returning to an idealized, pre-agricultural past is a form of primitivism that ignores the creational mandate to cultivate and develop the world (a post-Eden but pre-Fall command). It also fails to account for the reality that redemption is forward-looking (to the New Creation), not backward-looking (to a lost paradise).
    - **Application to All Diets:** Any diet that promises a return to a state of perfect health or an escape from the effects of the Fall is offering a false gospel. Our stewardship is a faithful holding action in a fallen world, not a quest for pre-lapsarian purity.
3. **The Lenses of Asceticism and Gluttony (Colossians 2:20-23, Philippians 3:19):** These are the twin ditches on either side of the path of wise stewardship.
    - **Asceticism:** Diets can easily become a new legalism, a "will-worship" that derives spiritual pride from its rigor and restriction. When dietary rules become a source of identity, judgment of others, and a means of earning righteousness, they have become a form of works-based religion that "is of no value in stopping the indulgence of the flesh" (Colossians 2:23).

   - **Gluttony:** Conversely, the modern Western diet, characterized by excess, processed foods, and a lack of discipline, is clearly a form of gluttony. It is the idolatry of appetite, the failure to steward the temple, and a direct violation of the principle that our bodies are for the Lord (1 Corinthians 6:13).
4. **The Lens of Ethical Consumption and Love of Neighbor (1 Corinthians 10:31-33):** How we eat has implications beyond our own bodies. It affects the global poor, the welfare of animals, and the health of the environment.
   - **Evaluation of Vegan/Vegetarian Diets:** The ethical impulse behind these diets to avoid animal cruelty and reduce environmental impact is often commendable and can be a valid application of the call to loving stewardship of creation and a desire for justice.
   - **Evaluation of Local/Sustainable Movements:** Diets that emphasize locally sourced, sustainably grown foods align well with the creational mandate to "keep" the garden (Genesis 2:15) and to love our global neighbors by supporting just agricultural practices.

A Christian Framework for Nutritional Evaluation:

Instead of asking "Which diet is the *right* one?", the theologically informed steward asks:

- **Does this way of eating foster gratitude for God's diverse creation, or does it promote fear and a critical spirit towards food?**

- **Does it help me steward my body for greater energy and vitality for God's service, or is its primary focus aesthetic vanity?**
- **Does it lead to a disordered obsession with food (either in restriction or indulgence), or does it promote freedom and self-control?**
- **How do my food choices impact the creation and my global neighbor? Can I make more ethically informed choices within my means?**
- The goal is not a universal "biblical diet," but a wise, discerning, and grateful approach to eating that honors God, cares for the temple, and loves our neighbor.

Appendix D: Lectio Divina and The Prayer of Examen: Detailed Guides

Beloved, we have repeatedly emphasized the renewal of the mind as the linchpin of holistic stewardship. These two ancient spiritual disciplines are the primary God-ordained tools for this very work. They are not esoteric practices for monastics, but practical, accessible exercises for every believer seeking to have the mind of Christ (1 Corinthians 2:16).

Lectio Divina ("Divine Reading"): Renewing the Mind with the Word

This is a slow, prayerful, immersive reading of Scripture, aimed not at information but at transformation. It involves four movements:

1. **Lectio (Reading):** Select a short passage of Scripture (a few verses). Read it slowly, aloud if possible. Listen for a word or a phrase that seems to shimmer, stand out, or attract your attention. Don't analyze it; simply receive it.

2. **Meditatio (Meditation):** Read the passage again, slowly. Now, gently repeat the word or phrase that struck you. Ruminate on it. "Chew" on it like a cow chews its cud. Let it sink in. Ask, "What is God saying to *me* through this word, today, in my current circumstance?" Allow the Holy Spirit to make connections to your life.
3. **Oratio (Prayer):** Read the passage a third time. Now, respond to God from the heart. This is a dialogue. If the word was "peace," you might pray, "Lord, you know my anxiety about this situation. I lack peace. I ask you to pour your peace into my heart." The prayer flows naturally from the meditation.
4. **Contemplatio (Contemplation):** Read the passage a final time. Now, move into a place of quiet rest. Let go of words and thoughts. Simply rest in the presence of God, holding the word you have received. Soak in the reality of His love and truth. This is a foretaste of the perfect communion of eternity.

The Prayer of Examen: Integrating the Soul and Cultivating Gratitude

This is a prayerful review of the day, designed to see God's activity in the ordinary and to bring our emotional and spiritual life into alignment with His presence. It is best practiced at the end of the day.

1. **Become Aware of God's Presence:** Begin by quieting yourself. Ask the Holy Spirit to guide you and to bring to light what He wants you to see.
2. **Review the Day with Gratitude:** Look back over the last 24 hours. What are you thankful for? Start with the small, simple gifts—a warm drink, a kind word, a moment of

beauty. Thank God for each one. This trains the heart in gratitude.

3. **Notice Your Emotions (The Affective Examen):** As you review the day, pay attention to the feelings that arise. Where did you feel joy, peace, love? These are *consolations*, places where God was likely present and active. Where did you feel anxiety, anger, resentment, boredom? These are *desolations*, places where you may have been distant from God's will. Don't judge the feelings; simply note them as data points about the state of your soul.
4. **Choose One Feature of the Day and Pray from It:** Select one moment of either consolation or desolation. Re-live it prayerfully. If it was a moment of consolation, savor it and thank God for it. If it was a moment of desolation, explore it. Why did you react that way? Is there something to confess? Do you need to ask for or extend forgiveness? Pray through this specific moment.
5. **Look Toward Tomorrow:** Having reviewed the day, ask God for the grace you will need for tomorrow. Conclude with the Lord's Prayer, offering the whole day—past, present, and future—back to Him.

Through these disciplines, the Word of God becomes the primary software for our mental operating system, and our daily experiences become the raw material for a deepening relationship with God. They are the practical, daily implementation of the command to "be transformed by the renewal of your mind" (Romans 12:2).

Bibliography

Beloved, as we bring this extensive treatise to its final formal section, it is incumbent upon us to acknowledge the great cloud of witnesses upon whose scholarly and spiritual shoulders we stand. A work of this scope and nature does not emerge from a vacuum, but is rather a conversation—a symphony of voices from across the centuries, each contributing a unique melody to the grand theme of God's truth as it relates to our embodied existence. This bibliography is not a mere list of sources; it is a theological map, a curated guide to the intellectual and spiritual traditions that have informed and shaped the arguments contained within these pages. It is an invitation for you, the diligent reader, to continue your exploration, to delve deeper into the rich soil from which this project has grown. We have organized this map into four distinct but overlapping territories: the foundational bedrock of Theological and Biblical Studies; the wisdom of the Historical Theology and Spirituality; the crucial dialogue partners from Psychology, Science, and Integration; and the practical outworking found in Pastoral and Practical Theology.

I. Theological and Biblical Studies

This first and most critical section provides the dogmatic architecture for our entire project. The works listed here grapple with the fundamental questions of who God is, what His creation is, and who we are as human beings within that creation. They provide the exegetical precision and theological depth without which our pursuit of holistic health would be merely a baptized form of secular humanism.

- **Brown, William P. *The Seven Pillars of Creation: The Bible, Science, and the Ecology of Wonder*. Oxford University Press, 2010.**

  Brown's work is indispensable for developing a robust theology of creation that takes both Scripture and modern science with profound seriousness. He moves beyond the tired debates of literalism versus liberalism and explores the seven primary creation accounts in the Hebrew Bible (e.g., Genesis 1 & 2, Job, Psalms, Proverbs) as complementary theological pillars. His work provides the exegetical foundation for understanding the natural world—including our own bodies—not as a mere stage for the drama of redemption, but as a central character in that drama, worthy of wonder, study, and care. His exploration of the *Imago Dei* as a vocation of representation and relationship deeply informs our understanding of Embodied Stewardship as a fulfillment of our creational mandate.

- **Green, Joel B. *Body, Soul, and Human Life: The Nature of Humanity in the Bible*. Baker Academic, 2008.**

If one were to select a single volume that most directly undergirds the anthropological foundation of this treatise, it would be Joel Green's masterful work. A New Testament scholar with a background in neuroscience, Green expertly dismantles the persistent body-soul dualism that has plagued Western Christianity. He argues compellingly for a holistic, monistic understanding of the human person—what we have referred to as the *nephesh*—demonstrating that this is the pervasive view of the biblical writers, particularly in the New Testament. His integration of neuroscientific insights with theological exegesis provides a powerful model for the kind of conversation we have attempted to foster between Special and General Revelation, showing that a physicalist (or non-reductive physicalist) view of human nature is not only biblically faithful but also scientifically coherent.

- **Middleton, J. Richard. *The Liberating Image: The Imago Dei in Genesis 1*. Brazos Press, 2005.**

Middleton's book is a tour de force in Old Testament theology that has revolutionized contemporary understanding of the *Imago Dei*. He convincingly argues, against a long tradition of intellectual or spiritual interpretations, that the Image of God in Genesis 1:26-28 is primarily a royal and functional concept. Humanity is created as God's idol or statue in the world, tasked with the vocation of representing His benevolent rule to all of creation. This "cultural mandate" provides the essential theological framework for understanding why our physical, cultural, and vocational lives matter to God. Our stewardship of our own bodies and the wider world is not an addendum to the spiritual life; it is the very outworking of what it means to be the *Imago Dei*.

- **Moltmann, Jürgen. *God in Creation: A New Theology of Creation and the Spirit of God.* Fortress Press, 1993.**

Moltmann, one of the most significant systematic theologians of the 20th century, offers a profound panentheistic vision of creation as the dwelling place of the divine Spirit. His development of the concept of the *Shekinah*—God's indwelling, suffering presence within creation—provides a powerful theological lens for understanding the Holy Spirit's presence within the "temple" of the human body. His emphasis on the Sabbath as the climax of creation and the hope of the eschatological redemption of all things infuses our discussion of rest and resurrection with deep theological resonance, connecting the microcosm of our personal stewardship to the macrocosm of God's cosmic redemption.

- **O'Donovan, Oliver. *Resurrection and Moral Order: An Outline for Evangelical Ethics.* InterVarsity Press, 1986.**

O'Donovan's seminal work is the bedrock for any Christian ethic that seeks to be both creational and redemptive. He argues that the resurrection of Jesus Christ is the vindication and renewal of the original created order. Therefore, Christian ethics is not about escaping creation or imposing an alien law upon it, but about discerning and living into the grain of the universe as restored in Christ. This principle is fundamental to our thesis: Embodied Stewardship is not a arbitrary set of rules, but a Spirit-enabled recovery of the creational design for the human body, a design definitively affirmed and redeemed in the resurrection of Jesus.

- **Plantinga, Alvin. *Where the Conflict Really Lies: Science, Religion, and Naturalism.* Oxford University Press, 2011.**

As a preeminent philosopher of religion, Plantinga provides a crucial philosophical defense for the entire project of integrating science and theology. He argues persuasively that the perceived conflict between science and Christian belief is superficial; the *deep* conflict is between science and metaphysical naturalism. He demonstrates that theism provides a more hospitable foundation for science than naturalism itself, as it grounds the rational intelligibility of the universe in a rational Creator. This work gives us the philosophical confidence to engage with nutritional science, neurobiology, and kinesiology not as threats to our faith, but as explorations of God's good and orderly creation.

- **Wright, N.T. *Surprised by Hope: Rethinking Heaven, the Resurrection, and the Mission of the Church.* HarperOne, 2008.**

Wright's accessible yet profound work has been instrumental in reorienting a generation of Christians away from a Platonic vision of "going to heaven" and toward a biblical hope of the resurrection of the body and the renewal of all creation. His robust eschatology is the necessary capstone for our doctrine of Embodied Stewardship. It provides the ultimate *telos*: we care for these bodies because God cares for them, and He will raise them anew. Our present stewardship is a hopeful, faithful participation in that future reality. His companion work, ***The Day the Revolution Began: Reconsidering the Meaning of Jesus's Crucifixion*** **(HarperOne, 2016)**, provides the complementary soteriological foundation, framing the cross not merely as a means for individual forgiveness but as the decisive victory over the powers of Sin and Death, the very forces that afflict our bodies and our world.

II. Historical Theology and Spirituality

To ignore history is to be condemned to repeat its errors. This section connects us to the wisdom and the warnings of the Christian tradition, showing that our contemporary concerns have deep roots and that the saints of old have much to teach us about the disciplined integration of faith and physicality.

- **Benedict of Nursia. *The Rule of St. Benedict.* Edited by Timothy Fry, O.S.B. Vintage Spiritual Classics, 1998.**

The Rule of St. Benedict is a masterpiece of practical wisdom for forming a whole human life around the worship of God. Its famous motto, *Ora et Labora* (Pray and Work), embodies the integration of the spiritual and the physical. Benedict's meticulous regulation of the daily horarium—with its balanced rhythm of prayer, manual labor, sacred reading, and rest—is a historical prototype for the "Rule of Life" we have proposed in Appendix A. It testifies to the ancient Christian conviction that holiness is cultivated through the sanctification of time and the disciplined stewardship of the body's energies.

- **Calvin, John. *Institutes of the Christian Religion.* Edited by John T. McNeill, translated by Ford Lewis Battles. Westminster John Knox Press, 1960.**
The magisterial systematic theology of the Protestant Reformation, Calvin's *Institutes* provides a deeply theocentric foundation for all of life. His doctrine of Providence—that God is sovereignly and intimately involved in the sustenance of every aspect of His creation—is the bedrock of trust that allows us to rest and sleep in peace. His emphasis on the noetic effects of sin cautions us against an uncritical reliance on human reason, including in the realms of science and health, while his affirmation of General Revelation encourages us to receive all truth as God's truth. His theology constantly drives the believer from a focus on self to a focus on the glory and goodness of God, which is the ultimate end of all stewardship.
- **Foster, Richard J. *Celebration of Discipline: The Path to Spiritual Growth.* Harper San Francisco, 1998.**
Foster's modern classic played a pivotal role in the late 20th-century recovery of the classical spiritual disciplines for the everyday Christian. By categorizing the disciplines into inward, outward, and corporate practices, he provides a holistic framework for spiritual formation that inherently involves the body. His chapters on disciplines such as fasting, solitude, and service directly inform our understanding of how physical practices are means of grace for shaping the soul and manifesting the life of Christ in the world.

- **Willard, Dallas. *The Spirit of the Disciplines: Understanding How God Changes Lives.* Harper San Francisco, 1988.**

Willard, building on Foster's work, provides the profound theological underpinning for the disciplines. He argues that spiritual transformation into Christlikeness is not a matter of mere intention but requires our intentional participation in practices that train our whole person—body, mind, and spirit—for life in the Kingdom of God. His work is essential for understanding why practices like fixed-hour prayer, Sabbath keeping, and dietary discipline are not legalistic but liberating—they are the "means of grace" through which we place ourselves before God for transformation. His concept of "the destruction of the body of sin through the re-embodiment of the person in Christ" is a powerful summary of the goal of Embodied Stewardship.

III. Psychology, Science, and Integration

A theology of embodiment that does not engage with the God-given insights of psychology and human biology is an abstraction. These works provide the crucial data and theoretical frameworks from General Revelation that help us understand the "how" of our psychosomatic unity, informing our pastoral practice and personal stewardship.

- **Collins, Gary R. *Christian Counseling: A Comprehensive Guide.* Thomas Nelson, 2007.**

As a foundational text in the field, Collins's work provides a broad overview of the issues, theories, and techniques relevant to a Christian approach to counseling. It helps to map the vast territory of human psychological suffering and health, offering a resource for pastors and caregivers to understand the landscape before them and to know when and how to refer to professional Christian counselors.

- **McMinn, Mark R. *Psychology, Theology, and Spirituality in Christian Counseling*. Tyndale House Publishers, 1996.**

McMinn's work is a more focused and integrative model than Collins's. He doesn't just place psychology and theology side-by-side; he thoughtfully weaves them together, showing how theological concepts like sin, grace, and redemption can and should inform the therapeutic process. His book is a practical guide for how to be a "theologian of the soul" in the counseling room, making it an invaluable resource for implementing the holistic discernment process outlined in Appendix B.

- **Siegel, Daniel J. *Mindsight: The New Science of Personal Transformation*. Bantam, 2010.**

A psychiatrist and leading voice in interpersonal neurobiology, Siegel provides the scientific framework for the "renewal of the mind." His concept of "mindsight"—the ability to perceive the internal world of oneself and others—is a powerful secular parallel to the biblical concept of self-examination and the healing power of presence and attuned relationships. His work explains the neurological mechanisms by which practices like prayer, meditation, and secure attachment literally re-wire the brain, providing a scientific validation for the transformative power of the spiritual disciplines.

- **Swenson, Richard A. *Margin: Restoring Emotional, Physical, Financial, and Time Reserves to Overloaded Lives.* NavPress, 2004.**
- Swenson, a medical doctor, diagnoses the central pathology of modern life: the systematic elimination of margin—the space between our load and our limits. His work is a prophetic call, grounded in both Scripture and medical science, to intentionally create space for rest, relationship, and reflection. It provides the practical, cultural critique that makes the disciplines of Sabbath and simplicity not just spiritually beneficial but essential for survival and health in the 21st century.
- **Van der Kolk, Bessel. *The Body Keeps the Score: Brain, Mind, and Body in the Healing of Trauma.* Penguin Books, 2015.**

This is arguably one of the most important books of the last decade for anyone in pastoral or caring ministry. Van der Kolk, a pioneering trauma researcher, presents overwhelming evidence for the profound psychosomatic unity of the human person. He demonstrates how trauma, and its healing, is not just a story in the mind but is etched into the physiology, posture, and nervous system of the body. This work forces a theological reckoning, compelling us to develop a pastoral theology that takes the physical, bodily dimensions of suffering and healing with absolute seriousness, and to recognize that some forms of "spiritual" brokenness require somatic, not just cognitive, pathways to healing.

IV. Practical and Pastoral Theology

Finally, we turn to resources that bridge the gap between theory and practice, providing concrete tools and frameworks for dealing with the specific, daily challenges of living as an embodied saint in a fallen world.

- **Carter, Dr. Les. *The Anger Workbook: An Interactive Guide to Anger Management.* Thomas Nelson, 2003.**

  Carter's workbook is an example of a practical, biblically-informed tool for addressing a specific, destructive emotional pattern. It guides the user through a process of understanding the roots of their anger, challenging distorted thinking, and developing healthier responses. It represents the kind of practical application that flows from a holistic anthropology, addressing the cognitive (*psyche*) and volitional dimensions of a problem with spiritual integrity.

- **Cloud, Dr. Henry, and Dr. John Townsend. *Boundaries: When to Say Yes, How to Say No to Take Control of Your Life.* Zondervan, 1992.**

  A landmark book that has shaped modern Christian thought on relationships and self-care. Cloud and Townsend provide a biblical and psychological framework for understanding and establishing healthy personal boundaries. This concept is absolutely essential for Embodied Stewardship, as it provides the relational "how-to" for protecting the temple of one's own life and energy from the draining demands and unhealthy patterns of others, thereby preserving the capacity for truly loving and sustainable service.

- **Powlison, David. *How Does Sanctification Work?* Crossway, 2017.**

Powlison, a leading voice in the biblical counseling movement, offers a wise and nuanced exploration of the diverse ways the Holy Spirit changes people. He avoids simplistic formulas and emphasizes the deeply personal, heart-oriented work of God that uses a variety of means—suffering, Scripture, community, insight, counseling. His work guards against the reductionism that can plague both secular therapeutic and overly simplistic religious approaches, reminding us that the Holy Spirit is the ultimate change agent who works through, but is not bound by, any single methodology.

- **Welch, Edward T. *Blame It on the Brain? Distinguishing Chemical Imbalances, Brain Disorders, and Disobedience.* P&R Publishing, 1998.**

This short but incredibly insightful book by Welch is a master class in the kind of nuanced discernment we advocated for in Appendix B. He provides a biblically faithful grid for navigating the complex relationship between the brain (the physical organ) and the mind/heart (the seat of personal responsibility and spiritual life). He helps the reader avoid the two errors of blaming all problems on biology or blaming all problems on sin, offering a more integrated, compassionate, and effective approach to problems like ADHD, depression, and addiction. His other work, ***Running Scared: Fear,***

Worry, and the God of Rest **(New Growth Press, 2007)**, is a deep, pastoral exploration of the anatomy of fear and the biblical pathway to the rest that comes from trusting in the character and promises of God, directly feeding into our discussions on mental and emotional well-being.

www.ingramcontent.com/pod-product-compliance
Lightning Source LLC
LaVergne TN
LVHW052212200926
848481LV00001B/83